Clinics in Developmental Medicine No. 136

DISABLED CHILDREN AND DEVELOPING COUNTRIES

© 1995 Mac Keith Press
526/529 High Holborn House, 52–54 High Holborn, London WC1V 6RL

Senior Editor: Martin C.O. Bax
Editor: Pamela A. Davies
Managing Editor: Michael Pountney
Sub Editor: Pat Chappelle

Set in Times and Avant Garde on QuarkXPress

First published in this edition 1995

British Library Cataloguing-in-Publication data:
A catalogue record for this book is available from the British Library

ISSN: 0069 4835
ISBN: 0 898683 04 2

Printed by The Lavenham Press Ltd, Water Street, Lavenham, Suffolk
Mac Keith Press is supported by **Scope** (formerly The Spastics Society)

Clinics in Developmental Medicine No. 136

Disabled Children & Developing Countries

Edited by
PAM ZINKIN
HELEN McCONACHIE
Institute of Child Health
London, England

with a Foreword by
ALFRED L. SCHERZER
Cornell University Medical Center
New York, USA

1995
Mac Keith Press

Distributed by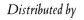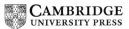

CONTENTS

CONTRIBUTORS

Anupam Ahuja

Lecturer in Special Education, National Council of Educational Research and Training, New Delhi, India

Mel Ainscow

Tutor in Special Educational Needs, University of Cambridge Institute of Education, Cambridge, England

Gillian Baird

Consultant Paediatrician, Newcomen Centre, Guy's Hospital, London, England

Gautam Chaudhury

Project Co-ordinator, Children in Need Institute, Calcutta; *and* Director, SANCHAR-AROD, West Bengal, India

Kevin Connolly

Professor of Psychology, University of Sheffield, England

Maureen Durkin

Assistant Professor of Public Health (Epidemiology), Gertrude H. Sergievsky Center, Columbia University, New York, USA

David Hall

Professor of Community Paediatrics, Children's Hospital, Sheffield, England

N.K. Jangira

Professor of Special Education *and* Head, Department of Teacher Education and Special Education, National Council of Educational Research and Training; *and* Basic Education Consultant, World Bank, New Delhi, India

Naila Khan

Consultant Paediatrician, Developmental Paediatrics and Child Neurology Unit, Dhaka Shishu Children's Hospital, Dhaka, Bangladesh

Joseph Kisanji	Lecturer in Special Education (International), University of Manchester, England
Stuart Logan	Senior Lecturer in Paediatric Epidemiology, Institute of Child Health, London, England
Margaret Martlew	Lecturer in Psychology, University of Sheffield, England
Michael P.A. Mathias	Honorary Secretary, Karnataka Parents' Association for Mentally Retarded Citizens; *and* Second Vice-President, International League of Societies for Persons with Mental Handicap, Bangalore, India
Helen McConachie	Senior Lecturer in Clinical Psychology, Institute of Child Health, London, England
Roy McConkey	Director of Training and Research, Brothers of Charity Services, Borders Region, Scotland
Kalyani Menon-Sen	Senior Programme Co-ordinator, SANCHAR-AROD, West Bengal, India
Kenneth C. Rankin	Consultant Orthopaedic Surgeon, Law Hospital, Carluke, Lanarkshire, Scotland
Naomi Richman	Emeritus Reader in Psychiatry, Hackney Community Child Health, London, England
Leonard Williams	President, Disabled Persons Rehabilitation Association, Honiara, Solomon Islands
Pam Zinkin	Senior Lecturer in International Child Health, Institute of Child Health, London, England

FOREWORD

A revolution in technology, diagnosis, treatment, management and program emphasis affecting children with disabilities has been in process over the past decade. Advances in obstetric management and intensive neonatal care have enabled survival of low-birthweight and at-risk infants as never before. Such survival is not alone the province of developed countries, for the developing areas are increasingly feeling the effects of the new technology. Moreover, follow-up data confirm that high-risk and low-birthweight survivors are likely to have significant developmental disabilities as they grow and mature. In addition, technology has also enabled increasing survival from malnutrition, infectious disease and traumatic injury—vastly adding to the population of children with potential developmental deficits.

An awareness and understanding of the earliest characteristics of developmental disabilities has led to an emphasis on infant diagnosis and early intervention programs. Increasingly there has been an appreciation that the focus of effort must be shifted from the affected child alone to the sphere of the family and beyond to the community itself.

Over many years there has also been a change in approach and emphasis to disabled people from disregarding their presence, employing segregation or institutionalization, to utilizing community resources to achieve integration and, more recently, working toward full potential (Helander 1993). Likewise, a shift has occurred from the model of Western 'experts' imposing their values and technology, to a more community-oriented culturally appropriate approach utilizing local personnel and resources with technical support.

All of these developments in direction and emphasis are in process simultaneously with monumental worldwide social, political and economic events which receive first priority. Yet emerging epidemiological data now suggest that perhaps some 7 per cent of the world's children have disabilities (Helander 1993)—predominantly in developing countries. This is a vast resource which must be viewed first in human then in social and economic terms and is a compelling basis for priority consideration. The 1990 United Nations Summit for Children put into perspective both the obligations of the international community toward this group and the rights of children to be assured the requirements needed for optimum growth and development. This is particularly relevant for children with special needs.

Now the challenge is how best to plan for and meet these special needs. Over many years of well-meaning aid programs, vast funding efforts and myriad professional approaches both by governmental and non-governmental organizations, there has often been considerable fragmentation, competition and conflicting aims in projects, with much resultant frustration. More recently, a definite consensus on principles has begun to emerge along with a more concerted and better communicated international effort.

This is reflected in *Disabled Children and Developing Countries*, which represents a broad range of current approaches, philosophy and technological experience in a field which is now beginning to achieve better international recognition but still cries out for more effective solutions to its complex problems. The work has the twin aims of providing information about this field to the developed countries and offering guidelines for those working in developing areas. The principles elicited will have significance wherever the disabled child can be found—whether in a rural village in an underdeveloped country or in a low-income neighborhood in a 'modern' metropolitan city.

What this work will do is provide much-needed current perspectives on the scope and dimensions of this population, principles and approaches to program planning and evaluation, and concepts on the place of technology and professional input. By pooling their expertise, sharing their varied experience and offering the benefit of this interdisciplinary outlook, the contributors have helped to move closer the day when efforts on behalf of the disabled child in developing countries will have greater relevance and long-lasting effectiveness.

ALFRED L. SCHERZER
Cornell University Medical Center;
and
Rehabilitation International Medical Commission,
New York

REFERENCE

Helander, E. (1993) *Prejudice and Dignity: an Introduction to Community-based Rehabilitation.* New York: United Nations Development Programme.

PREFACE

This book is intended to help professionals working in developed countries to understand the situation, needs and problems of disabled children who live in developing countries. It will help them to be more critical of what they contribute to effective interventions if working in or acting as a consultant to childhood disability services. The book also aims to be relevant to professionals in developing countries in choosing types of intervention and modes of service delivery appropriate for their own situation. Furthermore, professionals in developing countries have more experience of working cooperatively with families and communities, valuable for the development of child disability services internationally.

The majority of the authors are from or have worked in developing countries. Some contributions are further informed by personal experience of disability. We have asked the contributors to the book to address issues, rather than to describe services for children with particular types of impairment. Therefore the range of examples is not comprehensive or equally balanced across impairments, nor have we attempted complete geographical coverage. The principles derived from the discussion, however, have wide applicability.

There is a wide variety of terms concerning disabled children, and a lack of clarity and agreement about their use in the field. As editors we have preferred to use the definitions agreed by disabled people's organizations. In essence, 'impairment' is an individual limitation, whereas 'disability' is restriction imposed by the current organization of society. 'Impairment' is defined by WHO (1980) as 'any loss or abnormality of psychological, physiological, or anatomical structure or function'. Making descriptions at the level of impairment allows focus on the individual child and her/his needs as an individual. When the emphasis is on children with impairments as a *social group* we have used the term 'disabled children', defining disability as 'the disadvantage or restriction of activity caused by contemporary social organization which takes little or no account of people who have . . . impairments and thus excludes them from participation in the mainstream of social activities' (UPIAS 1976, Finkelstein 1993).

Ultimately the terms used in the chapters have been the choice of the author. For example, when dealing with medical issues authors have tended to use WHO definitions (impairment, disability and handicap), or wording is maintained from previously published work. Likewise we have not expected the authors to present a united view. If the differences stimulate questioning and debate, then the book will have achieved its purpose.

REFERENCES

Finkelstein, V. (1993) 'The commonality of disability.' *In:* Swain, J., Finkelstein, V., French, S., Oliver, M. (Eds.) *Disabling Barriers – Enabling Environments.* London: Sage in association with the Open University, pp. 9–16.
World Health Organization (1980) *International Classification of Impairments, Disabilities, and Handicaps. A Manual of Classification Relating to the Consequences of Disease.* Geneva: WHO.
UPIAS (1976) *Fundamental Principles of Disability.* London: Union of the Physically Impaired Against Segregation.

1
FRAMEWORK: PREVALENCE

Naila Khan and Maureen Durkin

It has been estimated that currently 85 per cent of the world's disabled children under 15 years of age live in developing countries (Helander 1993). However, most of these children receive scant attention, if any, from formal health services. There are several reasons for this. Often, the health care system is centralized, hospital-based and physician-oriented. The physician-to-population ratio is low, particularly in rural areas where the majority of the population live. Where health services are available, the focus is more on the prevention and treatment of common conditions with high fatality rates than on developmental disorders and disability (Walsh and Warren 1979, Evans *et al.* 1981). Lack of an appropriate infrastructure precludes monitoring universal developmental milestones and early identification of conditions with long-term implications for the health and abilities of children. Yet, for the sake of primary and secondary prevention, and rehabilitation, there is an increasing need to identify children at risk of disability (Marfo 1986).

Several United Nations programmes, including the International Year of the Child in 1979, the International Year of Disabled Persons in 1981 and the World Programme of Action Concerning Disabled Persons (United Nations 1982, Helander 1993) publicized the situation of disabled children in developing countries. It is now recognized that basic child health programmes in developing countries need to take into account the long-term consequences of diseases and injuries and to pay attention to child development. Documentation of the frequency and distribution of childhood disabilities through epidemiological studies has been undertaken in several developing countries in conjunction with programmes providing rehabilitation services (Stein and Susser 1980; Belmont 1981, 1986; Hammerman and Maikowski 1981; Durkin *et al.* 1990, 1991; Zaman *et al.* 1990; Stein *et al.* 1992; Thorburn *et al.* 1992).

To address the rehabilitation and medical needs of the large numbers of disabled children in developing countries will require simple methods of screening, assessment and rehabilitation. This chapter discusses an approach to screening and assessment that has been implemented on a wide scale in Bangladesh, and presents some estimates of the prevalence of disability.

Information on specific disabilities
Most information on the prevalence of childhood disabilities in developing countries has been generated from surveys on specific public health problems of which disability is an outcome. For example, there is considerable knowledge about the extent of nutritional blindness caused by vitamin A deficiency in Asia and Africa (Menon and Vijayaraghavan

1

1980, Sommer *et al.* 1981, Cohen *et al.* 1986, Foster and Sommer 1986). Studies have also confirmed that poliomyelitis is a major cause of lameness in many countries (Expanded Programme on Immunization 1977, Ofusu-Amaah *et al.* 1977, Soewarso 1978, Ulfah *et al.* 1981). Other public health conditions which lead to disability and which are well documented include the link between otitis media and hearing impairment (Holborow *et al.* 1981), effects of poverty and its consequences on mental functions (Cravioto and Robles 1965, Monckeberg 1968, Richardson *et al.* 1973, Townsend *et al.* 1982, Stein and Susser 1992), the effects of iodine deficiency disorders on peri- and postnatal development (Ramalingaswami *et al.* 1961, Delange *et al.* 1972, Hetzel 1983, Pharoah *et al.* 1984), and the neurological sequelae of intracranial infections such as meningitis, encephalitis and cerebral malaria (Schmutzhard and Gerstenbrand 1984, Phillips and Solomon 1990). Most studies and consequent intervention programmes have been centrally planned (Balasubrahmanyan 1991), and have been thwarted by unrealistic expectations and minimal professional interest, having failed to consider child health and morbidity against the social, cultural and economic backdrop (Vijayaraghavan *et al.* 1990). On the other hand, socio-cultural and economic factors such as parental awareness and access to information, parental (especially maternal) education, dietary and food preparation habits, and the general level and coverage of primary health care have been found to have a greater effect than any specific intervention (Belcher *et al.* 1978, Bachani *et al.* 1983, Tsou *et al.*1984, Bhuiya *et al.* 1987, Fauveau *et al.* 1990).

The increasing focus on disability
A focus in prevalence studies on the disease–impairment relationship stops short of acknowledging the consequences of the disease. The World Health Organization (1980*a*) classification suggested a spectrum of 'impairment – disability – handicap'. Disability, which is a failure of function or skill, may be caused by a multitude of impairments whose aetiologies vary greatly. Surveys of impairment will be useful for providing information for prevention; surveys of disability gauge the magnitude of the problem and suggest services that need to be provided.

Prioritizing serious disabilities
One consideration regarding the scope of any survey is whether to target severe disabilities or all grades of disability. An argument in favour of screening for milder disabilities is that they may have a highly favourable outcome after intervention. Mild mental retardation is thought to be a result of understimulation of children in disadvantaged societies (Stein *et al.* 1986). Supporting evidence for this view comes from Sweden where a rise in the general socio-economic level has lowered the rate of mild mental retardation (Hagberg *et al.* 1981). Identification of children with mild mental retardation is justified where appropriate intensive teaching can be made available (Templer and Galloway 1988) but not if little can be done for children so identified.

An argument in favour of focusing on children with more severe disabilities is that they are in greatest need and also their disability is recognized by the community. Surveys of severe disability are also likely to be more accurate because it is easier to distinguish severely disabled children than to distinguish mildly disabled from non-disabled children (Hirst and Cooke 1988). This argument also gains ground when paraprofessionals are doing the identifying.

Information on the prevalence of disability

The prevalence of childhood disability refers to the proportion of children in the community who are disabled at a given time. It is the function of two community parameters—one is the risk of becoming disabled and the other is the average duration of disabilities that occur. Duration, in turn, is influenced by the probability of surviving once disabled and by the availability of treatment for curable conditions. It is likely that the risk of impairment is elevated for children in developing countries because of the excess exposure of many children to serious infections (*e.g.* meningitis, poliomyelitis) and nutritional deficiencies (*e.g.* iodine, vitamin A). Increased mortality of children once disabled due to these conditions might, on the other hand, reduce the rate of serious disability in these communities. Appropriate screening programmes are needed to provide knowledge and insight into the magnitude of the problem (Durkin *et al.* 1991).

Methods of data collection

In developed countries systematic and valid epidemiological information on childhood disability is available from service records and registers containing information on all causes of a specific kind of disorder, or from organized studies that follow a birth cohort of several thousand children (Davie *et al.* 1972, Hagberg 1978, Drillien and Drummond 1983, Nelson and Ellenberg 1986, Stewart-Brown and Haslum 1988). In most developing countries these sources are not readily available, and special efforts have to be made to collect baseline information.

Two low-cost methods have been found unsatisfactory because too many children remain unidentified. One of these involves adding a question to the national census asking whether anyone in the household is disabled. This approach tends to under-enumerate disabilities that are not highly visible (*e.g.* hearing loss, mental retardation), and disabilities in women and children (Chamie 1986). The other low-cost method has been to ask key informants in the community (*e.g.* community leaders, teachers, healers, midwives) to identify all disabled persons in the community. This method was studied in several countries and again found to be inaccurate (Belmont 1984, Thorburn 1993), with serious under-enumeration especially of less physically obvious conditions.

A third approach involves door-to-door household surveys with screening of children for disabilities and follow-up professional evaluations of selected children. A survey based on this approach is described in the following section.

Population-based study of childhood disability

The 'Rapid Epidemiological Assessment of Childhood Disability' study was carried out in Bangladesh, Jamaica and Pakistan with the primary objective of developing a low-cost and rapid method of screening children with serious disabilities by community workers in populations where professional resources are scarce. A secondary objective was to

TABLE 1.1
The 'Ten Questions' screen

1. Compared with other children, did the child have any serious delay in sitting, standing or walking?

2. Compared with other children does the child have difficulty seeing, either in the daytime or at night?

3. Does the child appear to have difficulty hearing?

4. When you tell the child to do something, does he/she seem to understand what you are saying?

5. Does the child have difficulty in walking or moving his/her arms or does he/she have weakness and/or stiffness in the arms or legs?

6. Does the child sometimes have fits, become rigid, or lose consciousness?

7. Does the child learn to do things like other children his/her age?

8. Does the child speak at all (can he/she make himself/herself understood in words; can he/she say any recognizable words)?

9. *For 3- to 9-year-olds ask:*
Is the child's speech in any way different from normal (not clear enough to be understood by people other than his/her immediate family)?

For 2-year-olds ask:
Can he/she name at least one object (for example, an animal, a toy, a cup, a spoon)?

10. Compared with other children of his/her age, does the child appear in any way mentally backward, dull or slow?

ascertain the prevalence and distribution of various disabilities for the sake of prioritizing limited resources into rehabilitation work.

In Phase 1, 2- to 9-year-old children were screened for developmental disabilities using the 'Ten Questions' screening questionnaire (Table 1.1). In Phase 2, a proportion of these children were referred for clinical assessments.

The Ten Questions survey is designed to identify children in any culture who may have developmental disabilities, including seizures and cognitive, motor, vision and hearing disabilities. It is a low-cost screening procedure that makes use of resources available in the community. Thus it is intended to be administered by community workers who can read and write and who have participated in a brief interviewer training programme. The Ten Questions are presented as a personal interview with a parent or other adult who knows the child being screened. On the basis of the Ten Questions, each child is classified as screened positive (one or more problems reported of the ten inquired about) or negative (no problems reported).

All children who screened positive and a random sample of about 10 per cent of those who screened negative were referred for medical and psychological assessments. These assessments in Phase 2 provided a basis for determining whether or not a child was disabled, and thus for confirming the screening result. The psychologists and physicians performed their assessments without knowledge of the screening results. To determine cognitive disability, the physician and psychologist made their assessment of the child independently, and then reached a consensus judgement.

Standard and comprehensive medical assessment procedures and criteria were used, with a structured form developed for this study. As far as possible, diagnoses were given using ICD-9 codes (World Health Organization 1980b) in addition to the ratings of disability.

All forms used in the study were pre-coded to facilitate comparability and computerized data entry. In Bangladesh, forms administered as interviews were translated from English into Bangla. Translated forms were back-translated, pre-tested and revised before arriving at the final versions.

Estimates of the prevalence of childhood disability in Bangladesh

A total of 10,299 children were screened, about half of whom lived in urban and half in rural communities in Bangladesh. The proportion screening positive on the Ten Questions was 8.2 per cent, and did not differ between urban and rural areas.

The estimated prevalence of disabilities per 1000 children is shown overleaf in Tables 1.2 and 1.3. The overall prevalence of disability was greater in girls than in boys, which may reflect the priority given to the male child in Bangladeshi cultures (Bhuiya *et al.* 1989). However, the reasons for the gender difference in serious hearing disability are unclear. The differential rate for serious hearing disability in older versus younger children reflects difficulties in accurate assessment in the communities. The prevalence of serious motor disabilities was higher in the younger age group. The reasons for this were not clearly established by the study. It may be that children are achieving developmental milestones later than usual where large numbers suffer from some degree of malnutrition (Upadhyay *et al.* 1989). Lack of micronutrients such as iodine, zinc, manganese and copper have been shown to cause various types of motor delay (Walravens *et al.* 1983, DeLong 1990). The much lower prevalence of serious motor disability in the older age group may be a more stable estimate.

Hearing disability was far more common in the older (6–9 years) than in the younger (2–5 years) age group. Most was a result of suppurative otitis media, which is common in a chiefly riverine terrain within a tropical climate, where children are in and out of the water several times a day. It could also be a reflection of a general early under-identification of covert impairments. There was an urban–rural differential for vision and hearing problems, vision disability being more prevalent in the urban areas, and hearing disabilities overall more prevalent in rural communities.

Conclusion

In developing countries the problem of disability in children is great. Combining all grades and types of disabilities, we estimate that nearly 7 per cent of 2- to 9-year-old children in Bangladesh have developmental disabilities. The main focus should be on prevention so that fewer children need treatment and rehabilitation. Consensus has to be reached about methods for early identification of children requiring treatment and rehabilitation.

TABLE 1.2
Estimated prevalence per 1000 of disabilities among 2- to 9-year-old children in Bangladesh

Type of disability	Total (N=10,299)	Urban (N=5103)	Rural (N=5196)
Any disability			
Serious	15.68	19.90	11.75
Mild	52.84	45.26	59.98
Cognitive			
Serious	5.93	6.05	5.84
Mild	14.84	15.80	13.18
Motor			
Serious	3.79	3.58	4.01
Mild	2.17	2.02	2.32
Vision			
Serious	2.46	3.74	1.27
Mild	13.33	22.04	5.14
Hearing			
Serious	5.87	9.66	2.32
Mild	23.06	6.37	38.77
Seizures			
Serious	0.33	0.45	0.21
Mild	4.57	3.52	5.57

TABLE 1.3
Estimated prevalence per 1000 of serious disabilities among 2- to 9-year-old children in Bangladesh, by age and gender

Type of serious disability	2–5 years (N=4947)	6–9 years (N=5352)	All boys (N=5413)	All girls (N=4886)
Any serious disability	12.27	18.68	13.66	18.05
Cognitive	5.12	6.62	5.08	6.94
Motor	6.46	1.26	3.66	3.95
Vision	2.91	2.10	3.17	1.63
Hearing	1.34	9.96	3.98	8.08
Seizures	0.45	0.21	0.61	0.00

REFERENCES

Bachani, D., Singh, M.P., Yadav, S., Pawar, R.G. (1983) 'Utilisation of preventive services—an elaborative study of vaccine acceptors.' *Indian Journal of Preventive and Social Medicine*, **14**, 35–41.

Balasubrahmanyan, V. (1991) 'India: protests over salt iodisation.' *Lancet*, **337**, 226.

Belcher, D.W., Nicholas, D.D., Ofosu-Amaah, S., Wurapa, F.K. (1978) 'A mass immunization campaign in rural Ghana—factors affecting participation.' *Public Health Reports*, **93**, 170–176.

Belmont, L. (1981) 'The development of a questionnaire to screen for severe mental retardation in developing countries.' *International Journal of Mental Health*, **10**, 85–99.

— — (1984) *The International Pilot Study of Severe Childhood Disability. Final Report.* Utrecht, Netherlands: Bishop Bekkers Institute.

— — (1986) 'Screening for severe mental retardation in developing countries: the International Pilot Study of

Severe Childhood Disability.' *In:* Berg, J.M. (Ed.) *Science and Technology in Mental Retardation.* London: Methuen, pp. 389–395.

Bhuiya, A., Wojtyniak, B., D'Souza, S., Nahar, L., Shaikh, K. (1987) 'Measles case fatality among under-fives: a multivariate analysis of risk factors in a rural area of Bangladesh.' *Social Science and Medicine,* **24,** 439–443.

— — — Karim, R. (1989) 'Malnutrition and child mortality: are socioeconomic factors important?' *Journal of Biosocial Science,* **21,** 357–364.

Chamie, M. (1986) *Development of Statistics of Disabled Persons: Case Studies. United Nations Department of International Economic and Social Affairs, Statistics on Special Population Groups, Series Y, No 2.* New York: United Nations.

Cohen, N.A., Jalil, M.A., Rahman, H., Leemhuis de Regt, E., Sprague, J., Mitra, M. (1986) 'Blinding malnutrition in rural Bangladesh.' *Journal of Tropical Pediatrics,* **32,** 73–78.

Cravioto, J., Robles, B. (1965) 'Evolution of adaptive and motor behavior during rehabilitation from kwashiorkor.' *American Journal of Orthopsychiatry,* **35,** 449–464.

Davie, R., Butler, N., Goldstein, H. (1972) *From Birth to Seven: The Second Report of the National Child Development Study (1958 Cohort).* London: Longman.

Delange, F., Costa, A., Ermans, A.M., Ibbertson, H.K., Querido, A., Stanbury, J.B. (1972) 'A survey of the clinical and metabolic patterns of endemic cretinism.' *Advances in Experimental Medicine and Biology,* **30,** 175–187.

DeLong, R.G. (1990) 'The effect of iodine deficiency on neuromuscular development.' *IDD Newsletter,* **6,** 1–9.

Drillien, C., Drummond, M. (1983) *Development Screening and the Child with Special Needs. Clinics in Developmental Medicine No. 86.* London: Spastics International Medical Publications.

Durkin, M.S., Davidson, L.L., Hasan, M., Khan, N., Thorburn, M.J., Zaman, S.S. (1990) 'Screening for childhood disability in community settings.' *In:* Thorburn, M., Marfo, K. (Eds.) *Practical Approaches to Childhood Disability in Developing Countries: Insights From Experience and Research.* St Johns, Newfoundland: Memorial University, Project SEREDEC; Spanish Town, Jamaica: 3D Projects, pp. 179–197.

— — Zaman, S., Thorburn, M., Hasan, Z.M., Shrout, P.E., Davidson, L.L., Stein, Z.A. (1991) 'Screening for childhood disability in less developed countries: rationale and study design.' *International Journal of Mental Health,* **20,** 47–60.

Evans, J.R., Lashman Hall, K., Warford, J. (1981) 'Shattuck Lecture. Health care in the developing world: problems of scarcity and choice.' *New England Journal of Medicine,* **305,** 1117–1127.

Expanded Programme on Immunization (1977) 'Survey for residual poliomyelitis–paralysis—Egypt.' *Weekly Epidemiological Record,* **52,** 269–271.

Fauveau, V., Wojtyniak, B., Mostafa, G., Sarder, A.M., Chakraborty, J. (1990) 'Perinatal mortality in Matlab, Bangladesh: a community-based study.' *International Journal of Epidemiology,* **19,** 606–612.

Foster, A., Sommer, A. (1986) 'Childhood blindness from corneal ulceration in Africa: causes, prevention, and treatment.' *Bulletin of the World Health Organization,* **64,** 619–623.

Hagberg, B. (1978) 'Severe mental retardation in Swedish children born 1959–1970: epidemiologic panorama and causative factors.' *In:* Elliott, K., O'Connor, M. (Eds.) *Major Mental Handicap: Methods and Costs of Prevention. Ciba Foundation Symposium 59.* Amsterdam: Elsevier, pp. 29–51.

— — Hagberg, G., Lewerth, A., Lindberg, U. (1981) 'Mild mental retardation in Swedish school children. I. Prevalence.' *Acta Paediatrica Scandinavica,* **70,** 441–444.

Hammerman, S., Maikowski, S. (1981) *The Economics of Disability: International Perspectives.* New York: Rehabilitation International.

Helander, E.A.S. (1993) *Prejudice and Dignity: an Introduction of Community-based Rehabilitation.* New York: United Nations Development Programme.

Hetzel, B.S. (1983) 'Iodine deficiency disorders (IDD) and their eradication.' *Lancet,* **2,** 1126–1129.

Hirst, M., Cooke, K. (1988) 'Grading severity of childhood disablement: comparing survey measures with a paediatrician's assessment.' *Child: Care, Health and Development,* **14,** 111–126.

Holborow, C., Martinson, F., Anger, N. (1981) *A Study of Deafness in West Africa.* London: Commonwealth Society for the Deaf.

Marfo, K. (1986) 'Confronting childhood disability in developing countries.' *In:* Marfo, K., Walker, S., Charles, B. (Eds.) *Childhood Disability in Developing Countries.* New York: Praeger, pp. 3–26.

Menon, K., Vijayaraghavan, K. (1980) 'Sequelae of severe xerophthalmia—a follow-up study.' *American Journal of Clinical Nutrition,* **33,** 218–220.

Monckeberg, F. (1968) 'Effects of early marasmic malnutrition on subsequent physical and psychological development.' *In:* Scrimshaw, N.S., Gordon, L. (Eds.) *Malnutrition, Learning and Behavior.* Cambridge, MA: MIT Press, pp. 269–277.

Nelson, K.B., Ellenberg, J.H. (1986) 'Antecedents of cerebral palsy. Multivariate analysis of risk.' *New England Journal of Medicine*, **315**, 81–86.

Ofusu-Amaah, S., Kratzer, J.H., Nicholas, D.D. (1977) 'Is poliomyelitis a serious problem in developing countries?—lameness in Ghanaian schools.' *British Medical Journal*, **1**, 1012–1014.

Pharoah, P.O.D., Connolly, K.J., Ekins, R.P., Harding, A.G. (1984) 'Maternal thyroid hormone levels in pregnancy and the subsequent cognitive and motor performance of the children.' *Clinical Endocrinology*, **21**, 265–270.

Phillips, R.E., Solomon, T. (1990) 'Cerebral malaria in children.' *Lancet*, **336**, 1355–1360.

Ramalingaswami, V., Subramanian, T.A.V., Deo, M.G. (1961) 'The aetiology of Himalayan endemic goitre.' *Lancet*, **1**, 791–794.

Richardson, S.A., Birch, H.G., Hertzig, M.E. (1973) 'School performance of children who were severely malnourished in infancy.' *American Journal of Mental Deficiency*, **77**, 623–632.

Schmutzhard, E., Gerstenbrand, F. (1984) 'Cerebral malaria in Tanzania. Its epidemiology, clinical symptoms and neurological long term sequelae in the light of 66 cases.' *Transactions of the Royal Society of Tropical Medicine and Hygiene*, **78**, 351–353.

Soewarso, T.I. (1978) 'Poliomyelitis in Indonesia.' *Epidemiological Bulletin*, (Second Quarter), 25–32.

Sommer, A., Tarwotjo, I., Hussaini, G., Susanto, D., Soegiharto, T. (1981) 'Incidence, prevalence, and scale of blinding malnutrition.' *Lancet*, **1**, 1407–1408.

Stein, Z., Susser, M. (1980) 'The less developed world: south-east Asia as a paradigm.' *In:* Wortis, J. (Ed.) *Mental Retardation and Developmental Disabilities: an Annual Review. XI.* New York: Brunner/Mazel, pp. 227–240.

— — — — (1992) 'Mental retardation.' *In:* Last, J.M., Wallace, R.B. (Eds.) *Public Health and Preventive Medicine. 13th Edn.* Norwalk, CT: Appleton & Lange, pp. 963–972.

— — Belmont, L., Durkin, M. (1986) 'Mild mental retardation and severe mental retardation compared: experiences in the eight less developed countries.' *Paper presented to the 2nd European Symposium on Scientific Studies in Mental Retardation, Uppsala, Sweden.*

— — Durkin, M.S., Davidson, L.L., Hasan, Z.M., Thorburn, M.J., Zaman, S.S. (1992) 'Guidelines for identifying children with mental retardation in community settings.' *In: Assessment of People with Mental Retardation.* Geneva: World Health Organization, pp. 12–41.

Stewart-Brown, S.L., Haslum, M.N. (1988) 'Partial sight and blindness in children of the 1970 birth cohort at 10 years of age.' *Journal of Epidemiology and Community Health*, **42**, 17–23.

Templer, S.L., Galloway, B.M. (1988) 'Developing more effective teaching programmes for intellectually handicapped children.' *In:* Ross, D.H. (Ed.) *Educating Handicapped Young People in Eastern and Southern Africa.* Paris: Unesco, pp. 103–108.

Thorburn, M. (1993) 'Recent developments in low-cost screening and assessment of childhood disabilities in Jamaica. Part 1: screening.' *West Indian Medical Journal*, **42**, 10–12.

— — Desai, P., Paul, T.J., Malcolm, L., Durkin, M., Davidson, L. (1992) 'Identification of childhood disability in Jamaica: the Ten Question screen.' *International Journal of Rehabilitation Research*, **15**, 115–127.

Townsend, J.W., Klein, R.E., Irwin, M.H., Owens, W., Yarborough, C., Engle, P. (1982) 'Nutrition and pre-school mental development.' *In:* Wagner, D.A., Stevenson, H.W. (Eds.) *Cultural Perspectives on Child Development.* San Francisco: W.H. Freeman, pp. 124–145.

Tsou, S.C.S., Gershon, J., Simpson, K.L., Chichester, C.O. (1984) 'Promoting household gardens for nutrition improvement.' *In:* Tanphaichitr, V., Dahlan, W., Suphakarn, V., Valyasevi, A. (Eds.) *Human Nutrition: Better Nutrition, Better Life. Proceedings of the 4th Asian Congress on Nutrition, Bangkok, Thailand, November 1983.* Bangkok: Aksornsmai Press, pp. 179–185.

Ulfah, N.M., Parastho, S., Sadjimin, T., Rohde, J.E. (1981) 'Polio and lameness in Yogyakarta, Indonesia.' *International Journal of Epidemiology*, **10**, 171–175.

United Nations (1982) *World Program of Action Concerning Disabled Persons.* New York: United Nations.

Upadhyay, S.K., Agarwal, D.K., Agarwal, K.N. (1989) 'Influence of malnutrition on intellectual development.' *Indian Journal of Medical Research*, **90**, 430–441.

Vijayaraghavan, K., Radhaiah, G., Surya Prakasam, B., Rameshwar Sarma, K.V., Reddy, V. (1990) 'Effects of massive dose Vitamin A on morbidity and mortality in Indian children.' *Lancet*, **336**, 1342–1345.

Walravens, P.A., Krebs, N.F., Hambridge, K.M. (1983) 'Linear growth of low income preschool children receiving a zinc supplement.' *American Journal of Clinical Nutrition*, **38**, 195–201.

8

Walsh, J.A., Warren, K.S. (1979) 'Selective primary health care. An interim strategy for disease control in developing countries.' *New England Journal of Medicine*, **301**, 967–974.

WHO (1980*a*) *International Classification of Impairments, Disabilities, and Handicaps.* Geneva: World Health Organization.

— — (1980*b*) *International Classification of Diseases and Diagnostic Codes. 9th Edn.* Geneva: World Health Organization.

Zaman, S.S., Khan N.Z., Islam, S., Banu, S., Dixit, S., Shrout, P., Durkin, M. (1990) 'Validity of the "Ten Questions" for screening serious childhood disability: results from urban Bangladesh.' *International Journal of Epidemiology*, **19**, 613–620.

2
FRAMEWORK: PRIORITIES

Pam Zinkin

This chapter asks some questions about priorities for action in helping disabled children in developing countries. The first question must be 'whose priorities?'. Although prevention is the initial topic in this chapter, it cannot be the main need of a child whose impairment has not been prevented and from whom all resources may be diverted. It is of little support to a family to tell them that improved antenatal care might have prevented their child's impairment, when there is no culturally, economically or geographically accessible care even after the event. Prevention of impairment appears first since it seems logical and also because the causes of impairment in developing countries raise serious questions about poverty and country development.

The starting point in helping children must be to find out what is already happening, what parents are already doing, who loves and cares for the child, what games disabled children play with their families, what fun they have together and so on. We cannot assume that our professional intervention is necessarily appropriate nor that we know the priorities and the 'right' order to pursue them. When initiating discussion of priorities with those who will be most affected by decisions made and resources allocated, we have to bear in mind that communities rarely perceive the needs of disabled people as a priority. For the families of disabled children the issues surrounding disability are complex and so deeply felt that they are not easily understood or expressed (see Chapter 11).

The prevention of impairment
The causes of impairments in children in developing countries are mainly the same preventable conditions that cause the higher mortality and morbidity rates associated with poverty. Many different impairments may follow, including hearing, visual, intellectual, motor and multiple impairments and seizures. The major medical conditions are:
• *Conditions associated with pregnancy, childbirth and the neonatal period.* Women's health and maternity services are usually inadequate, as reflected in the huge discrepancy in maternal mortality rates (MMRs) between poor countries and industrialized ones. Although there is great variation between and within countries, the average MMR in developed countries is around 26/100,000 live births as compared with around 450/100,000 live births in developing countries. For example, AbouZahr and Royston (1991, 1992) reported an MMR for Australia of just 3, compared with 522 for Sudan and 874 for rural Andra Pradesh, India. Correspondingly high perinatal mortality rates of 81/1000 births in Africa compared with 7/1000 in the UK (WHO 1992) also reflect the health status of women before and during pregnancy and the care they receive during pregnancy and childbirth.

- *Infectious diseases.* These include poliomyelitis, measles, whooping cough, tuberculosis, meningitis, encephalitis, cerebral malaria, neglected otitis media and many other infections for which the causes, prevention and treatment are known but not implemented.

- *Malnutrition.* The relationship between malnutrition and intellectual impairment is not straightforward, but there is no doubt that the cluster of adverse factors related to under-nutrition is associated with intellectual impairment and poor school performance (Grantham McGregor 1992). Deficiency of micronutrients, such as vitamin A and iodine, occurs widely. Although there is debate about approaches to the problem (*e.g.* population synthetic vitamin A programmes *versus* a community nutrition approach—Gopolan 1990), there is no *scientific* reason why these conditions should continue to cause impairments in children.

- *Congenital anomalies.* The incidence of most congenital anomalies may be different in different parts of the world, but reported variation diminishes after services develop. The discrepancies reported may be genetic and related to intermarriage, but in poorer countries they are more often due to under-reporting, delayed diagnosis, or to early deaths of children with anomalies where facilities are not available or attitudes are different.

- *Violence and accidents.* Rising violence in relation to wars, civil strife and worsening economic conditions has massive impact on the children of developing countries, who increasingly are its victims. Many are killed and many more are injured, leading to perm-anent impairment. Children are also victims of domestic and street violence. Children's need to explore leads them into many dangerous situations, but hazards are increased in poor, uncontrolled environments and children are even more vulnerable in war. Children continue to be injured by land-mines in the aftermath of war (see Chapter 13).

- *Toxic substances and iatrogenic effects.* Toxic waste disposal and the use of pesticides, insecticides and pharmaceuticals are poorly controlled in developing countries and thus the risk of harm to children is elevated. With increased charges for medical care at health centres, many partly qualified doctors and nurses may set up in uncontrolled private practice. Parents of children with impairments are often duped into believing that there are medical cures and may try dangerous and unsuitable treatments.

Prevention is directed toward eradicating poverty and inequitable distribution of resources, the primary causes of both disease and impairment. Although this may seem idealistic, professionals could at the least examine whether any of their activities increase inequities. Professional support for banning land-mines, preventing toxic waste disposal, control of pharmaceuticals and so on may have a more significant impact than does their specific rehabilitation expertise.

Comprehensive primary health care and the promotion of country and community development (see Chapter 11) are essential for basic prevention.

The *early diagnosis and treatment* of conditions such as meningitis and tuberculosis which may lead to different types of impairment is a second priority. This treatment must be affordable and accessible to all. Increasingly, policy changes in health services inter-nationally imposed throughout developing countries have resulted in increased charges for medical treatment (Yoder 1989, Loewenson *et al.* 1991). This has meant that parents often delay seeking medical advice, buy drugs at shops and in markets, cannot afford to com-plete a course of treatment or forgo medical opinion and treatment altogether.

Basic needs for children with impairments

A child with a permanent impairment has the same basic needs as other children: adequate clean water, food, clothing, shelter, protection and consistent loving care. Children's psychological needs are addressed in Chapters 12 and 13.

Professionals concerned with impairment have to consider if their activities may make it more difficult for a child and her/his family's basic needs to be met. For example, encouraging parents to spend a high percentage of family income on equipment might mean the family do not have enough money for food. An example is a family in a village in Uganda, who were saving up for an operation and a special shoe for one of their children with a clubfoot; in the meantime, however, the child was hungry and her younger sister had developed kwashiorkor.

In all actions undertaken to meet the basic needs of all children, disabled children must also be included. In all actions which benefit the community, it is also important for disabled children that disabled adults are included as role models and advisers (see Chapter 11).

Is early detection of impairment a priority?

The obvious answer to this question is 'of course', but the money and energy put into early detection is often not matched by appropriate actions after detection. In some instances early detection has a negative effect and results in labelling causing anxiety to the family and stigmatizing the child, without any benefit. The consequences of false identification and false reassurance are referred to in Chapter 7.

Social integration

The 'individual personal tragedy' view of impairment shared by most professionals contributes to the poor self-esteem and negative self-image that most young disabled people have (Finkelstein and French 1993, Oliver 1993). It is of fundamental importance for a young child who has impairments to be a valued member of a family, and to belong to a social group. Medical rehabilitation and 'special' teaching may be helpful in themselves but their demands should not be allowed to prevent a child from building a positive social identity and way of life.

Are surveys a priority?

This is probably the wrong question: instead, the questions should be 'Who needs surveys?' and 'What purpose do they serve?'. For example, is it a priority to know how many children with conductive deafness there are if we know that there are no means for diagnosing and treating otitis media? (see Chapter 12).

Often surveys are carried out to inform planners and government about the extent of a problem, but well-conducted surveys are expensive and time-consuming.

WHO goes so far as to state that,

'No country needs to undertake censuses, surveys or registration to find out the needs of its disabled citizens. They are so well known that CBR [community-based rehabilitation] can go ahead without question–marks. Every dollar spent on further investigation is a dollar mis-spent' (WHO 1984).

When the situation is obvious to those living and working in the community, and it is equally obvious that adequate resources are simply not available, a preferable use of available resources may be to work out with all those involved how a sustainable, acceptable community-based service could be set up.

In some areas, children with certain conditions such as cerebral palsy and epilepsy may be kept hidden. In surveys carried out in Africa the reported prevalence of epilepsy varies widely from 1:1000 to 49:1000 (Baldwin *et al.* 1990, Meinardi 1993), and few children receive drug therapy. Some of the reasons for this are the widespread negative cultural attitudes both to the condition and to prolonged drug treatment, the preference for traditional measures, the high cost of drug therapy, and the woefully inadequate delivery systems. It would be pointless to carry out a survey including epilepsy unless some of these issues were addressed, for example through a community approach such as the Nakuru experiment (Feksi 1993). However, even in this project an excellent coverage of 82 per cent fell to 62 per cent over time and might have been associated with the reduction of community health workers from 16 to three. Sustainability has to be considered carefully before projects begin.

In these situations surveys are not only inaccurate and unnecessary but may actually do harm through lost alternative opportunities, and through families' disillusion and lack of trust in future ventures if their past experience is that little of value was achieved.

Adult disabled people criticize surveys, such as the OPCS survey (Abberley 1992), for focusing on the individual and on aspects that cannot be changed instead of asking questions about environmental barriers that could be changed (see Chapter 15). The relationship between the people carrying out the survey and those they are surveying is fundamental both to what questions are asked and how they are answered.

The problem of definition is complex. There are different medically based definitions, such as of the diagnosis or disease, the impairment or difficulties in daily living activities, and so on. There are also educational, social, administrative and legal definitions, all of which emanate from different viewpoints, use different criteria and produce different incidence and prevalence rates.

The approach of looking at difficulties in function, instead of medical conditions and impairments, as Khan and Durkin have done (Chapter 1), gives useful information and the methodology used is scientifically sound. Still, it may not be applicable everywhere and again may not give the quality of information required to inform policy and planning. A difficulty in walking may not be easily remediable, and it may be more important to know how happy the child is, what opportunities s/he has for education and how her/his family views priorities.

REFERENCES

Abberley, P. (1992) 'Counting us out: a discussion of the OPCS disability surveys.' *Disability, Handicap and Society*, **7**, 139–155.
AbouZahr, C., Royston E. (1991) *Maternal Mortality: a Global Factbook*. Geneva: WHO.
— — — — (1992) 'Excessive hazards of pregnancy and childbirth in the Third World.' *World Health Forum*, **13**, 343–345.

Baldwin, S., Asindua, S., Stanfield, P. (1990) *Survey of Childhood Disabilities within a Community-based Programme for the Rehabilitation of the Disabled in Kibwezi Division, Kenya*. Nairobi: African Medical and Research Foundation with Action Aid.

Feksi, A.T. (1993) 'Epilepsy. A community approach.' *Tropical and Geographical Medicine*, **45**, 221–222.

Finkelstein, V., French, S. (1993) 'Towards a psychology of disability.' *In:* Swain J., Finkelstein V., French S., Oliver M. (Eds.) *Disabling Barriers – Enabling Environments*. Milton Keynes and London: The Open University with Sage Publications, pp. 26–33.

Gopolan, C. (1990) 'Vitamin A and child mortality.' *Bulletin of the Nutrition Foundation of India*, **11** (3), 1–3.

Grantham McGregor, S. (1992) 'The effect of malnutrition on mental development.' *In:* Waterlow, J.C. (Ed.) *Protein–Energy Malnutriton*. London: Edward Arnold, pp. 344–360.

Loewenson, R., Sanders, D., Davies, R. (1991) 'Challenges to equity in health and health care. A Zimbabwean case study.' *Social Science and Medicine*, **32**, 1079–1088.

Meinardi, H. (1993) 'Epidemiology of epilepsy.' *Tropical and Geographical Medicine*, **45**, 218–221.

Oliver, M. (1993) 'Disability and dependency: a creation of industrial societies?' *In:* Swain, J., Finkelstein, V., French, S., Oliver, M. (Eds.) *Disabling Barriers – Enabling Environments*. Milton Keynes and London: The Open University with Sage Publications, pp. 49–60.

WHO (1984) 'Drop that census!' *World Health, the Magazine of the World Health Organization* (May issue: *Rehabilitation for All*), p. 4.

—— (1992) *Child Health: the Newborn. Report to the World Health Assembly*. Geneva: World Health Organization.

Yoder, R.A. (1989) 'Are people willing and able to pay for health services?' *Social Science and Medicine*, **29**, 35–42.

14

3
CHILD DISABILITY SERVICES AND INTERVENTIONS

Gillian Baird and Helen McConachie

This chapter describes current services in developed countries, particularly Britain, and is mainly concerned with children who have a biological impairment. However, it should not be forgotten that the major disabling factors for most children are environmental. In the western world most biologically based impairment is genetic; elsewhere in the world, disease and malnutrition are more important in causation, and the need for primary prevention is paramount. In Western countries the macro-environmental risks are those of the wider economic scene; unemployment, housing and financial problems have impacts on families and family functioning which require political solutions. The task of the government funded and voluntary services is to identify and respond to children's and families' needs, to aim to prevent potential complications of the impairment and to counter disabling effects of the psychosocial environment.

Overview of philosophy and service structures in Britain
Attitudes and philosophy
In this country, over the last 20–30 years, there have been many changes in the approach of the professional services toward disabled people. However, those who are disabled, or who support disabled people, may feel that changes in the attitude of society in general toward disability are of greater importance.

There are cultural expectations of 'normality' in our society which have profound implications for the development of personal identity, and therefore put particular pressure on those who have an obvious impairment. The main modes for transmission of social–cultural values are social behaviour and language through discourse (Shotter and Gergen 1990). Women and Black people are recognized as being frequent recipients of discrimination in our society, but disabled people also attract a vocabulary with clear social implications, such as 'dumb', 'moron', and 'spastic'. Others have written of the 'stigma of handicap'.

Changing negative attitudes requires more than legislation, though that too is important. Examples of positive efforts are appointing a Minister for the Disabled at government level, and showing disabled people in ordinary situations on television, *e.g.* a person with Down syndrome in a popular 'soap opera', and in films like *Children of a Lesser God* and *Rain Man*.

The availability of prenatal testing for certain genetic conditions, such as Down syndrome, can lead to an assumption that abortion is then a preferred option. This makes value judgements about the quality of a life, and assumes that it depends only on the nature and severity of the impairment(s) or lack of them. The quality of life, however, is determined primarily by parents' attitudes and feelings and by the social and physical barriers the child and family encounter. Achieving a balance that respects parents' feelings while valuing disabled people is not easy, and is the topic of popular ethical debate in newspapers and on television.

'Normalization of the disabled' has been the guiding philosophy of some of the changes in the last 20 years. But this is often not the same as valuing a person for themself and is a view that some disabled people feel neglects the very special perspectives and individuality that they have. An obvious example is the lack of understanding of Deaf culture, and the obstacles put in the way of full recognition of British Sign Language.

Educational philosophy (*e.g.* the Warnock Report 1978, and particularly the Fish Report 1985) has moved toward a policy of integration of disabled children into ordinary schools, despite problems of resources. Vital to successful integration are the views of the teachers and parents and of the children who are not disabled. King *et al.* (1989) studied non-disabled children's views of disability. They confirmed previous findings of the important effect of maternal views, and that the children's views were positively related to having either a disabled relative or recent contact with a disabled person. The non-disabled children's attitudes were not associated with their own perceived self-esteem or social status. The characteristics of the disabled child were not evaluated in this study, but another source (Bak and Siperstein 1986) suggests social competence has a favourable impact. The structure of the contact also matters, as was found in a controlled trial of a 'buddy' programme (Armstrong *et al.* 1987) wherein a non-disabled classmate (preferably a popular child in the class) volunteers to befriend the newly integrated disabled child, and receives some pre-training. Rosenbaum *et al.* (1988) give a full review of children's attitudes to disability.

Within the health and social services, there has been a shift from care in large institutions to care in the community, with small houses, local work, etc. This encompasses the aim of more diverse experiences and ability to make choices for those whose lives were previously severely limited. However, the policy requires to be balanced by ensuring that the very real practical needs that disabled people have are met. Professional services need to be flexible in encouraging self-advocacy.

Legislative change and services
To professionals working with disabled people, one of the biggest changes in England and Wales was the Education Act 1971, which offered education to all children. This not only altered the provision for severely intellectually impaired children (previously excluded from education, in Junior Training Centres) but moved them to a system where progress was expected, and educational principles applied. The removal of labels (*e.g.* 'subnormal') for both children and schools, and the substitution of the term 'learning difficulties' with an assessment of needs and the provision of facilities to meet those needs, was intended to foster a change from negative attitudes. The Warnock Report (1978) on special education made explicit recommendations concerning the need for services for preschool children.

The Education Act 1981 also enshrined the important principle of incorporating parental views in the assessment process, which results in a written statement of a child's special educational needs.

During the same period, reorganization of the child health services meant that nearly every health district now has a Child Development Team (Bax and Whitmore 1991), which usually includes therapists, community paediatricians and health visitors, and sometimes psychologists, child psychiatrists, social workers, etc. The team aims to identify and meet the needs of every disabled child and her/his family. Most districts are setting up registers of children with special needs using the World Health Organization's International Classification of Diseases. However, the ICD codes as they stand are medical diagnostic categories, not functional ones. Therefore they are not easily applied to developmental conditions in a way that can be used for identifying their impact on function, for service planning or for audit of services.

The social services departments of local councils also have a major role to play in meeting the needs of disabled children and their families. The Children Act 1989 has given the social services the task of identifying and making a register of all children in need, and of making appropriate provision for them. This group includes those more traditionally thought of as disabled in the medico-pathological sense, but definitions are not clear, and the definition of 'disabled' used derives from a previous Act dated 1948. The special needs registers of social services and health should, in theory, be broadly compatible if they are oriented toward 'service needs'. In practice, medical preference for diagnostic categories and the difficulties of agreed cross-professional terminologies may slow down the process of achieving compatibility. The importance of the Children Act is as a piece of legislation with children's rights and needs as central. The child's views must be taken into account in placement decisions and consent to examination. The Act also emphasizes the obligations and responsibilities of parents.

From this brief account, it will be clear that many agencies have the responsibility of responding to the needs of a child with an impairment—primarily the parents, but also the health, social and education services. The Care in the Community legislation which came into operation in April 1993 implied the possibility that disabled people would have control over a budget to purchase services as they saw appropriate. It was to be hoped that the government might have proposed a joint agency composed of the three main services, with ring-fenced monies, but this now appears unlikely. Effective working will depend on inter-agency co-operation with all the difficulties of different personalities, responsibilities, philosophies, budgets, and often geographic boundaries. One of the major challenges in developed countries like Britain is not the lack of agencies but their multiplicity, and the difficulty of creating effective inter-agency working in continuing support of a child and her/his family (see Chapter 11).

Disability agencies
Voluntary societies such as the National Autistic Society and Scope (formerly called The Spastics Society), frequently founded by parents, have made a major contribution toward recognition of the needs of families and also have set a lead in service provision (such as

schools, sheltered residences and work places). They provide information and a point of contact for parents to meet each other. It is mandatory for professionals to make parents aware of the voluntary society most relevant to them.

Independent agencies (rather like the Citizens Advice Bureaux) funded by central government and local services are now being developed in several counties. These agencies are sources of advice about what is available and where to find it for the disabled person (*e.g.* DISS—Disability Information Service Surrey).

Now in a time of reducing central resources, voluntary agencies are being asked to plan, manage and implement a range of services, with attendant dangers such as incomplete coverage (both of types of condition and of types of family needs), and also inadequate management and professional support. Collectively the voluntary agencies represent a powerful voice in shaping government policy and professional practice.

Rationing
Within health care, we are becoming much more aware of being forced to make choices between different services, treatments and patients (Smith 1991). Who should do it, and how should it be done?—by public and democratic discussion, as in the Oregon experiment where the population is grappling with decisions about ranking medical problems and deciding on treatment priorities (Oregon Health Services Commission 1991)? or by using other measures such as QALY (quality-adjusted life years)? Whereas it may be necessary to decide which services or treatments should be prioritized, access to these services and treatments must be equitable. For disabled people who rely on care in the community for their lifetime, essential services are already sparse and haphazard. Adequately meeting their needs has cost implications in staffing, equipment and, most importantly, in the training of health and other care professionals.

The financial cost to individual families when a child has an impairment can be immense and this is recognized in the benefits system. Discussions about compensation in Britain have considered the 'no fault' schemes in operation in other countries. To date it has been decided that the best system is to concentrate resources via benefits from the social services department, regardless of the cause of disablement (Smith 1992). What disabled people and their families endure, however, is constantly being assessed for one thing after another.

The effects of a disabled child on families
Early research adopted a 'pathological' model, assuming that the impact of a child with impairment upon the family was likely to be negative, involving greater or lesser psychological trauma. Research focused on measures of pathological effect in family members, particularly mothers, for example looking at psychiatric morbidity and relationship problems (Wishart *et al.* 1981, Romans-Clarkson *et al.* 1986; for a conceptual review, see Byrne and Cunningham 1985).

The feelings and behaviours of parents of children with impairments, after the time of being told the diagnosis, have been likened to a bereavement process (Mac Keith 1973, Bicknell 1983). The way in which the parents are given 'bad news' has been found to have an impact which goes beyond immediate parental feelings. Lack of information and lack of warmth on the part of the giver of bad news have been found to be the most important sources of dissatisfaction (Sloper and Turner 1993). For most parents, there is a period of shock followed by sadness, and frequently anger and sometimes denial. Time is needed for parental adjustment; this is not a 'once-and-for-all' adjustment process, but tends to recur at times of family life changes, anniversaries, etc. But one must be aware as a professional of psychological stereotypes and presumed negative family effects. For some parents, diagnosis can be a positive relief (Sloper and Turner 1990, Urey and Viar 1990). The primary need of families at this stage is for emotional support (Cunningham 1975, Davis 1993), and another parent of a child with a similar diagnosis may be the best person to offer that support.

In more recent research on families, the 'pathological' model has been left behind and family members' strengths as well as needs have been explored. A wide range of adaptation over time is recognized; for many families with a child with impairment many aspects of outcome may be positive. Many studies have adopted as a theoretical framework a model of stress and coping (Lazarus and Folkman 1984). Stress is seen when coping strategies are outweighed by the demands of the situation, which will of course change over time in response to a variety of factors. Some stressors are child-related such as behaviour problems; others are concerned with life events and day-to-day hassles. Coping resources include family finances; personality, including morale and coping style; family relationships; social support; and adequacy of services (McConachie 1994).

Knussen and Sloper (1992) have summarized recent studies concerning families whose children have a variety of impairments. The differences between the studies could be related to the type of impairment and its severity, but there are many common features. In general, the actual characteristics of the child affect mothers' stress levels more than they do the fathers'. Positive outcomes for both parents are associated with financial security; with good social support, especially within the family; and with confiding relationships. Personality factors were shown as increasing parents' vulnerability to stress. Coping strategies which were high in perceived ability to manage the situation, and low in wishful thinking and self-blame, were also associated with a favourable outcome. Being well-adjusted to the child, having few other life events to cope with, and being at work were all factors which modified for mothers the effects of a child's impairment and behaviour. One could postulate that a common factor in many of these findings is the importance of bolstering maternal self-esteem (Frey *et al.* 1989; Wallander *et al.* 1989, 1990; Quine and Pahl 1991; Sloper *et al.* 1991).

Cultural differences in responses to disability
Cultural groups may differ radically in their views of medicine and health care, in the meaning they attach to disability and its causation, and in child-rearing practices (see Chapters 5 and 12; also Hanson *et al.* 1990 for a review of issues). The need for sensitivity to cultural differences grows in importance in developed countries as the demography changes. What tends to happen is that ethnic minority groups receive less adequate services, as professionals make assumptions about needs (*e.g.* for respite care) and information is not disseminated appropriately (Shah 1992).

Designing services to respond to needs

Although service provision has been conceptualized as important to family coping and stress, studies have often not found any clear relationship between the two. Both research and everyday experience suggest that for most families there is a feeling of having to fight for everything. Sloper and Turner (1992) provide evidence that many families with a physically disabled child have clear unmet needs despite high frequency of professional contact. Those families already coping with other stresses were most likely to have needs not being met by services. Trying to get services added to the stress!

Coordination between service departments is generally poor, and arguments about which is responsible for provision and payment are common. Many commentators have suggested that it is essential to have someone recognized as the coordinator of care who would bridge the family/professional service gap, and is particularly needed where families have fewest resources of their own.

In summary, the service needs of families are:

(1) Information about diagnosis and aetiology, and genetic advice, and the opportunity to discuss these as frequently as necessary.
(2) Information about services: health, social, education and voluntary. (Some districts produce a booklet, regularly updated.)
(3) Social and psychological support, firstly in the stage of primary adaptation and then in the secondary phase of longer-term adaptation. Recognizing existing supportive social networks and parent groups is as important as providing direct professional support.
(4) Specific resources, including: financial; housing; transport; respite care; medication; help with behaviour problems; personal help or family relationship help; specific teaching and therapy; and educational advice, support in school and modifications to the national curriculum.

Families with a disabled child have a right to have their needs met by local authorities. It is a general responsibility, which therefore does not require the same proofs of effectiveness as must be sought for specific types of intervention.

Parents and professionals

There are various models of parent–professional partnership (Mittler and Mittler 1983, Cunningham 1985, Cunningham and Davis 1985). Parents must feel they are equal partners, but with a unique contribution (Wolfendale 1983). The Fish Report (1985) commented that parents who had been in contact with a child development centre were more confident about their participation in educational assessment (although the committee also commented that health service assessments tended to stress what children could not do, rather than describe their skills). Most intervention programmes try to work through parents, particularly at the preschool age, either individually or in groups.

There are good theoretical reasons why parents should be involved quite apart from the fact that this is their expressed wish: economy, generalization of skills and effectiveness. However, care needs to be taken in linking outcome to amount of therapy and thereby engendering guilt in parents that they 'haven't done enough'.

Models of individual parent–professional relationships have been characterized as follows:

(1) *The expert model.* The expert professional designs and carries out the programme, with an assumed high level of technical competence. The problem with this model is that it deskills parents and fails to negotiate parent and professional goals.

(2) *The 'transplant' model.* This assumes that the professional knows how to design the best programme; the professional then shows the parent what to do and the parent carries it out. It assumes that the professional can transfer her/his skills, and that the parents can learn and carry them out. This is a familiar model covering physiotherapy, speech and language therapy, and home-based teaching such as Portage. Potential problems are lack of attention to family differences, lack of recognition of parents' knowledge and inventiveness, and continued dependence on professionals.

(3) *The consumer model.* This model assumes that a choice of services is available, and that parents have sufficient information to choose amongst those options. Parent choice would come before professional opinion; a potential problem is lack of attention to building up the child's autonomy and choice.

(4) *The partnership model.* The needs of the child and the family within their wider social network are assessed, and mutually agreed aims are set. Variable support is given, depending on changing needs. This may at times include parents fully entrusting their child's education or treatment to the professionals. The aim is to empower parents, to help them to develop confidence in dealing with service systems, both as individuals and in groups (Cochran 1986, Appleton and Minchom 1991).

Ensuring effective inter-professional relationships is crucial to building parent–professional partnerships. Many parents will testify to the lack of communication between the multiple agencies with which they are involved. Case conferences and team meetings are intended to improve professional coordination.

Two methods of coping with the problem of multiple advice are:

(1) The *single therapist*, as in the Conductor of the Peto method of conductive education (Hari and Akos 1988) and the transdisciplinary home visitor (Brynelsen 1983). Problems with this model arise because of the level and amount of knowledge expected of any one individual.

(2) The *key worker* model, whereby a member of the district team is named and designated as the person who liaises between parents and all the other agencies, but who is not necessarily the person who is the sole worker with the child and family. The Sloper and Turner (1992) study suggested that this model was not being implemented well. Child development teams have found that it is a difficult model to put into operation. However, it can prove very effective in the case of children with multiple impairments with carefully managed support from the team (Brimblecombe and Russell 1988).

Child development theory and assessment philosophy

The history of early childhood intervention is built on educational philosophies and on a framework of legislation backed by changing philosophies of child development. The impact of longitudinal studies, notably that of Werner (1985) describing the children of

Kauai, challenged traditional views of the invincibility of genetic influences on intelligence, and emphasized social and family influences on outcome. The studies also highlighted factors leading to individual vulnerability or resilience. Recent research using twin, family and adoption studies has demonstrated a very strong genetic influence in conditions such as autism (Rutter *et al.* 1990, Bailey *et al.* 1995) while also confirming the importance of environmental factors in most psychological problems and gene–environment interactions (Scarr 1992, Plomin *et al.* 1993).

Child development research has similarly shifted the emphasis from cognitive assessments built on the fixed, genetically determined, maturational views of development to aspects of social and emotional development. The theoretical focus has been moving toward attachment theories, affective development (emotional matching and attunement) and homeostatic skills (those of internal physical state adaptation and self-regulation).

These basic processes are mediated by the child–caregiver relationship, and the importance of this transaction as well as of the interactions between family members has been increasingly recognized. The emphasis on intervention has moved from the child alone to include the family.

Rutter (1982), in a discussion of psycho-social risk, pointed to the fallacy of thinking that single child-centred interventions would deal with either cause or outcome. Other studies of development in biologically at-risk children confirm this view; that is, perinatal risk factors are overtaken by environmental factors in predicting outcome (intellectual or social), although some specific cognitive deficits may be persistent.

Two concepts stand out which have evolved in the last 20 years in the field of child development research. The first is the *ecological model* articulated by Bronfenbrenner (1979, 1986). He describes the interaction between the levels of environment which surround the child. There is the immediate environment of the individual, including patterns of parent–child interaction (the microsystem), the local and wider world, including legislation (the macrosystem), and, intermediate between the two, elements such as local facilities (the mesosystem). Changes in the macrosystem (for example, general economic circumstances, the prevailing social culture) all influence the microsystem. The systems interact with each other, and thus provide a model for considering risks and stresses.

The second concept, propounded by Sameroff and Chandler (1975), is the *transactional model* of biological and social–environmental factors continuously interacting and exerting changing effects on each other. This model allows for the severity of any one factor exerting a great influence, but more importantly that multiple risk factors are cumulative. Sameroff *et al.* (1987) in a study of 4-year-old children found that social–emotional and cognitive outcomes were determined by the number of risk factors (but in varying combinations). The risk variables studied were maternal anxiety, mental illness, education and attitude to child development, maternal interactions with the child, family size, minority status, family support, occupation, and stressful life events. The transactional model can also take account of protective factors for the individual and increased resilience allowing better adaptation. For example, the temperamentally difficult baby, also at risk because of preterm birth, may have exceptionally good parents with no other stresses in their lives who can adapt to the need of the baby for diminished stimulation and achieve successful interaction. Also the active, temperamentally easy but assertive child who elicits positive affective responses from caregivers may overcome risk factors that in other children lead to learning and behaviour problems (Werner 1985).

It follows from the above discussion that identification of risk is very complex. The classification of 'at-risk' children which is commonly used is that of Tjossem (1976):

(1) Children in whom there is an established diagnosis, *e.g.* Down syndrome, spina bifida.

(2) The biologically vulnerable, low birthweight babies and the nutritionally disadvantaged.

(3) Children whose environment or early childhood experiences put them at risk, *i.e.* abused or neglected children and those with chaotic and disorganized family relationships.

(Children may, of course, fall into two or all three categories.)

In Britain the Children Act 1989 requires local authorities to identify children in need and uses the term 'significant harm' as a criterion for legal intervention. This can be ill-treatment or impairment of health or development, and the test will be a comparison with a similar child and the expectation of 'reasonable parental care'. Over-identification is likely in the biological risk group (2) if perinatal factors alone are used. Protective factors also need to be considered for the individual.

Meisels and Wasik (1990) argue against a single factor assessment, such as a psychometric screening test or perinatal factor (the first is poorly predictive in the first two years of life and the second a poor predictor of cognitive and language outcome). Instead they favour multifactor or contextual assessment so that biological risks and individual impairments are combined with environmental factors which can be cumulative and, of course, change over time. Traditional assessment methods would be linked with the assessment of aspects of parenting (interaction, attachment, affective and communicative behaviour) and the assessment of family ecology (Bee *et al.* 1982) (see Chapter 8).

Part H of USA Public Law 99-457 (Education of the Handicapped Act Amendments 1986) required states to have in place by 1993 a system of intervention services focusing on supporting the family in providing an optimum environment for infants and toddlers at risk of developmental problems. Services are to be based on an Individual Family Service Plan. This requirement highlighted gaps in existing assessment strategies, and moved service providers toward developing assessments of family members' needs and strengths (Seligman and Darling 1989, Dunst and Trivette 1990). Blackman *et al.* (1992) discuss the role of paediatricians and highlight the obstacles of agency politics and funding, as well as paediatric awareness and training.

Both in Britain and in the USA there have recently been published views on screening and surveillance (Committee on Children with Disabilities 1986, Hall 1991). Both sets of recommendations emphasize the need for parental participation and an approach to screening which looks at the context of the child when coming to conclusions about her/his development (for a reconciliation of the apparent differences between the American and British approaches, see Dworkin 1989). Controversy still surrounds the use of developmental screening tests, which have the merit of giving a norm-based measurement but with limited specificity and sensitivity (Frankenburg *et al.* 1992, Glascoe *et al.* 1992). Most severe defects are detected by parents, who are still too frequently wrongly reassured by professionals that there is no problem (see Chapter 7).

The theoretical basis for intervention

Some basic assumptions are common to many neurodevelopmental intervention programmes, although the evidence for their validity is mixed. It is held that:

(1) infancy represents a sensitive period for development, so that early intervention is likely to be important. There is some good evidence for this view, *e.g.* for vision and hearing defects, but much less good evidence in respect of developmental delays where environment has more influence;

(2) genetic and biological problems can be overcome or at least ameliorated. However, severity and associated cognition are important factors. Initial cognitive status has been shown in studies of many different impairments to be strongly predictive of outcome (*e.g.* Brinker *et al.* 1994);

(3) disabled children have different experiences from other children, and need special programmes and trained people. However, this is controversial, and many programmes instead emphasize the needs which all children have in common.

Recent child developmental research further suggests that:

(4) developmental programmes for children must (a) include arousal and the focusing of attention, (b) be based on active as opposed to passive participation, and (c) recognize that learning occurs where the child must accommodate to and assimilate new types of information (Bricker and Veltman 1990);

(5) a child with impairment(s) must be treated as a total person; there is interdependence between different domains of development. Some impairments can impinge on social and emotional growth, but need not do so;

(6) a positive caregiver-to-child relationship is crucial;

(7) multiple and changing caregivers interfere with the development of secure adult–child relationships;

(8) intervention must take account of the child being part of a family;

(9) specific neuropsychological pathology should lead to specific treatment strategies (although there is limited evidence in the literature of the validity of this statement);

(10) and finally, a balanced analysis of the benefits and problems of intervention should be made, particularly in situations where it might be assumed that intensive intervention leads to greatest improvement.

The theoretical bases for intervention are proposed at six different levels within a systems model: (1) physiological processing; (2) information processing and specific deficit model; (3) behavioural learning; (4) interaction-based learning; (5) family context; (6) social context. These are discussed below. Change in any one level is likely to have consequent effects at other levels in the system.

Physiological processing

Some approaches have a specifically neural theoretical basis. The question has been raised of whether it is possible to stimulate regrowth of damaged axons (Ferry 1981); what is more likely is an increase in synaptic connections from undamaged neighbouring axons (Kolb 1992). There has also been observation of the retention of parallel neural pathways which would otherwise have been expected to decay during the child's development.

Clear prescriptions for rehabilitation therapy with children have yet to emerge from such research.

There is well-established evidence that deprivation, particularly in sensory areas, leads to anatomical change, *e.g.* in the visual cortex (see Goodman 1989). Some therapies aim to treat the primary deficit, *e.g.* the use of cochlear implants in deafness and programmes for visual development (see the section on specific impairments, below). This is a different theoretical approach from teaching a compensating strategy such as sign language.

Information processing and specific deficit model
Another theoretical approach is to use an information processing model of development, including the control and direction of attention, perceptual discrimination and integration, immediate memory, learning and affective responses (Gaussen and Stratton 1985). Therapy aims to alleviate problems in children who process information slowly, or have difficulty taking in information from multiple channels simultaneously, or who have difficulty in reasoning flexibly. This model could make use of a knowledge of specific deficits in syndromes. Gibson (1991) discusses the profile of specific strengths and weaknesses in children who have Down syndrome and suggests, for example, building on strengths in motor imitation to enhance early cognitive exploration and learning. It is also important to emphasize time for play activities to give repeated experiences of combining, grouping and comparing objects, in order to underpin real understanding of basic concepts of size, shape, etc., so that there is not just imitation learning without comprehension.

Behavioural learning
The behavioural model of learning has formed the basis for many early educational interventions, including the Portage project (Shearer and Shearer 1976). Portage is a home-based educational programme taught to the child by the parent (Clements *et al.* 1980). A target behaviour (or behaviours) is selected for the week from the developmental checklist. Parents are shown how to teach their child through demonstration by a home visitor. The approach was originally developed in the USA for rural children with mild to moderate delays in development. This has become one of the most internationally used of the developmental programmes. In Britain the curriculum is seldom adhered to in the ways laid out. Much of the benefit to parents probably derives from the personal support of the home visitor (for a review of Portage use in Britain, India and Jamaica, see Sturmey *et al.* 1992; see also Chapter 5).

Some behavioural approaches are applied to the management of difficult behaviour (*e.g.* Yule and Carr 1987). Such approaches demand precise measurement of behaviour both at the stage of functional analysis of the problem, and in recording outcome. Carefully controlled intervention of this sort has been shown to be effective, and the new social skills taught shown to generalize across situations (Zifferblatt *et al.* 1977).

Interaction-based learning
The importance of parent–child interaction is emphasized within a model of intervention based on social–cognitive development, where intellectual progress is dependent on

meaningful shared social experiences in the context of a close affectional relationship. Interaction-based teaching specifically aims to increase the mutual enjoyment of the parent and child, and responsiveness of the parent to the child's cues. Various techniques have been used, such as encouraging imitation of the baby, or setting up communicative situations which increase the necessity for the child to produce a reciprocal response (Girolametto 1988). However, the number of studies which have looked at developmental changes over a long period of time in children who have had interaction intervention are limited, and show complex results.

The problems addressed by intervention at the level of parent–child interaction may include the following:

(1) the parent may be depressed, which will affect the frequency and type of contingent responding to the child (Murray 1992);

(2) the parent's own experiences of childhood may affect her/his skills in social inter-action with an infant;

(3) there may be some aspect of a child's impairment that specifically alters the ease and reciprocity of interaction, *e.g.* in deaf or blind children, in autism, or in very low birth-weight children who are irritable and not able to cope with too great a level of stimulus (Field 1983). Multiply impaired children may show more limited developmental gains than other children, but greater improvement in the home caretaking environment (Barrera 1991).

The question of whether parents of children who have impairments are overly directive in their interactions with their children has been commented on frequently in the literature (Mahoney *et al.* 1985) with the implication that this is detrimental (see review by Marfo 1990). However, studies of children with Down syndrome show that they use less social initiation than children without impairments of the same developmental level, and this pattern is echoed in studies of young children with cerebral palsy. Parents therefore seem to have to work harder to establish interaction. Some descriptive studies have shown that parents can be both directive and sensitive to the child's attempts at communication (Crawley and Spiker 1983). Parental language has been shown to adjust in a develop-mentally sensitive way over time as children progress (*e.g.* Conti-Ramsden and Friel-Patti 1983, Snow *et al.* 1987).

Family context

There has been considerable discussion of problems in the simplistic use of the interaction intervention model, and also of the behavioural teaching model. Research on family func-tioning suggests that studies of whether parent–child interactions are successful must take into account wider family issues (McCollum 1991). This implies broader assessment methods, and not just measuring face-to-face encounters. It is also necessary to take a longer time perspective. Several studies have shown a decline in systematic teaching by parents after direct professional support has ceased, and failure to maintain the child's new skills (Baker 1984, Cunningham 1987). It has also been shown that vulnerable families, *e.g.* single parents, find it particularly hard to take part in intervention programmes. There has been insufficient study of which families benefit from particular approaches, and concerns are voiced that some parents have other overwhelming needs. The aim of intervention should be not to increase the burden, but to help parents make the best use of the time they already spend together with their child (McConkey 1985). It has been noted that the combination of mothering and teaching roles may create conflict for some mothers (McConachie 1991), and that the isolation of some fathers may be accentuated by professionals narrowly focusing their attention on interventions by the mother (McConachie 1982).

The findings of the Manchester Down syndrome cohort studies have been influential. Cunningham (1986) commented that one of the most striking findings was that the significant correlates or predictors of later development for the children with Down syndrome, *i.e.* social class, birth order, family size, parental education and gender, were those found for ordinary children. In contrast the specific elements of the intervention programmes seem to have only a limited and short-lived influence on outcome measures such as developmental progress.

Social context
The theoretical void of many intervention studies in ignoring the family's social context is made clear in approaches such as that of Davis and Rushton (1991). They describe a parent counselling approach, the Parent Adviser Scheme, which was introduced in a deprived area of London. Their model uses personal construct psychology as the framework for understanding how the family can come to adapt to the circumstances—emotional, material and financial—in which they find themselves. It is proposed that the mother's self-esteem and perceptions of her child and of the child's father have a crucial impact on interactions in the family, and thus on the child's social environment for development. The parent advisers were mostly local professionals already involved with families of children with impairments, who received special training so that they could offer psycho-social support. A local Bangladeshi mother was also recruited and trained. In a well-controlled study, it was shown that mothers who had a parent adviser showed significant positive changes in their feelings about themselves, their families and their children compared with mothers who received simply the usual services of the local child development team. Their children also showed significant developmental gains even though no specific systematic teaching was included in the intervention. The programme was especially successful for the substantial number of parents of Bangladeshi origin who were included (Davis and Ali Choudhury 1988).

The appropriateness of transferring any of these models of parent intervention to a developing country is open to question. For example, O'Toole (1989) (see also Chapter 11) has described applying the behavioural learning approach within Guyana. He examines three beliefs of the model: that child development needs to be understood as a series of orderly stages; that teaching helps; and that changes in parental behaviour will help the child. He found that parents in Guyana did understand development as an orderly progression, and believed that teaching helped, but expected a teacher to do it. Culturally, parents and children did not play with toys together, so different ways were devised to involve parents in helping their children.

It seems clear that any intervention programme must take account of specific cultural and social contexts, so that appropriate goals for child development are agreed with the families, rather than trying to use aims and techniques transferred directly from Western cultures (Chamberlin 1987).

Specific impairments

The general model evolved above is relevant to any of the different impairments in children. In the individual sections below, the discussion concentrates on interventions specific to each impairment. However, the published literature on each topic increasingly is emphasizing other aspects of intervention such as improvements in parental under-standing, confidence, support, etc.

Intervention studies that are successful are more likely to be reported and published than those which show no improvement. In most reports, outcome will be described for groups of children, rather than describing individuals. Nevertheless, a specific and well-timed intervention can make very great differences for an individual child (or family) which might be lost within group variability or by a failure to apply the appropriate out-come measure, *e.g.* the child who has persistent glue ear for whom surgery restores hearing at a crucial time, and enhanced functioning of the family system which might be overlooked if measures taken in a research study are only of child progress (see Chapter 4).

Biological impairments
GENERAL DEVELOPMENTAL DELAYS
Thorough reviews of intervention studies are presented by Denhoff (1981), Simeonsson *et al.* (1982), Guralnick and Bricker (1987) and Farran (1990). All of these authors draw attention to the short-term nature of many of the studies, and the statistical difficulties of using pre- and post-intervention measurements on standard IQ tests. In the main, inter-ventions have proved beneficial in halting decline in IQ in children with Down syndrome and in increasing the rate of development in children with other aetiologies of develop-mental delay, but only for the duration of the intervention. Generally outcomes are narrowly focused, gains are reported but not always generalized across place or activity, and the best predictor of post-intervention outcome is the pre-intervention test score.

One well-conducted study of intervention in Down syndrome by Piper and Pless (1980) found no short- or long-term effects. However, later studies have given evidence of other types of effects in the intervention group; for example, the parents of children who have Down syndrome may be more able to use facilities, they may be more confident of themselves, and the intervention can be found to have altered their attitudes to their child (Byrne *et al.* 1988). This then raises the question of whether child development oriented interventions are the primary way to proceed, or whether direct parent support strategies are of equal or greater importance.

THE SEVERELY VISUALLY IMPAIRED CHILD
Visual impairment may result from an abnormality of the orbit, the optic nerve or the visual cortex, or a combination of these. In developed countries the most frequent causes

of severe visual impairment are genetic, of which congenital cataract, inherited retinal dystrophies and albinism are the most common, and perinatal disorders, the most important of which is visual pathway damage often with more extensive neurological impairment. Retinopathy of prematurity used to be more common but is now both prevented and treated more successfully (Baird and Moore 1993). A particular difficulty with evaluation of Western studies of blind children is this heterogeneity of ophthalmological diagnoses, and the associated cognitive and other impairments in at least two thirds of visually impaired children. It is even difficult to establish the level of visual competence in 'blind' children, especially if they are 'cortically' blind.

There are sound developmental reasons for thinking that the first few months of life are the optimal and possibly critical time for establishing the neuro-anatomical basis for vision at cortical level, and for ensuring optimal vision at this time, for example by performing early cataract surgery (Taylor *et al.* 1979, Garey 1984).

One particular developmental treatment approach for visually impaired babies has as its basis the provision of visual images known to be interesting in early development, *i.e.* those with colour, contour or contrast (Sonksen *et al.* 1991). In addition, multi-sensory support of visual information is used. Parents are instructed in the programme, and asked to carry it out several times a day. The results of a one year controlled evaluation study showed improved vision in the treatment group as compared with controls who had a general developmental programme only. Initial visual level and visual diagnosis were also important independent variables. A useful book for parents and professionals, *Show Me What My Friends Can See* (Sonksen and Stiff 1991), describes the visual programme used in the study.

One of the first intervention studies with blind infants was conducted by Fraiberg and co-workers. As a psychoanalyst, Fraiberg made detailed observations of the infant's responses to events, and by interpreting these to the parents helped them to understand their child better. The published studies show developmental gains from the intervention (Adelson and Fraiberg 1974, Fraiberg 1977).

The importance of parent–child reciprocal social interaction is illuminated by Preisler's (1991) study of blind babies. This is based on a social–cognitive child development approach and describes detailed observation of mutual responsiveness and harmonious timing of interaction; it also illustrates the importance of different adaptive techniques on the part of the caregiver of a blind infant, *i.e.* using tactile cues as well as words to convey pleasure or to warn the child of an impending change. Preisler (1993) has gone on to describe the experiences of blind children on entering nursery class.

The Vancouver group who have been involved in intervention programmes with the visually impaired have contributed a rare longitudinal perspective (Freeman *et al.* 1989). They suggest that emotional or psychiatric difficulties experienced by blind children in childhood are less likely to persist as problems in adulthood than would be the case for children who are sighted.

SEVERE HEARING IMPAIRMENT
There is evidence to suggest benefits from the earliest possible correction of hearing

impairment, although the neurophysiological basis for critical periods is not as clear as in the visual system. The trend has been for earlier diagnosis by objective technical means rather than waiting for the behavioural responses of deficit, *i.e.* a shift from diagnosis relying on the eight month distraction hearing test to neonatal screening (in Britain of high-risk infants only) by brainstem evoked responses and cochlear echo (see Chapter 7). Lately, the possibility of prenatal screening has been demonstrated (Shahidullah and Hepper 1993).

Treatment strategies for children with severe sensorineural hearing loss have been transformed firstly with sophisticated hearing aids, and latterly with multi-channel cochlear implants. If the children are carefully selected for surgery, and if post-implant teaching is given, then the improvement in hearing is impressive (Quittner *et al.* 1991). Current guidelines for referral, which may change as more experience is gained, are: (i) priority to children aged 2–5 years; (ii) profound or total hearing loss with lack of benefit from a hearing aid (aided responses >70dB over the full frequency range); (iii) no other significant learning difficulties; (iv) strong parental support; (v) good teaching services available to the child and family.

For most children, the emphasis in the preschool period is on early diagnosis, the provision of hearing aids, and specialist teaching which focuses on parent–child interaction (Stokes and Bamford 1990). High quality technical support is required, particularly to ensure well-fitting moulds and correct amplification as the child grows. In school-age children, there is a similar emphasis on the importance of technical support combined with an approach to language teaching based on the more recent social–cognitive literature (Wood *et al.* 1989). For example, children will learn to communicate better if adults ask them questions to which they genuinely want to know the answer, rather than relying on more directive questions and comments.

Studies of deaf children from deaf families show that they have a positive advantage in early expressive communication compared with deaf children in hearing families (Gregory and Barlow 1989). The advantages of 'total communication', *i.e.* encouraging both signing and speech, are increasingly being recognized (Meadow-Orleans 1987), though many schools still pursue auditory training alone.

In interventions for children with severe hearing impairment, one can confidently state that early diagnosis, good technical back-up for hearing aids, and a total communication approach together with family counselling and support have been shown to make substantial differences to outcome (and we can now add referral, where suitable, for cochlear implant).

CHILDREN WITH MOTOR IMPAIRMENTS

The causes of motor impairments include: myelomeningoceles, muscle disorders, motor delays associated with intellectual impairment (*e.g.* in Down syndrome), and other central neurological disorders of which cerebral palsy is the most common.

• *Cerebral palsy.* Cerebral palsy is an umbrella term for a variety of disorders of movement and posture in children, which evolve over time, but have their origin in a nonprogressive cerebral malformation or lesion. Studies of therapy in cerebral palsy have focused on physiotherapy but have been bedevilled by rather simplistic notions of 'Does physiotherapy work?'. There are many different physiotherapy methods including positive promotion of functional skill attainment, sensory stimulation and muscle strengthening, as well as prevention of further impairment such as fixed deformities due to muscle imbalance, positional deformity and motor delay. Furthermore, those intervention studies which have been reported have considerable problems of study design, including the selection of appropriate control groups, and difficulties with assessment scales including the question of their validity as measures. No study seems to have used a wider ecological model to look more broadly at child and family responses to intervention (Wright and Nicholson 1973, Scherzer *et al.* 1976, Palmer *et al.* 1988). None of these studies found evidence to support the particular physical intervention used.

In a recent study of the effect of intensive physiotherapy, Bower and McLellan (1992) used Goal Attainment Scaling (Kiresuk and Sherman 1968), plus a validated norm-referenced measure (the Gross Motor Function Measure—Russell *et al.* 1989) and a parent–teacher questionnaire. They showed that motor skills could be increased and that non-motor goals could be attained during intensive physiotherapy, but that maintenance of the skills depends on a high level of continued use and requires building into the child's daily routine. Bower (1994) subsequently showed that the specific method used in the therapy (Bobath, Peto or Eclectic) did not affect the outcome.

Conductive education has attracted a great deal of attention in the last decade as a treatment method for children who have cerebral palsy. It was developed in Hungary at the Peto Institute (Hari and Akos 1988). Conductive education is carried out by 'conductors' who are responsible for all aspects of a child's education and development, though the main short-term aim is to achieve independent motor functioning without the use of physical aids. Wide public interest in conductive education in Britain, fed by the media, led to great pressure on parents. An Institute for Conductive Education opened in Birmingham in 1988 in close collaboration with the Hungarian Institute, and the Department for Education funded a controlled study of the progress of the 17 children in the first two intakes. The control group, selected by the Hungarian consultants as equally appropriate candidates for conductive education, were attending special schools for children with physical disorder in another city (Bairstow *et al.* 1991). Both groups made progress over a two year period on a wide range of functional and physical measures. The only evidence of differences in rate of progress was in favour of the special school group. The research team concluded that parents of children with cerebral palsy should regard with caution the promises made on behalf of conductive education, and that they should not feel they are failing if they do not secure conductive education for their child (Bairstow *et al.* 1993). Many therapists are concerned about the emphasis on sitting and walking in conductive education, to the relative neglect of approriate strategies for encouraging self-feeding, communication and learning. Children require adequately supportive seating at some times of the day in order to be able to use their hands, eyes and thinking capacity effectively (Green 1992).

The role of the overseeing physician and physiotherapist is to negotiate the long-term goals for the child, which may require a largely preventive programme, while promoting the short-term goals and meeting family needs. Physical management may require the judicious use of physiotherapy techniques, the use of orthoses and the use of surgery (Bleck 1987, Scrutton 1989). Recently, gait laboratories have begun to measure with great precision the movements which children make in walking, allowing more detailed decisions to be made about orthopaedic surgery, and thus reducing the number of operations required (Gage 1991). However, the techniques still are largely confined to the research laboratory. An important paper by Tardieu *et al.* (1988) looks at the effect of length of time on muscle stretch and can be used as a guide for the amount of time, for example, that a child might need to be in a fixed brace. These researchers found that there was no progressive contracture in children with and without cerebral palsy when the soleus muscle was stretched for at least six hours per day, but there was if the stretch was for two hours per day.

• *Developmental 'clumsiness'.* This developmental problem, difficult to diagnose in the first years of life, has been shown to be associated with other attentional, learning and behavioural difficulties. Long-term follow-up of children with perceptuomotor disorder has shown firstly the heterogeneity of the children identified, and secondly that for many children their difficulties persist throughout school years and beyond (for a review, see Henderson 1993). Various treatment regimes depend on the originators' theoretical stance. Some emphasize a perceptual deficit such as poor kinaesthetic awareness or memory, so that the treatment approach is highly focused (Laszlo and Bairstow 1985). Postulation of a perceptual and cross-modal processing deficit is the basis for sensory integration therapy (Ayres 1987). More traditional therapy adopts a target skills training approach, *e.g.* teaching dressing, writing, or whatever the child finds difficult.

CHILDREN WITH LANGUAGE AND COMMUNICATION DISORDERS INCLUDING AUTISM

The first problem that besets any review of this topic is that of definition. The most common way of subdividing is to consider whether there is a speech (the production of recognizably and conventionally articulated words) or language problem, and then to consider whether this is a specific deficit or part of a more general disorder such as autism or intellectual impairment (Lees and Urwin 1991).

In this field, comparison of different interventions is difficult because of the influence of maturational effects upon outcome, the association of language disorders with other cognitive deficits, and the use of widely varying assessment tools to define the groups of children studied. Most interventions have been short-term, and directed at specific language targets (*e.g.* acquisition of syntactic rules) where it is hoped that generalization of new skills will follow. Few studies have used adequate control groups (Cooper *et al.* 1979, Stevenson *et al.* 1982).

Published studies support the value of early intervention (Snyder-McLean and McClean 1987). There is convincing evidence of the efficacy of treatment of specific speech disorders in individual children or groups using a variety of methods (behavioural and cognitive) but usually in clinic surroundings (Weiner 1981). Interaction-based teaching (see pp. 25–26) has been found useful, but needs careful evaluation (Girolametto 1988, McCollum 1991).

Longitudinal studies of children with language disorders emphasize that they are not a homogenous group. However, as with many other biologically based impairments, the severity of the disorder and the child's cognitive skills are important predictors of outcome. Deficits have been identified in representational and symbolic thinking, and short-term memory. Follow-up to adult life shows that some children continue to experience major problems in personal social relationships and in finding employment (Rutter and Mawhood 1991).

• *Autism.* In children with autism the use of agreed schedules for diagnosis (*e.g.* the ADI—LeCouteur *et al.* 1989) should in future make comparisons between studies easier. Howlin and Rutter (1989) describe an individualized home-based programme which was effective in altering children's behaviour and management by the parents. In the USA, the intervention approach developed by Lovaas and colleagues is characterized by its intensiveness, structured targeting of new behaviour, and the involvement of parents both to teach the new skills and to generalize their use to different settings, a particularly difficult task for autistic children. The long-term outcome of this approach looks encouraging (McEachin *et al.* 1993), though there are criticisms of the study design. There is also emerging evidence that there are advantages in involving other young non-disabled children in teaching social skills (Strain *et al.* 1985).

Specialist teaching for children with autism includes many different approaches. TEACCH (Schopler *et al.* 1984) is a system capitalizing on the fact that children with autism frequently have better visual than auditory skills. It uses a physically structured environment and visual cues to aid understanding, tolerance to change and independence. The Higashi school, originating in Japan, uses a very high staff–pupil ratio and incorporates programmes of physical exercise performed in groups (Gould *et al.* 1991). Music therapy to promote interpersonal communication and social timing is yet another approach to show apparently promising results with such children (Christie *et al.* 1992).

OTHER TREATMENTS

Drug treatments have a limited role in interventions for children with biological impairments. Much work has been done on looking for a neurochemical marker in autism, and various drug treatments have been tried with variable effects, more on specific behaviours than on cognition (Gordon *et al.* 1992). Drug treatment has more convincingly been shown effective in the treatment of hyperactive behaviour, and Taylor (1991) finds evidence of the possibility that diet could also be influential in some children.

Biologically at-risk babies

Low birthweight babies and those born early are biologically at risk. Long-term follow-up studies have confirmed that as a group low birthweight survivors have an increased risk of educational and behavioural problems, and the lower the birthweight the greater the risk (Wolke 1991). Intrauterine growth retardation, or other causes of the baby being small for gestational age, also increase the likelihood of impairment. However, for the individual child who has not been exposed to major neonatal complications, the outlook should be cautious optimism. Many specific minor impairments are being reported: increased problems of attention control, perceptual problems, speech dysfunction and language delays.

Studies of intervention for low birthweight babies have used the transactional model first put forward by Sameroff and Chandler (1975). However, as Bradley and Casey point out in a recent annotation (1992), the focus of research has moved from more distant ecological markers like socio-economic status to 'proximal' ones looking precisely at the experiences of children in their environments. Measures of the home and parent–child interaction such as the HOME inventory (Bradley and Caldwell 1984) are found to correlate well with development measured by cognitive scales (Siegel 1984, Bradley *et al.* 1987).

The complex interaction of child factors influencing quality of caregiving was carefully assessed in the Infant Health and Development Program (1990), a multicentre trial in the USA focusing on low birthweight babies. There were significant effects on child measures like IQ and adaptive behaviour as a result of the intervention. Children with higher birthweights showed greater gains. The quality of caregiving was also improved by the programme, which consisted of home visits, a daily children's and parent's group focusing on support, increasing knowledge, an educational curriculum and enhancing problem solving skills. Other studies with neurodevelopmental therapy and physiotherapy but without the more intensive home support failed to show altered patterns of development or altered outcome (Goodman *et al.* 1985). Bennett (1987) gives a useful review of the intervention studies.

The environmentally at-risk group
Detailed consideration of this group is beyond the scope of this chapter. Farran (1990), after reviewing the many mainly American studies, concluded 'that available data support the notion of benefits from carefully planned and well implemented intervention efforts but that they must be continued longer term if short-term gains are to be sustained, *e.g.* for cognitive gains it is better to provide an improved educational program for the four years of elementary school than one year only of preschool experience.' Follow-up of children from the Perry Preschool Project found a number of long-term positive effects in the intervention group in terms of social outcomes, delinquency, etc. (Berrueta-Clement *et al.* 1984).

Conclusions

This chapter has attempted to outline some of the complex issues involved in analysing and planning services for disabled children and their families. The 'medical model' of an impairment which can be cured or ameliorated (*cf.* prescribing spectacles) has held back the development of appropriate interventions. Disability is a complex transaction between a child's physical make-up and the environment. Thus appropriate professional support to children and their families must encompass a range from specific information on diagnosis to advocacy in the community, based on optimism and enjoyment of the child's uniqueness.

REFERENCES

Adelson, E., Fraiberg, S. (1974) 'Gross motor development in infants blind from birth.' *Child Development*, **45**, 114–126.

Appleton, P.L., Minchom, P.E. (1991) 'Models of parent partnership and child development centres.' *Child: Care, Health and Development*, **17**, 27–38.

Armstrong, R.W., Rosenbaum, P.L., King, S.M. (1987) 'A randomized controlled trial of a 'buddy' programme to improve children's attitudes toward the disabled.' *Developmental Medicine and Child Neurology*, **29**, 327–336.

Ayres, A.J. (1987) *Sensory Integration and the Child.* Los Angeles: Western Psychological Services.

Bailey, A., Le Couteur, A., Gottesman, I., Bolton, P., Simonoff, E., Yazuda, E., Rutter, M. (1995) 'Autism as a strongly genetic disorder: Evidence from a British twin study.' *Psychological Medicine. (In press.)*

Baird, G., Moore, A.T. (1993) 'Epidemiology of childhood blindness'. *In:* Fielder, A.R., Best, A.B., Bax, M.C.O. (Eds.) *The Management of Visual Impairment in Childhood. Clinics in Developmental Medicine No. 128.* London: Mac Keith Press, pp. 1–8.

Bairstow, P., Cochrane, R., Rusk, I. (1991) 'Selection of children with cerebral palsy for conductive education and the characteristics of children judged suitable and unsuitable.' *Developmental Medicine and Child Neurology*, **33**, 984–992.

Bairstow, P., Cochrane, R., Hur, J. (1993) *Evaluation of Conductive Education for Children with Cerebral Palsy: Final Report.* London: HMSO.

Bak, J.J., Siperstein, G.N. (1986) 'Protective effects of the label "mentally retarded" on children's attitudes towards mentally retarded peers.' *American Journal of Mental Deficiency*, **91**, 95–97.

Baker, B.L. (1984) 'Intervention with families with young severely handicapped children'. *In:* Blacher, J. (Ed.) *Families of Severely Handicapped Children: Research in Review.* New York: Academic Press, pp. 319–375.

Barrera, M.E. (1991) 'The transactional model of early home intervention: application with developmentally delayed children and their families.' *In:* Marfo, K. (Ed.) *Early Intervention in Transition: Current Perspectives on Programs for Handicapped Children.* New York: Praeger, pp. 109–146.

Bax, M.C.O., Whitmore, K. (1991) 'District handicap teams in England: 1983–8.' *Archives of Disease in Childhood*, **66**, 656–664.

Bee, H.L., Barnard, K.E., Eyres, S.J., Gray, C.A., Hammond, M.A., Spietz, A.L., Snyder, C., Clark, B. (1982) 'Prediction of IQ and language skill from perinatal status, child performance, family characteristics, and mother–infant interaction.' *Child Development*, **53**, 1134–1156.

Bennett, F.C. (1987) 'The effectiveness of early intervention for infants at increased biological risk.' *In:* Guralnick, M.J., Bennett, F.C. (Eds.) *The Effectiveness of Early Intervention for At-risk and Handicapped Children.* Orlando, FL: Academic Press, pp. 79–109.

Berrueta-Clement, J.R., Schweinhart, L.J., Barnett, W.S., Epstein, A.S., Weikart, D.P. (1984) *Changed Lives: The Effects of the Perry Preschool Program on Youths Through Age 19.* Ypsilanti, MI: High/Scope.

Bicknell, J. (1983) 'The psychopathology of handicap.' *British Journal of Medical Psychology*, **56**, 167–178.

Blackman, J.A., Healy, A., Ruppert, E.S. (1992) 'Participation by pediatricians in early intervention: impetus from Public Law 99–457.' *Pediatrics*, **89**, 98–102.

Bleck, E.E. (1987) *The Orthopaedic Management of Cerebral Palsy. Clinics in Developmental Medicine No. 99/100.* London: Mac Keith Press.

Bower, E. (1994) 'Assessing motor skill acquisition in four centres for the treatment of children with cerebral palsy'. *Developmental Medicine and Child Neurology*, **36**, 902–909.

—— McLellan, D.L. (1992) 'Effect of increased exposure to physiotherapy on skill acquisition of children with cerebral palsy.' *Developmental Medicine and Child Neurology*, **34**, 25–39.

Bradley, R.H., Caldwell, B.M. (1984) '174 children: a study of the relationship between home environment and cognitive development during the first five years.' *In:* Gottfried, A.W. (Eds.) *Home Environment and Early Cognitive Development.* New York: Academic Press, pp. 5–56.

—— Casey, P.H. (1992) 'Family environment and behavioral development of low-birthweight children.' *Developmental Medicine and Child Neurology*, **34**, 822–826.

—— Caldwell, B.M., Rock, S.L., Casey, P.H., Nelson, J.M. (1987) 'The early development of low birthweight infants: relationship to health, family status, family context, family processes and parenting.' *International Journal of Behavioral Development*, **10**, 1–18.

Bricker, D., Veltman, M. (1990) 'Early intervention programs: child-focused approaches.' *In:* Meisels, S.J., Shonkoff, J.P. (Eds.) *Handbook of Early Childhood Intervention.* Cambridge: Cambridge University Press, pp. 373–399.

Brimblecombe, F., Russell, P. (1988) *Honeylands: Developing a Service for Families with Handicapped Children.* London: National Children's Bureau.

35

Brinker, R.P., Seifer, R., Sameroff, A.J. (1994) 'Relations among maternal stress, cognitive development, and early intervention in middle- and low-SES infants with developmental disabilities.' *American Journal on Mental Retardation*, **98**, 463–480.

Bronfenbrenner, U. (1979) *The Ecology of Human Development: Experiments by Nature and Design*. Cambridge, MA: Harvard University Press.

—— (1986) 'Ecology of the family as a context for human developmental research perspectives.' *Developmental Psychology*, **22**, 723–742.

Brynelsen, D. (1983) 'Infant development programmes in British Columbia.' *In:* Mittler, P., McConachie, H. (Eds.) *Parents, Professionals and Mentally Handicapped People: Approaches to Partnership*. London: Croom Helm, pp. 77–90.

Byrne, E.A., Cunningham, C.C. (1985) 'The effects of mentally handicapped children on families—a conceptual review.' *Journal of Child Psychology and Psychiatry*, **26**, 847–864.

—— —— Sloper, P. (1988) *Families and Their Children with Down's Syndrome: One Feature in Common*. London: Routledge.

Chamberlin, R.W. (1987) 'Developmental assessment and early intervention programs for young children: lessons learned from longitudinal research.' *Pediatrics in Review*, **8**, 237–247.

Christie, P., Newson, E., Newson, J., Prevezer, W. (1992) 'An interactive approach to language and communication for non-speaking children.' *In:* Lane, D.A., Miller, A. (Eds.) *Child and Adolescent Therapy: a Handbook*. Milton Keynes: Open University Press, pp. 67–88.

Clements, J.C., Bidder, R.T., Gardner, S., Bryant, G., Gray, O.P. (1980) 'A home advisory service for preschool children with developmental delays'. *Child: Care, Health and Development*, **6**, 25–33.

Cochran, M. (1986) 'The parental empowerment process, building on family strengths.' *In:* Harris, J. (Ed.) *Child Psychology in Action, Linking Research to Practice. Part 1: Families*. London: Croom Helm, pp. 12–33.

Committee on Children with Disabilities (1986) 'Screening for developmental disability.' *Pediatrics*, **78**, 526–528.

Conti-Ramsden, G., Friel-Patti, S. (1983) 'Mothers' discourse adjustments to language-impaired and non-language-impaired children.' *Journal of Speech and Hearing Disorders*, **48**, 360–367.

Cooper, J., Moodley, M., Reynell, J. (1979) 'The developmental language programme. Results from a five year study.' *British Journal of Disorders of Communication*, **14**, 57–69.

Crawley, S.B., Spiker, D. (1983) 'Mother–child interactions involving two-year-olds with Down syndrome: a look at individual differences.' *Child Development*, **54**, 1312–1323.

Cunningham, C.C. (1975) 'Parents as therapists and educators.' *In:* Kiernan, C., Woodford, F.P. (Eds.) *Behaviour Modification with the Severely Mentally Retarded*. Amsterdam: Associated Scientific Publishers, pp. 175–193.

—— (1985) 'Training and education approaches for parents of children with special needs.' *British Journal of Medical Psychology*, **58**, 285–305.

—— (1986) 'Early intervention: some findings from the Manchester cohort of children with Down's syndrome.' *In:* Bishop, M., Copley, M., Porter, J. (Eds.) *Portage: More Than a Teaching Programme?* Windsor: NFER–Nelson, pp. 89–106.

—— (1987) 'Early intervention in Down's syndrome.' *In:* Hosking, G., Murphy, G. (Eds.) *Prevention of Mental Handicap: a World View. Royal Society of Medicine International Congress and Sympsium Series No. 112*. London: Royal Society of Medicine, pp. 169–188.

—— Davis, H. (1985) *Working with Parents: Frameworks for Collaboration*. Milton Keynes: Open University Press.

Davis, H. (1993) *Counselling Parents of Children with Chronic Illness or Disability*. Leicester: BPS Books.

—— Ali Choudhury, P. (1988) 'Helping Bangladeshi families: Tower Hamlets parent adviser scheme.' *Mental Handicap*, **16**, 48–51.

—— Rushton, R. (1991) 'Counselling and supporting parents of children with developmental delay: a research evaluation.' *Journal of Mental Deficiency Research*, **35**, 89–112.

Denhoff, E. (1981) 'Current status of infant stimulation or enrichment programs for children with developmental disabilities.' *Pediatrics*, **67**, 32–37.

Dunst, C.J., Trivette, C.M. (1990) 'Assessment of social support in early intervention programs.' *In:* Meisels, S.J., Shonkoff, J.P. (Eds.) *Handbook of Early Childhood Intervention*. Cambridge: Cambridge University Press, pp. 326–349.

Dworkin, P.H. (1989) 'Developmental screening—expecting the impossible?' *Pediatrics*, **83**, 619–622.

Farran, D.C. (1990) 'Effects of intervention with disadvantaged and disabled children: a decade review.' *In:* Meisels, S.J., Shonkoff, J.P. (Eds.) *Handbook of Early Childhood Intervention.* Cambridge: Cambridge University Press, pp. 501–539.

Ferry, P.C. (1981) 'On growing new neurons: are early intervention programs effective.' *Pediatrics,* **67,** 38–41.

Field, T. (1983) 'Distress syndrome and post-term postmaturity syndrome infants.' *In:* Field, T., Sostek, A. (Eds.) *Infants Born at Risk: Physiological, Perceptual and Cognitive Processes.* New York: Grune & Stratton, pp. 333–356.

Fish Report (1985) *Equal Educational Opportunities for All? Report of the Committee of Enquiry into Special Educational Needs.* London: Inner London Education Authority.

Fraiberg, S. (1977) *Insights from the Blind.* London: Souvenir Press; New York: Basic Books.

Frankenburg, W.K., Dodds, J., Archer, P., Shapiro, H., Bresnick, B. (1992) 'The Denver II: a major revision and restandardization of the Denver Developmental Screening Test.' *Pediatrics,* **89,** 91–97.

Freeman, R.D.. Goetz, E., Richards, D.P., Groenvald, H., Blockberger, S., Jan, J.E., Sykanda, A.M. (1989) 'Blind children's early emotional development, do we know enough to help?' *Child: Care, Health and Development,* **15,** 3–28.

Frey, K.S., Greenberg, M.T., Fewell, R.R. (1989) 'Stress and coping among parents of handicapped children: a multidimensional approach.' *American Journal on Mental Retardation,* **94,** 240–249.

Gage, J.R. (1991) *Gait Analysis in Cerebral Palsy. Clinics in Developmental Medicine No. 121.* London: Mac Keith Press.

Garey, L.J. (1984) 'Structural development of the visual system of man.' *Human Neurobiology,* **3,** 75–80.

Gaussen, T., Stratton, P. (1985) 'Beyond the milestone model—a systems framework for alternative infant assessment procedures.' *Child: Care, Health and Development,* **11,** 131–150.

Gibson, D. (1991) 'Down syndrome and cognitive enhancement: not like the others.' *In:* Marfo, K. (Ed.) *Early Intervention in Transition: Current Perspectives on Programs for Handicapped Children.* New York: Praeger, pp. 61–90.

Girolametto, L.E. (1988) 'Improving the social–conversational skills of developmentally delayed children: an intervention study.' *Journal of Speech and Hearing Disorders,* **53,** 156–167.

Glascoe, F.P., Byrne, K.E., Ashford, L.G., Johnson, K.L., Chang, B., Strickland, B. (1992) 'Accuracy of the Denver-II in developmental screening.' *Pediatrics,* **89,** 1221–1225.

Goodman, M., Rothberg, A.D., Houston-McMillan, J.E., Cooper, P.A., Cartwright, J.D., van der Velde, M.A. (1985) 'Effect of early neurodevelopmental therapy in normal and at-risk survivors of neonatal intensive care'. *Lancet,* **2,** 1327–1330.

Goodman, R. (1989) 'Limits to cerebral plasticity.' *In:* Johnson, D., Uttley, D., Wyke, M. (Eds.) *Children's Head Injury: Who Cares?* London: Taylor & Francis, pp. 12–22.

Gordon, C.T., Rapoport, J.L., Hamburger, S.D., State, R.C., Mannheim, G.B. (1992) 'Differential response of seven subjects with autistic disorder to clomipramine and desipramine.' *American Journal of Psychiatry,* **149,** 363–366.

Gould, J., Rigg, M., Bignell, L. (1991) *The Higashi Experience. The Report of a Visit to the Boston Higashi School, 23–28 January 1991.* London: National Autistic Society.

Green, E.M. (1992) 'Cerebral palsy: postural stabilisation.' *In:* McCarthy, G. (Ed.) *Physical Disability in Childhood.* Edinburgh: Churchill Livingstone, pp. 159–162.

Gregory, S., Barlow, S. (1989) 'Interaction betwen deaf babies and their deaf and hearing mothers.' *In:* Woll, B. (Ed.) *Language Development and Sign Language.* Bristol: University of Bristol Centre for Deaf Studies, pp. 23–35.

Guralnick, M.J., Bricker, D.B. (1987) 'The effectiveness of early intervention for children with cognitive and general developmental delays.' *In:* Guralnick, M.J., Bennett, F.C. (Eds.) *The Effectiveness of Early Intervention for At-risk and Handicapped Children.* Orlando, FL: Academic Press, pp.115–168.

Hanson, M.J., Lynch, E.W., Wayman, K.I. (1990) 'Honoring the cultural diversity of families when gathering data'. *Topics in Early Childhood Special Education,* **10,** 112–131.

Hall, D.M.B. (1991) *Health for All Children.* Oxford: Oxford University Press.

Hari, M., Akos, C (1988) *Conductive Education.* London: Routledge.

Henderson, S. (1993) 'Motor development and minor handicap.' *In:* Kalverboer, A.F., Hopkins, B., Geuze, R. (Eds.) *Motor Development in Early and Later Childhood: Longitudinal Approaches.* Cambridge University Press, pp. 286–306.

Howlin, P., Rutter, M. (1989) *Treatment of Austistic Children.* London: Wiley.

Infant Health and Development Program (1990) 'Enhancing the outcomes of low-birth-weight, premature infants. A multisite, randomized trial.' *Journal of the American Medical Association*, **263**, 3035–3042.

King, S.M., Rosenbaum, P., Armstrong, R.W., Milner, R. (1989) 'An epidemiological study of children's attitudes toward disability.' *Developmental Medicine and Child Neurology*, **31**, 237–245.

Kiresuk, T., Sherman, R. (1968) 'Goal attainment scaling: a general method for evaluating comprehensive community mental health programs.' *Community Mental Health Journal*, **4**, 443–453.

Knussen, C., Sloper, P. (1992) 'Stress in families of children with disability: a review of risk factors.' *Journal of Mental Health*, **1**, 241–256.

Kolb, B. (1992) 'Mechanisms underlying recovery from cortical injury: Reflections on progress and directions for the future.' *In:* Rose, F.D., Johnson, D.A. (Eds.) *Recovery from Brain Damage.* New York: Plenum Press, pp. 169–186.

Laszlo, J.I., Bairstow, P.J. (1985) *Perceptual–Motor Behaviour: Developmental Assessment and Therapy.* London: Holt, Rinehart & Winston.

Lazarus, R.S., Folkman, S. (1984) *Stress, Appraisal and Coping.* New York: Springer.

Le Couteur, A., Rutter, M., Lord, C., Rios, P., Robertson, S., Holdgrapter, M., Maclennan, J. (1989) 'Autism diagnostic interview: a standardised investigator based interview.' *Journal of Autism and Developmental Disorders*, **19**, 363–387.

Lees, J., Urwin, S. (1991) *Children with Language Disorders.* London: Whurr.

Mac Keith, R. (1973) 'The feelings and behaviour of parents of handicapped children.' *Developmental Medicine and Child Neurology*, **15**, 524–527.

Mahoney, G., Finger, I., Powell, A. (1985) 'Relationship of maternal behavioral style to the development of organically impaired mentally retarded infants.' *American Journal of Mental Deficiency*, **90**, 296–302.

Marfo, K. (1990) 'Maternal directiveness in interactions with mentally handicapped children: an analytical commentary.' *Journal of Child Psychology and Psychiatry*, **31**, 531–549.

McCollum, J.A. (1991) 'At the cross-road: reviewing and rethinking interaction coaching.' *In:* Marfo, K. (Ed.) *Early Intervention in Transition: Current Perspectives on Programs for Handicapped Children.* New York: Praeger, pp. 147–175.

McConachie, H.R. (1982) 'Fathers of mentally handicapped children.' *In:* Beail, N., McGuire, J. (Eds.) *Fathers: Psychological Perspectives.* London: Junction Books, pp. 144–173.

—— (1991) 'Home-based teaching: what are we asking of parents?' *Child: Care, Health and Development*, **17**, 123–136.

—— (1994) 'Implications of a model of stress and coping for services to families of young disabled children.' *Child: Care, Health and Development*, **20**, 37–46.

McConkey, R. (1985) *Working with Parents: A Practical Guide for Teachers and Therapists.* London: Croom Helm.

McEachin, J.J., Smith, T., Lovaas, O.I. (1993) 'Long-term outcome for children with autism who received early intensive behavioral treatment.' *American Journal on Mental Retardation*, **97**, 359–372.

Meadow-Orleans, K.P. (1987) 'An analysis of the effectiveness of early intervention programs for hearing impaired children.' *In:* Guralnick, M.J., Bennett, F.C. (Eds.) *The Effectiveness of Early Intervention for At-risk and Handicapped Children.* Orlando, FL: Academic Press, pp. 325–362.

Meisels, S.J., Wasik, B.A. (1990) 'Identifying children in need of early intervention.' *In:* Meisels, S.J., Shonkoff, J.P. (Eds.) *Handbook of Early Childhood Intervention.* Cambridge: Cambridge University Press, pp. 605–632.

Mittler, P.J., Mittler, H. (1983) 'Partnership with parents: an overview.' *In:* Mittler, P., McConachie, H. (Eds.) *Parents, Professionals and Mentally Handicapped People: Approaches to Partnership.* Beckenham: Croom Helm, pp. 8–43.

Murray, L. (1992) 'The impact of postnatal depression on infant development.' *Journal of Child Psychology and Psychiatry*, **33**, 543–561.

Oregon Health Services Commission (1991) *Prioritization of Health Services.* Portland, OR: O.H.S.C.

O'Toole, B. (1989) 'The relevance of parental involvement programmes in developing countries.' *Child: Care, Health and Development*, **15**, 329–342.

Palmer, F.B., Shapiro, B.K., Wachtel, R.C., Allen, M.C., Hiller, J.E., Harryman, S.E., Mosher, B.S., Meinert, C.L., Capute, A.J. (1988) 'The effects of physical therapy on cerebral palsy. A controlled trial in infants with spastic diplegia.' *New England Journal of Medicine*, **318**, 803–808.

Piper, M.C., Pless, I.B. (1980) 'Early intervention for infants with Down syndrome: a controlled trial.' *Pediatrics*, **65**, 463–468.

Plomin, R., Emde, R.N., Braungart, J.M., Campos, J., Corley, R., Fulker, D.W., Kagan, J., Reznick, J.S.,

Robinson, J., *et al.* (1993) 'Genetic change and continuity from fourteen to twenty months: the MacArthur longitudinal twin study.' *Child Development*, **64**, 1354–1376.

Preisler, G.M. (1991) 'Early patterns of interaction between blind infants and their sighted mothers.' *Child: Care, Health and Development*, **17**, 65–90.

—— (1993) 'A descriptive study of blind children in nurseries with sighted children.' *Child: Care, Health and Development*, **19**, 295–315.

Quine, L., Pahl, J. (1991) 'Stress and coping in mothers caring for a child with severe learning difficulties: a test of Lazarus' Transactional Model of Coping.' *Journal of Community and Applied Social Psychology*, **1**, 57–70.

Quittner, A.L., Steck, J.L., Rouiller, R.L. (1991) 'Cochlear implants in children—a study of parental stress and adjustment.' *American Journal of Otology*, **12** (Suppl.), 95–104.

Romans-Clarkson, S.E., Clarkson, J.E., Dittmer, I.D., Flett, R., Linsell, C., Mullen, P.E., Mullin, B. (1986) 'Impact of a handicapped child on mental health of parents.' *British Medical Journal*, **293**, 1395–1397.

Rosenbaum, P., Armstrong, R.W. and King, S.M. (1988) 'Determinants of children's attitudes to disability: a review of the evidence.' *Children's Health Care*, **17**, 32–39.

Russell, D.J., Rosenbaum, P.L., Cadman, D.T., Gowland, C., Hardy, S., Jarvis, S. (1989) 'The Gross Motor Function Measure: a means to evaluate the effects of physical therapy.' *Developmental Medicine and Child Neurology*, **31**, 341–352.

Rutter, M. (1982) 'Prevention of children's psychosocial disorders: myth and substance.' *Pediatrics*, **70**, 883–894.

—— Mawhood, L. (1991) 'The long-term psychosocial sequelae of specific developmental disorders of speech and language.' *In:* Rutter, M., Casaer, P. (Eds.) *Biological Risk Factors for Psychosocial Disorders*. Cambridge: Cambridge University Press, pp. 233–259.

—— Macdonald, H., Le Couteur, A., Harrington, R., Bolton, P., Bailey, A. (1990) 'Genetic factors in child psychiatric disorders—II. Empirical findings.' *Journal of Child Psychology and Psychiatry*, **31**, 39–83.

Sameroff, A.J., Chandler, M.J. (1975) 'Reproductive risk and the continuum of caretaking casualty.' *In:* Horowitz, F.D., Harrington, M., Scarr-Salatapek, S., Siegel, G. (Eds.) *Review of Child Development Research, Vol.4*. Chicago: University of Chicago Press, pp. 187–244.

—— Seifer, R., Barocas, R., Zax, M., Greenspan, S. (1987) 'Intelligence quotient scores of 4-year-old children: social–environmental risk factors.' *Pediatrics*, **79**, 343–350.

Scarr, S. (1992) 'Developmental theories for the 1990s: development and individual differences.' *Child Development*, **63**, 1–19.

Scherzer, A.L., Mike, V., Ilson, J. (1976) 'Physical therapy as a determinant of change in the cerebral palsied infant.' *Pediatrics*, **58**, 47–52.

Schopler, E., Mesibov, G.B., Shipley, R.H., Bashford, A. (1984) 'Helping autistic children through their parents: the TEACCH model.' *In:* Schopler, E., Mesibov, G.B. (Eds.) *The Effects of Autism on the Family*. New York: Plenum, pp. 65–81.

Scrutton, D. (1989) 'The early management of hips in cerebral palsy.' *Developmental Medicine and Child Neurology*, **31**, 108–116.

Seligman, M., Darling, R.B. (1989) *Ordinary Families, Special Children: a Systems Approach to Childhood Disability*. New York: The Guilford Press.

Shah, R. (1992) *The Silent Minority: Children with Disabilities in Asian Families*. London: National Children's Bureau.

Shahidullah, S., Hepper, P. (1993) 'Prenatal hearing tests?' *Journal of Reproductive and Infant Psychology*, **11**, 143–146.

Shearer, D.E., Shearer, M.S. (1976) 'The Portage Project: a model for early childhood education.' *In:* Tjossem, T.D. (Ed.) *Intervention Strategies for High Risk Infants and Young Children*. Baltimore: University Park Press, pp. 335–350.

Shotter, J., Gergen, K.J. (1990) *Texts of Identity. Inquiries in Social Construction Series, Vol. 2*. London: Sage.

Siegel, L. (1984) 'Home environment influences on cognitive development in preterm and full-term children during the first five years.' *In:* Gottfried, A.W. (Ed.) *Home Environment and Early Cognitive Development*. New York: Academic Press, pp. 197–234.

Siméonsson, R.J., Cooper, D.H., Scheiner, A.P. (1982) 'A review and analysis of the effectiveness of early intervention programs.' *Pediatrics*, **69**, 635–641.

Sloper, P., Turner, S. (1990) 'Parental and professional views of the needs of families with a child with severe disability.' *Psychology Quarterly*, **4**, 323–330.

—— —— (1992) 'Service needs of families of children with severe physical disability.' *Child: Care, Health and Development*, **18**, 259–282.

—— —— (1993) 'Determinants of parental satisfaction with disclosure of disability.' *Developmental Medicine and Child Neurology*, **35**, 816–825.

—— Knussen, C., Turner, S., Cunningham, C. (1991) 'Factors related to stress and satisfaction with life in families of children with Down's syndrome.' *Journal of Child Psychology and Psychiatry*, **32**, 655–676.

Smith, R. (1991) 'Rationing: the search for sunlight. Rationing decisions should be explicit and rational.' *British Medical Journal*, **303**, 1561–1562. *(Editorial.)*

—— (1992) 'Reconsidering compensation for medical accidents. Concentrate on those with the severest disabilities, whatever the cause.' *British Medical Journal*, **304**, 1066–1067. *(Editorial.)*

Snow, C.E., Perlman, R., Nathan, D. (1987) 'Why routines are different: toward a multiple-factors model of the relation between input and language acquisition.' *In:* Nelson, K.E., van Kleek, A. (Eds.) *Children's Language. Vol. 6.* London: Lawrence Erlbaum, pp. 65–97.

Snyder-McClean, L., McLean, J.E. (1987) 'Effectiveness of early intervention for children with language and communication disorders.' *In:* Guralnick, M.J., Bennett, F.C. (Eds.) *The Effectiveness of Early Intervention for At-risk and Handicapped Children.* Orlando, FL: Academic Press, pp. 213–272.

Sonksen, P.M., Stiff, B. (1991) *Show Me What My Friends Can See. A Developmental Guide for Parents of Babies with Severely Impaired Sight and their Professional Advisors.* London: Institute of Child Health.

—— Petrie, A., Drew, K.J. (1991) 'Promotion of visual development of severely visually impaired babies: evaluation of a developmentally based programme.' *Developmental Medicine and Child Neurology*, **33**, 320–335.

Stevenson, P., Bax, M., Stevenson, J. (1982) 'The evaluation of home based speech therapy for language delayed pre-school children in an inner city area.' *British Journal of Disorders of Communication*, **17**, 141–148.

Stokes, J., Bamford, J.M. (1990) 'Transition from pre-linguistic to linguistic communication in hearing-impaired infants.' *British Journal of Audiology*, **24**, 217–222.

Strain, P.S., Hoyson, M.H., Jamieson, B.J. (1985) 'Normally developing preschoolers as intervention agents for autistic-like children: effects on class deportment and social interaction.' *Journal of the Division for Early Childhood*, **9**, 105–115.

Sturmey, P., Thorburn, M.J., Brown, J.M., Reed, J., Kaur, J., King, G. (1992) 'Portage guide to early intervention: cross-cultural aspects and intra-cultural variability.' *Child: Care, Health and Development*, **18**, 377–394.

Tardieu, C., Lespargot, A., Tabary, C., Bret, M.D. (1988) 'For how long must the soleus muscle be stretched each day to prevent contracture?' *Developmental Medicine and Child Neurology*, **30**, 3–10.

Taylor, D., Vaegan, Morris, J.A., Rogers, J.E., Warland, J. (1979) 'Amblyopia in bilateral infantile and juvenile cataract. Relationship to timing of treatment.' *Transactions of the Ophthalmological Society of the United Kingdom*, **99**, 170–175.

Taylor, E. (1991) 'Toxins and allergens.' *In:* Rutter, M., Casaer, P. (Eds.) *Biological Risk Factors for Psychosocial Disorders.* Cambridge: Cambridge University Press, pp. 199–232.

Tjossem, T. (1976) 'Early intervention: issues and approaches.' *In:* Tjossem, T. (Ed.) *Intervention Strategies for High Risk Infants and Young Children.* Baltimore: University Park Press, pp. 3–33.

Urey, J.R., Viar, V. (1990) 'Use of mental health support services among families of children with disabilities: discrepant views of parents and paediatricians.' *Mental Handicap Research*, **3**, 81–88.

Wallander, J.L., Varni, J.W., Babani, L., DeHaan, C.B., Wilcox, K.T., Banis, H.T. (1989) 'The social environment and the adaptation of mothers of physically handicapped children.' *Journal of Pediatric Psychology*, **14**, 371–387.

—— Pitt, L.C., Mellins, C.A. (1990) 'Child functional independence and maternal psychosocial stress as risk factors threatening adaptation in mothers of physically or sensorially handicapped children.' *Journal of Consulting and Clinical Psychology*, **58**, 818–824.

Warnock, H.M. (1978) *Special Educational Needs. Report of the Committee of Enquiry into the Education of Handicapped Children and Young People.* London: HMSO.

Weiner, F. (1981) 'Treatment of phonological disability using the method of meaningful minimal contrast: two case studies.' *Journal of Speech and Hearing Disorders*, **46**, 97–103.

Werner, E.E. (1985) 'Stress and protective factors in children's lives.' *In:* Nicol, A.R. (Ed.) *Longitudinal Studies in Child Psychology and Psychiatry.* Chichester: Wiley, pp. 335–355.

Wishart, M.C., Bidder, R.T., Gray, O.P. (1981) 'Parents' report of family life with a developmentally delayed child.' *Child: Care, Health and Development*, **7**, 267–279.

Wolfendale, S. (1983) *Parental Participation in Children's Development and Education.* London: Gordon & Breach Scientific.

Wolke, D. (1991) 'Supporting the development of low birthweight infants.' *Journal of Child Psychology and Psychiatry*, **32**, 723–741.

Wood, D., Wood, H., Griffiths, A., Howarth, I. (1989) *Teaching and Talking to Deaf Children.* Chichester: Wiley.

Wright, T., Nicholson, J. (1973) 'Physiotherapy for the spastic child: an evaluation.' *Developmental Medicine and Child Neurology*, **15**, 146–163.

Yule, W., Carr, J. (Eds.) (1987) *Behaviour Modification for People with Mental Handicaps. 2nd Edn.* London: Croom Helm.

Zifferblatt, S.M., Burton, S.D., Horner, R., White, T. (1977) 'Establishing generalization effects among autistic children.' *Journal of Autism and Childhood Schizophrenia*, **7**, 337–347.

4
THE EVALUATION OF INTERVENTIONS

Margaret Martlew and Kevin Connolly

Introduction

The dictionary defines evaluation as a process which is directed at finding the *worth* or *value* of something. In simple terms, it is an attempt to answer the·question, 'Does it work?', the 'it' here being some treatment or intervention designed to produce a specified effect. Whether a given intervention works is usually the first and principal thing we want to know about a treatment, whether it be chemotherapy, physiotherapy or psychotherapy. If it does not work under certain conditions or if it does not work with some people then we want to know whether the circumstances apply to the case in hand. On the face of it, discovering whether something works might seem straightforward, but in fact the question is complex and can be quite difficult to answer.

Attempts to evaluate a medical treatment or the effectiveness of an educational scheme have ancient roots. Over the 20th century these concerns have developed into a specialist discipline known as evaluation research which has its own textbooks, courses and specialist journals. Evaluations are undertaken for a variety of reasons. They may be carried out for the purposes of management and administration; as a part of planning and policy making; or to decide between one treatment regimen and another; to assess the efficacy of a particular form of therapy; or to measure the success of a particular educational scheme. In essence, evaluation is a process designed to obtain knowledge about a particular intervention the purpose of which is to influence in a specified way a present or future state.

Like all disciplines, evaluation research, or evaluation as it is commonly called, has developed its own vocabulary, concepts and procedures. It also has specialists skilled in different areas. However, there is a basic set of principles which lie at the heart of all evaluations and this chapter is concerned with this set of principles. Some of the points may seem obvious, even banal, but we make no apology for listing these. All too often the obvious is overlooked. Our aim is to provide a brief but systematic account of the issues and questions that are fundamental to the evaluation of intervention programmes.

The process of evaluation is best seen as a series of questions, which serve as a guide or a key to systematic assessment. The existence of a key of this kind implies an *objective* structured process with specified criteria; however, there are constraints and problems which may restrict the extent of any objective process at a particular time. In such circumstances it is common for people to make subjective evaluations. Subjective evaluations, that is evaluations which are not made on the basis of specified objective criteria, can be useful in a number of ways, and the distinction between subjective and objective processes is not always as sharp as one might suppose.

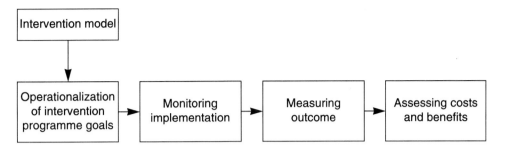

Fig. 4.1. The principle components of evaluation.

The development of an intervention model

The term 'model' relates to the underlying theory on which the programme is based (see Warr 1980). Sometimes this consists of nothing more than a set of implicit assumptions drawn from experience and perhaps supported by some small scale study or by data gathered informally. An intervention model, whether it is implicit or explicit, is based on some notion of cause and effect. Often, especially in dealing with complex and highly variable conditions and situations, there is only a very crudely operationalized hypothesis about cause and effect (that is, one having only poorly defined validation procedures).* A sound theoretical base gives coherence and consistency to an intervention programme. Broad theoretical assumptions, for example the importance of early learning, can give a general rationale. Other theoretical guidelines may then be brought in, such as the importance of attentional states and active participation in the process of learning (Bricker and Veltman 1990). In the absence of an explicitly stated intervention model it is extremely difficult if not impossible to replicate an intervention programme. The opportunities for quality control and for monitoring effectiveness are severely curtailed.

The first rule for evaluating an intervention of whatever kind is a precise specification of the programme in operational terms. Unless the required conditions are specified and the goal(s) made clear it is really not possible to evaluate its efficacy. Of course, the precision with which these requirements are met varies and is subject to change as the model is developed and modified, but unless we know what an intervention is it cannot be implemented and consequently it cannot be tested. This is an obvious and compelling point, but many therapeutic and educational schemes are shrouded in mystery. For example, Bairstow

*The concept of operationism was introduced in 1927 by P.W. Bridgman in his influential book *The Logic of Modern Physics* (New York: Macmillan). The principle of operationism is simply a formal statement of a basic rule of scientific communication to the effect that the empirical basis for each term used must be made clear. A construct is defined in terms of the operations carried out in measuring it—an operational definition. The principle of operationism in an objective in scientific communication, an ultimate requirement rather than one which must be satisfied here and now. As the precision of the operations is improved, the definition becomes clearer. (See S.S. Stevens, 'Psychology and the science of science.' *Psychological Bulletin*, 1939, **36**, 221–263; and M.H. Marx, 'Formal theory.' *In:* Marx, M.H., Goodson, F.E. (Eds.) *Theories in Contemporary Psychology, 2nd Edn.* New York: Macmillan, 1976, pp. 234–260.)

et al. (1993) found it 'impossible to identify which of the implied principles of conductive education might be crucial to its effective implementation'.

Evaluating an intervention involves four basic components. First, there must be something which is to be evaluated, that is an intervention of some kind. This derives from the underlying theory and must be precisely specified. Second, the intervention must be correctly delivered, which entails monitoring its implementation. Third, the outcome of the intervention must be assessed and measured. Finally, the costs and benefits associated with the intervention programme must be ascertained and examined as part of the overall process. The links between the principal components are shown in Figure 4.1.

The intervention programme
The term 'programme' means any systematic attempt to influence and change in a specified way the situation and condition of others. This is a very broad definition encompassing medicine, education, social services, and a whole range of general and particular human activities designed to produce particular outcomes.

Intervention programmes, of course, vary greatly in their scope and size (*e.g.* Meisels and Shonkoff 1990). Some have limited, specific and quite precise goals. For example, a training programme may have as its goal teaching a disabled child a specific skill such as using a cup or a spoon. While these commonplace activities are enormously complicated, the goal is specific and can be quite precisely specified. Other programmes are extensive and define their goals in very broad terms. For example, the 1960s Head Start programme in the USA was directed at facilitating the development of young children through intervention in areas such as health, education and community development (Zigler and Berman 1983).

Goals and objectives
In the case of intervention programmes with broad and rather generally defined goals, it is useful to draw a distinction between goals and objectives. Large programmes usually define their goals in very broad terms. In Europe and North America there has been great concern over the past 25 years about the separate and segregated education of disabled children. This concern led to the movement for the integration or mainstreaming of disabled children into the regular school system. In practical terms alone, integration or mainstreaming is an enormous undertaking and constitutes a very broad goal (Guralnick 1986, Meisel 1986). The attainment of such a goal and the process of working towards it is helped by identifying specific objectives. For example, an objective which constitutes a sub-set of the general goal would be to specify that all disabled children who are mobile, who do not have severe behaviour problems, and whose IQs are greater than 85 should attend a mainstream school within a period of five years. The attainment of this objective, as a reflection of the general goals of integration, could be more easily quantified (Swann 1985).

Objectives and requirements
Once the objective or objectives of a programme have been identified, a number of questions follow. With respect to each of these, the closer they are to operational statements,

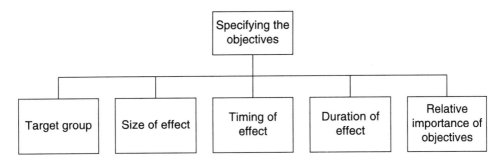

Fig. 4.2. Principal questions following specification of central objective.

that is to phenomena that can be measured, the more likely it is that an evaluation can be undertaken. Unless goals can be clarified and objectives operationally defined, it is unlikely that any adequate or satisfactory evaluation can be made. The principal questions which follow once the central objective is identified are shown in Figure 4.2.

THE TARGET GROUP

It is obviously essential to be clear and to specify the nature of the individuals for whom the programme was devised. For example, an educational programme may require that the individuals undertaking it have a measured IQ within the average range, or have acquired certain skills, *e.g.* the ability to read at a given level. Unless these prerequisites of the target group are met it will not be possible to conclude that the intervention does or does not work since it will not have been given a fair test. It would be a serious mistake to expect the programme to do something for which it was not designed. The Perry Preschool Project, which was designed to enhance the cognitive abilities of disadvantaged children, is a good example of the careful selection of a target group involving several variables (Schweinhart and Weikart 1983).

THE SIZE OF EFFECT

How great a change is required before we conclude that an intervention has worked satisfactorily? The question can be applied to individuals, in which case we might, for example, specify a change of at least 5 per cent improvement on some measured variable. Alternatively the question can be applied to a population. In this instance we must indicate what proportion of the population must show a change of a given magnitude in the desired direction. In each case it is a matter for the programme designer and those using it to decide on an acceptable magnitude of effect which may vary as a function of alternatives and relative costs. However, before beginning an evaluation the size of effect expected should be explicitly stated.

TIMING OF EFFECT

Another important issue associated with an intervention programme is how quickly an effect is expected. Effects may be rapid as with the administration of a drug (*e.g.* an anti-biotic) or the protection afforded by vaccination, or they may take much longer to produce as may be the case with some educational programmes. For example, Seitz *et al.* (1985) contend that the effects of an intensive caregiver-focused programme can be greater after ten years than immediately after the programme ends. In setting up an intervention some indication of when effects will occur should be specified, as in the case of the better Head Start programmes (Bronfenbrenner 1974). Subsequent and different effects are not precluded and indeed were found in some Head Start programmes (Lazar and Darlington 1982).

DURATION OF THE EFFECT

An important property of any change is how long it lasts. A change brought about by an intervention may be quite short lived or it may be long term. This is sometimes called the stability of an effect. In the case of short-term changes the individual will revert to an earlier pre-treatment stage after some relatively brief period. An alternative is that the change produced is effectively permanent when the state following intervention is main-tained for a specified period, perhaps several years. Another possibility is that the change produced by the intervention is sustained just as long as the intervention programme con-tinues. In this case the programme both produces a change and maintains it. Without the programme the person reverts to the earlier pre-treatment state. An example of this kind of situation is provided by drugs used to control a chronic syndrome, for example, asthma. It is necessary to indicate how long an effect must last for it to be regarded as successful.

IMPORTANCE OF OBJECTIVES

Many intervention programmes have more than one objective. These objectives may be related or they may be dissimilar. For example, involving parents in programmes for learning-disabled children may have as one objective recruiting the parents to teach specific skills, and, as another, bringing about changes in the roles and attitudes to one another of the parents and professionals (*e.g.* McConachie 1986). Where there is more than a single objective, different persons, or professions, may place different emphases on them. For example, some consequences of impairments may cause more distress than others but individuals often differ markedly in their assessment of these effects. Similarly, in caring for people with intellectual impairment a psychologist may give primary emphasis to the educational consequences of an intervention whereas the nurses or care staff may emphasize its effect on the family of the client. Both of these are legitimate, and in order to incorporate such differences into the evaluation it is necessary to specify and, where possible, arrange in order of priority the various objectives linked in an intervention. Plainly, it is important to ensure that all those involved in service provision are aware of the objectives (see also Chapter 15).

Monitoring programme implementation

In simple terms this amounts to making sure that what is presumed to be happening—what is presumed in the intervention model and what is specified by the programme design and requirements—is actually taking place. This cannot just be assumed; it must be checked. In relation to this issue there are two key questions to be answered. The first of these relates to the population receiving the intervention: is it the population for which it was designed? Unless this question can be answered affirmatively the programme cannot be evaluated because a fundamental and necessary condition is not being met. The second key question is concerned with the delivery of the programme and whether it is consistent with the programme specifications. Again, unless this is ensured the test would not be a fair one and consequently would not be helpful.

Establishing the appropriateness of the target group
In monitoring implementation, the first requirement is thus to ensure that the population which is to receive the intervention meets any necessary specifications of the programme. There are various ways in which the suitability of a population for a particular intervention can be established. This is not a matter of selecting an 'easy' or 'difficult' target group but of ensuring that the group meets any requirements which are specified in the intervention model. For example, let us consider an intervention for children with moderate intellectual impairment and poor speech intelligibility. These children are to be trained in the use of Makaton signing. However, if some are dyspraxic and unable to make the fine movements required for effective communication, the intervention will be inappropriate for them.

USE OF RECORDS
An obvious source of information about a person is from records. It is customary to keep records on both children and adults. Obvious examples are educational and medical records. Records of course vary from the skeletal, sometimes little more than name, age, and major experiences, to detailed, accurate and up to date accounts of medical, educational or social history which include the results of various tests and assessments dealing with a range of a person's attributes. If reliable and sufficiently detailed records exist they may provide a satisfactory basis on which to decide the suitability of individuals.

The adequacy of records varies greatly. Information that is important with respect to an intervention programme may not have been recorded or it may never have been gathered. If required information is not available from the records, *e.g.* the child's precise age may not be known, it will be necessary to find another means of confirming a child's suitability for the programme.

DIRECT ASSESSMENT OF PARTICIPANTS
If there are no satisfactory records on which to decide the suitability of potential participants, other means must be found. An obvious way of proceeding may be to make a survey of all, or an adequate sample of, the potential participants to determine by direct assessment whether they meet the requirements stipulated by the intervention model. In the case of projects in special education, children may have to be tested on relevant dimensions. For example, admission into a remedial reading programme may be determined by performance on a reading test. The assessment of children with severe impairments presents special

difficulties and there are problems in obtaining a valid assessment (Simeonsson *et al.* 1980). Inevitably, from time to time the information available is not of the standard required, and sometimes there are insurmountable practical difficulties. In such circumstances compromises have to be made, but they should not be accepted lightly and certainly should not lead to any erosion of the high standards to which all professionals should aspire or of the basic standards to which they work in all but the most exceptional circumstances.

COMMUNITY SURVEY

When a project is not narrowly targeted on a restricted and tightly specified set of individuals, it is possible to survey a whole group. For example, we might want to know what proportion of children in special schools would be appropriate for a particular intervention. The necessary information may be obtained from a questionnaire completed by teachers.

DANGER OF BIAS IN PROGRAMME PARTICIPANTS

Correctly recruiting into programmes is plainly a necessary condition for evaluating any intervention. Once this is achieved, the question of maintenance in and completion of a programme becomes important. To ensure that the data collected are not biased it is necessary to be sure that those who drop out from an intervention are not systematically different on any essential dimension from those who stay in the programme. Assuming 'drop outs' and 'stayers' both continue to be eligible for the programme, any differences between them may indicate a bias in the evaluation which would prevent a satisfactory analysis.

Checking programme delivery

One cannot assume that issuing instructions to carry out a particular programme will result in this being done in the prescribed manner. It is necessary to check carefully and systematically that what is supposed to have been done has actually been done. Failure to achieve the outcome predicted by the intervention model may reflect a failure to deliver the programme correctly and this possibility must be accounted for in any evaluation. From a review of a number of interventions with learning disabled children, Marfo and Kysela (1985) found that only two checked on programme delivery. There are three main ways in which this aspect of the process may go wrong. First, the treatment may simply not be delivered, or less than that specified may be given; second, the wrong treatment may be given; and third, the process may be unstandardized and may vary across the target population. Any of these possibilities would rule out a proper test of the intervention.

To ensure the adequate and correct delivery of an intervention it is necessary to specify precisely the operations involved in carrying out the programme. To do this, the activities and actions required must be defined. Consider an educational programme; the first requirement is to specify the *context* in which it takes place. This involves the location, the school or classroom where the programme will be run; the staff, teachers, care assistants and so forth; the necessary resources, the materials and equipment, etc. This is then followed by the *activities* which make up the programme. It is obviously important to ensure that the appropriate materials are used as intended and with the prescribed frequency for the specified period of time. From this it follows that the procedures which teachers should use in their interactions with children must be described. If other people are involved in aspects of the programme delivery, it is necessary to ensure that they too play their part in the specified way.

Methods of monitoring

Various methods for monitoring implementation are available. The appropriateness of each in relation to any given programme depends on a number of factors. Four principal methods are used. Their suitability depends on the nature of the programme, its size and its complexity. Some methods are inherently difficult where issues of privacy and confidentiality are important. For example, direct observations of implementation may well not be appropriate in relation to a programme involving counselling or to one giving family planning advice. The four main methods are briefly as follows.

DIRECT OBSERVATION

As the name implies, this method entails making systematic direct observations on the implementation of the programme, that is, the intervention in process. Making observations is a difficult, technical process; they must be systematic, the sampling scheme must satisfy a number of considerations, specific behaviours/events must be operationally defined, recording techniques be specified, observers carefully trained and checked, and so forth (see Connolly 1973, Martin and Bateson 1986). It is necessary to have a detailed plan which deals with these considerations, and the data collected should be quantitative. Rating schemes, including check lists to ensure that certain questions are answered, are often valuable in this context. The possibility that the presence of an observer may interfere with the programme implementation must also be considered (Connolly and Smith 1972, Martin and Bateson 1986).

SERVICE RECORDS

In certain cases the records of service delivery, where the intervention is simple, discrete and specific, may be sufficient to monitor delivery. For example, if the administration of a drug and the dosage are routinely and reliably recorded, this should be sufficient to check that the intervention was made if supported by random occasional direct observation. It may of course be necessary to note additional information such as the time when the drug was given. The accuracy and reliability of the data obtained are a concern whatever method is used. There are three general rules which are worth bearing in mind. First, it is generally the case that a few data items collected and recorded reliably are better for monitoring purposes than a much larger and more comprehensive data set which is not reliable. Second, whenever possible it is sensible to use structured data collecting forms which can be quickly and efficiently used, perhaps in the form of a check list. Third, it is important to review completed records to check for consistency and accuracy; of course this should be done as soon as possible after the records have been completed.

Needless to say, there are risks in using routine service records and these should be considered in selecting an appropriate method of monitoring the delivery of an intervention. The accuracy of records must always be considered. The possibility that they may exaggerate the effects of an intervention, especially when the person providing the service is also responsible for recording the data, is a real one that must be guarded against. The accuracy of record keeping may also fall victim to the pressures of providing a service.

INFORMATION FROM THE PROGRAMME PROVIDER

Rather than rely on the information contained in service records, it is possible to ask the providers (*e.g.* teachers and therapists) for an account of the process. This may vary from a narrative diary account of the implementation of the programme to a carefully structured questionnaire, or even an interview conducted by the evaluation team. For long or complex intervention programmes, asking the person who is conducting the intervention may give access to a rich source of information. However, there are a number of caveats which must be applied. What of the validity and reliability of the information obtained? For the informant this may also be a time consuming and burdensome process.

DATA FROM PATIENTS/CLIENTS

Depending on the nature of the programme and on the individuals involved it may be possible to obtain satisfactory information on implementation from the recipients themselves. This is less likely in cases where young children are involved, or where the intervention is complex or where a great deal of detail is involved. For the purpose of obtaining information from disabled children or their parents or carers, check lists or interviews may be useful. Information from those receiving services is of particular importance because professionals may not be aware of some features which are of great concern to children and their parents. Also it is generally valuable to have some idea of client satisfaction. In some circumstances, asking those who receive an intervention may prove to be the only way of finding out what was actually delivered (Turnbull and Winton 1984).

Using the data from programme monitoring

The information obtained from monitoring the implementation of an intervention can be used in various ways, but there are three particular issues which need to be addressed. The first is to determine to what extent the programme, as delivered, resembles in essential details the programme as designed. This may be dealt with by a statement in narrative form, though considerations such as coverage, adequacy and any bias which may be introduced in the implementation of the intervention are best dealt with quantitatively.

Frequently, programmes and methods of treatment are implemented in more than one centre. In this case, different staff will be involved and there may be special local factors which create further differences. Implementation monitoring should provide some estimate of diversity in staff, equipment, exact procedures and local culture (Schweinhart and Weikart 1983). The evaluation of a programme requires that variability in implementation between centres be taken into account.

The third important consideration is programme continuity. Interventions, especially complex ones, tend to change over time; they both drift and are modified informally as a result of experience and feedback. Ensuring that the implementation of a programme matches the designed programme at a given time is not a guarantee that this state of affairs will continue indefinitely to a later time: this must be empirically confirmed.

Assessment of outcome

The purpose of evaluation is to establish whether or not an intervention has worked, that is, whether the intended and specified outcome or outcomes were achieved. The measurement of outcome is rarely simple or easy because of the inevitable complexity of the situation in which most interventions are undertaken. Fundamentally the question is about causality: has the intervention which was carried out been the cause of the changes that were observed? More precisely, the issue is one of probability: what is the probability that the observed outcome is a consequence of the intervention? Often this results in statements of the kind, 'This works in x per cent of such cases.'

Establishing whether an intervention has worked entails dealing with three issues. First and obviously is the need to rule out other explanations for any changes seen following the intervention. The second issue is the size or extent of change following an intervention; this is likely to be variable, and it is important to devise a means of measuring or estimating the magnitude of any effect. Finally, there is the question of any unintended or unexpected effects. These side-effects, as they are often called, may be positive or negative. Because they are undesirable, negative consequences are our principal concern.

The aim of an investigation is to estimate the effect or outcome which can be attributed specifically to the treatment. These effects, sometimes called net outcomes, are those which are free of any other variable in the situation. Before this can be done, two prerequisites must be met. These seem, on the face of it, straightforward, but they are probably the conditions which are most often not fulfilled and as such present the greatest threat to the evaluation of a treatment programme. They are often not easy conditions but they are *essential*. The first of these concerns the goals of the intervention itself. These must be sufficiently well articulated to make it possible to identify a satisfactory measure of whether the goal is attained or of the degree to which it is achieved. Unless an outcome can be specified and operationally defined, an intervention cannot be evaluated because there simply is no criterion (Bairstow *et al.* 1993). In the case of a drug the goal may be to produce a physiological change such as reducing a patient's temperature, or to kill infective agents such as parasites. In cases like these, operationalizing outcomes is not too difficult. But, with respect to various forms of therapy for disabled children it is not an easy task. Nevertheless it must be done. Goals can be adapted and refined but they must be explicitly specified and operationalized. The second prerequisite is of course to ensure that the treatment is correctly carried out; no essential features must be missing or incorrectly applied. This is the issue of monitoring programme implementation dealt with in the previous section.

Once the goals of an intervention are clearly established, an outcome measure must be found or devised. The outcome measure is in fact the operationalization of the goal. For example, let us suppose that we wanted to measure the efficacy of a scheme for teaching reading to children between 9 and 10 years of age. A reasonable outcome measure would be in terms of children's scores on a standardized reading test. An outcome is thus a change in the level of a measurable variable. The basic process of measuring outcome entails measuring the relevant variable before intervention and following the intervention in an attempt to establish whether any change has taken place. This can be expressed symbolically as:

$$O = E_2 - E_1$$

where O is the outcome, E_1 is the initial measure taken before intervention and E_2 is that taken after the intervention.

This simple design is of limited value because it does not include controls and it is therefore difficult to be confident that any observed change is due to the intervention and not some other unknown variable. If a control group, that is a group in all important respects similar to the experimental group, is included and treated identically to the experimental group except that they do not receive the intervention itself then a more satisfactory comparison can be made. Again, the process can be expressed symbolically as follows:

$$O = (E_2 - E_1) - (C_2 - C_1)$$

where C_1 and C_2 are the measures for the control group coincident with the initial and post-intervention measures respectively for the treatment group. Differences between C_2 and C_1 cannot be caused by the intervention and therefore they provide an estimate of change due to other unknown variables.

The choice of an outcome measure is often not easy and there are advantages in using several different measures. This is especially so in cases where the period needed for the intervention to show effects is long or perhaps both unknown and variable. For example, the initial enthusiasm for the Head Start programmes was tempered by the fact that the early gains reported were not sustained (Bronfenbrenner 1974). A much later follow-up by the Consortium for Longitudinal Studies (1983) traced the progress of children who had taken part in eleven of these programmes. Using different measures they found sustained long-term effects. For example, children who had increased IQ scores at age 6 years were less likely to be in need of remedial education and more likely to satisfy the school's performance requirements. The mothers of children in the programmes were more satisfied with their children's performance and reported higher aspirations for their children. Preschool programmes of comparatively short duration may show long-term effects if appropriate outcome measures are selected.

The validity and reliability of measures
To be of use in the evaluation of an intervention, the outcome measures used must be both valid and reliable. Validity is in some respects the more difficult to establish. In essence, it refers to truth and is concerned with whether the measuring instrument *actually* measures what it purports to measure. Using more than one measure of a construct and looking for good correlations between measures is a useful way to explore whether a measure is satisfactory. With regard to psychological tests various ways of estimating validity have been developed (Ghiselli *et al.* 1981). Several different forms of validity have been dis-

tinguished. *Face validity* refers to whether or not the test appears to measure the construct in question. If it does not have face validity those taking the test are unlikely to treat it seriously or be adequately motivated. *Content validity* refers to the content of the test in question. For example, a test of spelling would by definition need to consist of a range of spelling tasks. *Criterion validity* is concerned with whether a test produces scores which match some independent and agreed criterion.

Reliability is a property of a specific instrument used in a prescribed way on a specified population. In essence, reliability refers to whether or not repeated measurements made on the same individual on successive occasions, or measures of the same population made by others, would yield the same results. Formally, reliability relates to the proportion of variance that is true variance, *i.e.* that due to differences between individuals and not to error variance. There are various ways of estimating reliability; one of the most widely used is *test–retest reliability* which refers to the reproducibility of results over time. *Split-half reliability* provides a check for internal consistency and *inter-observer agreement* is a way of assessing the agreement on a set of criteria between examiners.

Outcome measures must be both valid and reliable, and the extent to which they are not is a limitation on the evaluation process itself. It is necessary to measure accurately and reliably the variables used in the outcome measure; limitations on accuracy or on reliability are serious constraints. It is not sufficient to assume that a measure is valid and reliable. Both constructs should be explicitly and critically examined in the context of deciding upon and testing outcome measures.

Factors which act as constraints on assessing outcome

The overall changes which occur in a population following an intervention, that is, changes between 'before' and 'after' measurements, are called gross outcome effects. These gross outcome effects include effects caused by the intervention programme itself and effects caused by other, confounding factors. When the effects of any confounding factors are subtracted from the gross outcome effects, what remains is due to the intervention itself. Sometimes these are called net outcome effects. There are various kinds of contaminating or confounding factors or effects and these should be considered both in designing an evaluation and in the interpretation of results. Among the principal contaminating effects are the following.

ENDOGENOUS CHANGES

These are changes in an outcome measure which occur irrespective of the intervention programme itself. An example is provided by patterns of recovery from common infections such as colds and influenza. Most people will recover from such an illness without any medical intervention.

SECULAR DRIFT

Secular changes are those which occur slowly over a long period of time. In any population there is usually some evidence of long-term changes. For example, increases in the height and weight of children in almost all European countries, Japan and North America have been reported (Roche 1979). On the other hand, in parts of India, Africa and Chile affected by famine, disease and poverty, there has been a decrease in adult stature (Tobias 1975). Depending on the variables involved and the duration of an intervention programme, secular drift may produce significant confounding effects.

MATURATIONAL TRENDS

Interventions which are directed toward producing changes in infancy or childhood must take into account that these are periods in the life cycle when rapid and extensive changes take place. Maturational changes which have nothing to do with the intervention itself may produce serious confounding effects in studies on children. Specific account should be taken of this in designing an evaluation study. In everyday language, this is a case of children who are said to 'grow out of it'.

SAMPLE BIAS

Many intervention studies are dependent on the voluntary cooperation of patients or clients, which raises the possibility that they are not representative of the population as a whole. The danger of bias in circumstances where the participants are self-selected is well known, but because of the voluntary nature of many intervention programmes it is difficult to avoid. It is important to consider this question and take such action as is appropriate at the design stage and again in the analysis and interpretation of results. Obvious risks are that only extreme cases, severe or mild, will be represented in the sample treated. A further risk is that postive outcome effects may be due more to the enthusiasm of participants than to the programme itself, and thus the magnitude of the outcome cannot be generalized beyond this initial group.

CHANCE EFFECTS

These are random fluctuations which occur while the intervention is in progress and which are difficult to identify. The possibility that any effects on the outcome measures are due to chance is dealt with by the appropriate statistical treatment of the data. This enables the investigator to estimate the significance of an effect, that is, the probability of it occurring by chance. For further discussion the reader should refer to an introductory text on experimental design and analysis.

PROGRAMME-RELATED EFFECTS

The evaluation process itself may result in contamination. It may, for example, draw the attention of those taking part in it to factors or behaviours which have opposite or inhibitory effects. An example of a programme-related effect, known as the Hawthorn effect, was described in the 1930s. This related to an experiment on worker productivity. The productivity of six average women workers was measured and a wide range of factors was varied. The results were surprising. No matter what was changed (number of rest periods increased or decreased, lengthening or shortening of the working day, increasing or reducing factory light levels, etc.), the women's productivity increased. The explanation for this surprising effect is simply that it resulted from the attention paid to the workers by the experimenter

(Homans 1965). In many therapeutic interventions there is a danger that the person who is responsible for the therapy and for deciding to undertake the intervention, for example, parents, become psychologically committed to it. This conviction about the value of a particular therapy or intervention is often in proportion to the cognitive and emotional investment made. As often as not this conviction does not match changes in the selected outcome measures (Cottam 1985).

DIFFUSION EFFECTS

The outcome of an intervention can sometimes be masked by diffusion effects. If the experimental and control groups are drawn from the same locality, elements of the intervention given to the experimental subject may seep into the care and treatment of the controls. Mothers in parental training schemes, for example, exchange information and ideas, or some idea is picked up from the media and unbeknown to the investigators is incorporated into regular practices. There is also the possibility that controls adopt what has been called 'compensatory rivalry' and find alternative methods of coping (Cook *et al.* 1977).

Methods of outcome assessment

Methods for assessing the outcome of an intervention can be divided roughly into two kinds, the rigorous and the approximate or informal. Of the two, rigorous methods are always preferable but not always possible. The most satisfactory approach is to design an experiment which enables any difference in the outcome measure to be attributed specifically to the effect of the treatment. In essence, an experiment entails manipulating one variable (the independent variable) and measuring the effects of this on a dependent variable (the outcome measure) while controlling for other factors. It is often difficult or impossible to keep all the relevant variables constant while manipulating the treatment, and so careful designs are needed.

RIGOROUS METHODS

• *Randomized designs.* The most satisfactory design is the randomized experiment which requires that experimental (treatment) and control (no treatment) groups be formed from a common population. This is achieved by randomly allocating individuals to experimental or control sets. Random here does not mean haphazard, but rather that an individual has an equal *chance* of being assigned to the experimental or control group. Experimental and control groups constructed in this way should differ from one another by chance only. Following the random assignment, treatment is given only to the experimental group. It is essential to ensure that only the specific treatment variable is different in the group's experience. If this is done, any differences in the outcome measure between the control and experimental groups can be attributed to the intervention. The randomized allocation of individuals to control or experimental groups is a very powerful method which is extensively used in drug trials. Despite its power in enabling valid conclusions to be drawn, there are many circumstances where, because of practical or ethical difficulties, the randomized design is not really feasible. Dunst and Rheingrover (1981) reviewed 49 educational intervention studies and found only one that used random assignment.

• *Matched controls.* When a randomized design cannot be used, it is necessary to construct experimental and control groups in other ways. Devising a constructed control group is by no means an easy task, and it is dependent upon prior knowledge and theoretical understanding. Essentially, constructing a control group entails matching it on important variables to the experimental group which will receive the treatment. But what are the relevant variables and to what extent is matching possible? Often matching is only attempted on a few variables, *e.g.* age, sex, social class and IQ, which have effects on many measures. In some cases, individual, *i.e.* subject to subject, matching is undertaken in order to provide a partner for each member of the experimental group. This is rarely possible with children who have multiple impairments. In other cases, aggregate matching is employed. In this case the overall distribution of variables considered important is matched between groups. Individual matching is usually considered to be more satisfactory, but it is invariably more expensive in money and time. The greatest limitations with this method, however, are (i) deciding on the important variables on which the groups must be matched, and (ii) the practical limitations of attempts at matching when more than one or two variables are involved. Studies which involve matching control and experimental groups are called quasi-experiments.

• *Reflexive controls.* Another method of obtaining control observations is to use subjects in the intervention as their own controls: these are known as reflexive controls. This can be a powerful method when substantial longitudinal data are available. In essence, the approach entails obtaining measurements on the outcome variable before any intervention takes place—the baseline condition—and again following the intervention. It is, of course, essential to ensure that the only important difference with respect to the conditions in which outcome measures were made is the presence of the intervention or treatment itself. Threats to the validity of this method are the existence of order effects, difficulties associated with withdrawing or withholding treatment once given in certain circumstances, and secular effects, especially if treatment needs to be prolonged.

A problem associated with group designs is that they do not take account of inter-subject variability, and consequently treatment effects may be masked. Group comparisons provide an estimate of the overall value and applicability of the intervention. More detailed examination of within-group effects may reveal other differences: the programme may produce significant effects for some but not for others. In the case of more complex interventions, some of the recipients may benefit from one aspect but not others. Sandow *et al.* (1981) found such differences in their evaluation of a home intervention programme for learning impaired children. For the less impaired children gains were found on measures of social and intellectual function, whereas in the case of the more profoundly impaired children, success was measured in terms of the personal support and access to information that the intervention afforded to the families.

Irrespective of the design used, there are other important considerations. Unless steps are specifically taken to avoid it there is always a risk of experimenter bias. The investigators' expectations concerning outcome may influence the results even if they are not consciously aware of these influences. This potential source of bias can be controlled by ensuring that the person collecting the data is not aware of which individuals are from the control group and which from the experimental. The procedure is commonly referred to as conducting a *blind* experiment. This method of eliminating bias can be improved still further if it is possible to prevent the subject from knowing whether s/he has received the control or experimental treatment. When neither the subject nor the person making the outcome measures knows which is control and which experimental, the experiment is said to be *double blind*.

Another general factor that is independent of the experimental design employed is the need for replication. The results of an experiment always have to be checked. Failure to replicate previous findings does not prove that the initial results were wrong, but repeated failure to replicate certainly leads one to look for some alternative explanation such as the influence of a contaminating variable. If the successful outcome of an intervention cannot be replicated its value is questionable and under such circumstances its use as a form of treatment in general, as distinct from experimental use, is not justified.

APPROXIMATE METHODS

Approximate methods for assessing the outcome of an intervention are not a substitute for rigorous methods but they can be a useful first attempt (see Chapter 15). The central purpose of evaluation is to obtain accurate information on the nature and magnitude of any changes which are a consequence of the specified intervention. Approximate or informal methods depend on the judgements of individuals and are inevitably subjective, though the use of experts who are themselves independent of the intervention will limit this to some extent. However, the degree of expertise is inevitably variable. From medical, educational or administrative records it may be possible to make a preliminary assessment of the outcome of some interventions.

Costs and benefits

These notes have been concerned primarily with the technical side of evaluation, that is with deciding whether a particular intervention, correctly carried out on an appropriate population, produces the specified effect. If interventions have been operationalized, the evaluation itself carefully designed, and assuming that rigorous methods have been used, there should be evidence concerning possible causal connections between the treatment and the outcome. The size of any effect may be great or small but the magnitude of the effect itself will not be the only factor which determines its significance. Anyone offering a therapy or an intervention of some kind would like the outcome to be large and wholly positive. However, in many cases small effects in the desired direction are very important, and sometimes an intervention which produces large positive effects may be abandoned because along with the positive effects are unacceptable negative consequences.

Any intervention, irrespective of the form it takes and whether it is medical, educational, behavioural, social or administrative, entails some cost. As part of deciding the value and efficacy of an intervention programme some account must be taken of the costs entailed and the benefits that accrue; do the benefits outweigh the costs, or does the balance fall the other way? This is an extremely difficult judgement to make in many cases. How much is an intervention worth if it substantially improves the quality of life of an individual, and who will decide whether that is so? How much pain and distress can be tolerated in order to prolong a life for ten years? How are we to decide such a question and who will make the decision? Costs and benefits are like chalk and cheese, weighing and evaluating them entails assessing qualitative opposites. We have no satisfactory calculus for this but somehow it must be done.

There are potentially many costs and many benefits associated with an intervention, and each case must necessarily be considered on its merits. It is possible to identify some classes of cost and these should be examined in connection with an intervention. Not all will be relevant but some will, and the possibility of other kinds of cost should also be borne in mind. Examples of classes of cost are as follows.

• *Financial costs.* What expenditure is involved in mounting the intervention? For example, the economic value of costs and benefits to the state was estimated for the Perry Pre-school Project. The costs of implementing the programme were examined along with the estimated savings achieved by a reduction in special education needs, delinquency, etc. The conclusion suggests that the programme was a sound financial investment (Barnett 1985).

• *Time.* How much time is required to carry out the intervention? Given the amount of time demanded, what activities/alternatives must be given up by children, parents and professionals? A physical therapy programme which demanded five hours per day from a child would leave little time or energy for anything else.

• *Equipment and material.* What equipment and materials are needed, are they available, and what are the financial implications? What must be given up to obtain them?

• *Professional expertise.* What does the intervention demand in terms of expert professional support to run it? Is that expertise available, and if it is deployed in one way, what alternatives have to be sacrificed? In the Milwaukee Project (Garber 1987) a number of disadvantaged infants were given home care for 18 months followed by an intensive centre-based programme. Their mothers were also given training in child care and job skills. When tested at 5 and 10 years the children who had received this very expensive treatment (high ratio of professionals to each child/mother) showed above average intelligence but they displayed just as many behavioural problems as the untreated controls.

• *Alternatives.* Often, taking up a particular intervention entails not following others. Interventions are often mutually incompatible, so choosing one implicitly means rejecting others.

• *Pain and quality of life.* Particular treatments designed to produce specific outcomes may carry with them negative consequences; pain, distress, severe limitation on activities, or a reduction in quality of life for the individual involved.

58

• *Family consequences.* Treatments and interventions for individual children often have consequences for members of their families. For example, electing for a particular form of treatment for a disabled child may well have consequences on siblings, or create added stress for the parents (Blacher 1984).

• *Side-effects.* It is always necessary to look carefully for any unexpected negative side-effects of a treatment. Indeed, one has to be alert to possible negative outcomes over quite an extended period. Karnes *et al.* (1970) found the results of an intervention involving mothers surprisingly disappointing and attributed this to the mothers perceiving visiting teachers as having responsibility for training their children, which led to their own interactions being inhibited. In another example, Sandler *et al.* (1983) found that fathers became less confident in dealing with their developmentallly delayed preschool child as mothers became more confident.

Alongside the list of potential costs, another of benefits can be identified. Potential benefits from an intervention programme may include the following.

• *Direct benefits.* These are the benefits for which the treatment is specifically designed and which the outcome measure is designed to assess, for example, any improvement in skill level following a speech therapy programme.

• *Unexpected benefits*, involving improvements in the performance of other skills. This implies the use of other outcome measures to decide that such change has taken place (see Consortium for Longitudinal Studies 1983).

• *Secondary benefits.* These are outcomes which are an indirect consequence of the intervention. For example, improvements in the level of performance of a particular skill may lead to improved self-esteem which in turn can foster cognitive competence. Fraiberg's (1977) intervention programme to establish sound/touch relationships in blind infants resulted in self-initiated mobility and earlier onset of walking.

• *Satisfaction to parents/family members.* Simply doing something designed to improve the conditions of a child can bring comfort and confidence to parents. The direct effect of many intervention programmes for learning disabled children is not evident in long-term developmental gains. The immediate impact is often more evident on mediator variables such as parental attitudes, caring skills, access to community support and so forth (Marfo and Kysela 1985).

• *Professional morale.* Professionals need to be committed to the therapy or the intervention they are providing. One of the potential benefits of an intervention, especially when linked to positive outcomes, is that it helps to sustain the belief that professionals have in their skills and in their capacity to effect desirable change. This at least will help them to maintain their efforts and give a high level of commitment.

TABLE 4.1
Basic questions associated with evaluation

	Monitoring implementation	*Measuring outcome*	*Assessing costs and benefits*
Purpose	To ensure that the implementation is as specified by the programme design	To examine effectiveness in attaining specified goals	To determine costs of programme on various resources and relate to benefits
Questions	Is the intervention being delivered to those for whom it was devised?	Does the intervention produce intended changes?	What are the costs? (staff, time, equipment, on family, etc.)
	Is the intervention being delivered in the specified way?	Are the changes significant or only trivial?	How do the total costs and benefits compare?

• *Social visibility.* The existence of an intervention programme, especially if there are attendant successes, will draw the attention of society to the issues involved in a positive light.

These examples of potential costs and benefits, and others, have to be integrated into a decision on the overall outcome—was the intervention beneficial or was it not? In essence, the professional must be satisfied that the balance of costs and benefits is such that it is worth continuing with the intervention programme. This is a difficult decision because the practitioner is almost invariably committed to a belief in the value of the intervention. We should expect this; someone who is not committed to the intervention will probably not be its best exponent, but here also lies danger. Without a belief in the value of the intervention it is likely to be half-hearted, but it must be counterbalanced by a determination to carry out a systematic evaluation and to *specifically* assess costs and benefits.

There is no simple formula that can be applied. The weighing of costs and benefits demands expert knowledge, experience and, above all, the criticism of experienced experts who are themselves independent of the specific intervention scheme. Costs and benefits analysis is usually done in monetary terms which makes integrating them easier, but there are many important factors which it is difficult to convert into cash values and we must be careful to ensure that these are not ignored.

Concluding comments

What we have sought to do in these notes is to sketch out the basic features of evaluation and consider their relationship to one another. The purposes and main questions associated with the basic components are summarized in Table 4.1. The rules we have outlined are in some senses idealized because different problems are associated with different interventions, but the requirements for all are broadly similar. Frequently, the most difficult aspect is specifying the programme itself with the necessary degree of precision. The process, from the initial theory to the implementation of an intervention, is shown in Figure 4.3.

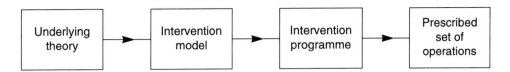

Fig. 4.3. Link between underlying theory and operations which constitute an intervention.

The underlying theory is the basis from which any treatment is derived, but the intervention itself must be expressed as a set of operations, *exactly* what the doctor, teacher or therapist has to do in delivering the programme. Correct and adequate delivery of the intervention is, of course, essential. However, it is almost inevitable that difficulties arise and from time to time compromises may have to be made. When changes are introduced, even minor adaptations to local conditions, they should be fully described and recorded because they may have important consequences for the outcome of the intervention.

Some intervention programmes are carefully designed, well resourced and undertaken within a well established organizational infrastructure. Others are less clearly specified, must be developed with limited resources and have to cope with many diverse problems in generally difficult circumstances. A good rule of thumb is to avoid, where possible, all-embracing schemes and stick to more limited and clearly specified interventions. Clarity and objectivity are the watchwords, and much excellent work can be done with limited resources.

REFERENCES

Bairstow, P., Cochrane, R., Hur, I. (1993) *Evaluation of Conductive Education for Children with Cerebral Palsy: Final Report.* London: HMSO.

Barnett, W.S. (1985) 'Benefit–cost analysis of the Perry Preschool Program and its policy implications.' *Educational Evaluation and Policy Analysis,* **7,** 333–342.

Blacher, J. (Ed.) (1984) *Severely Handicapped Young Children and their Families: Research in Review.* New York: Academic Press.

Bricker, D., Veltman, Y. (1990) 'Early intervention programs: child focused approaches.' *In:* Meisels, S.J., Shonkoff, J.P. (Eds.) *Handbook of Early Childhood Intervention.* Cambridge: Cambridge University Press, pp. 373–399.

Bronfenbrenner, U. (1974) *A Report of Longitudinal Evaluations of Preschool Programs. Vol II. Is Early Intervention Effective?* Washington: Department of Health, Education and Welfare. (Pubn. no. (OMD) 74–25.)

Connolly, K.J. (1973) 'Ethological techniques and the direct observation of behaviour.' *In:* Mittler, P. (Ed.) *Assessment for Learning in the Mentally Handicapped.* London: Churchill Livingstone, pp. 25–33.

—— Smith, P.K. (1972) 'Reactions of preschool children to a strange observer.' *In:* Blurton Jones, N. (Ed.) *Ethological Studies of Child Behaviour.* Cambridge: Cambridge University Press, pp. 157–172.

Consortium for Longitudinal Studies (1983) *As the Twig is Bent.* Hillsdale, NJ: Lawrence Erlbaum.

Cook, T.D., Cook, F.L., Mark, M.M. (1977) Randomized and quasi-experimental designs in evaluation research: an introduction.' *In:* Rutman, L. (Ed.) *Evaluation in Research Methods: a Basic Guide.* Beverly Hills: Sage, pp. 103–139.

Cottam, P. (1985) 'The effectiveness of conductive education principles with profoundly handicapped children.' *British Journal of Communication Disorders,* **20,** 45–60.

Dunst, C.J., Rheingrover, R. (1981) 'An analysis of the efficacy of infant intervention programs with organically handicapped children.' *Evaluation and Program Planning,* **4,** 287–323.

Fraiberg, S. (1977) *Insights from the Blind.* London: Souvenir Press; New York: Basic Books.

Garber, H. (1987) *The Milwaukee Project: Preventing Retardation in Children at Risk.* Washington, DC: American Association of Mental Retardation.

Ghiselli, E.E., Campbell, J.P., Zedeck, S. (1981) *Measurement Theory for the Behavioral Sciences.* San Francisco: Freeman.

Guralnick, M. (1986) *Mainstreaming Handicapped Children: Outcomes, Controversies and New Directions.* Hillsdale, NJ: Lawrence Erlbaum.

Homans, G.C. (1965) 'Group factors in worker productivity.' *In:* Proshansky, H., Seidenberg, L. (Eds.) *Basic Studies in Social Psychology.* New York: Holt, pp. 592–604.

Karnes, M.B., Teska, J.A., Hodgins, A.S., Badger, E.D. (1970) 'Educational intervention at home by mothers of disadvantaged infants.' *Child Development,* **41,** 925–935.

Lazar, I., Darlington, R. (1982) *Lasting Effects of Early Education: a Report from the Consortium for Longitudinal Studies. Monographs of the Society for Research in Child Development. Serial No. 195, Vol. 47, Nos. 2–3.*

Marfo, K., Kysela, G.M. (1985) 'Early intervention with mentally handicapped children: a critical appraisal of applied research.' *Journal of Pediatric Psychology,* **10,** 305–324.

Martin, P., Bateson, P. (1986) *Measuring Behaviour.* Cambridge: Cambridge University Press.

McConachie, H. (1986) *Parents and Young Mentally Handicapped Children: a Review of Research Issues.* London: Croom Helm.

Meisel, C. (1986) *Mainstreaming Handicapped Children: Outcomes, Controversies and New Directions.* Hillsdale, NJ: Lawrence Erlbaum.

Meisels, S.J., Shonkoff, J.P. (Eds.) (1990) *Handbook of Early Childhood Intervention.* Cambridge: Cambridge University Press.

Roche, A.F. (1979) *Secular Trends in Human Growth, Maturation, and Development. Monographs of the Society for Research in Child Development. Serial No. 179, Vol. 44, Nos. 3–4.*

Sandler, A., Coren, A., Thurman, S.K. (1983) 'A training program for parents of handicapped preschool children: effects upon mother, father and child.' *Exceptional Children,* **49,** 355–358.

Sandow, S.A., Clark, A.D., Cox, M.V., Stewart, F.L. (1981) 'Home intervention with parents of severely subnormal pre-school children: a. final report.' *Child: Care, Health and Development,* **7,** 135–144.

Schweinhart, L.J., Weikart, D.P. (1983) 'The effects of the Perry Preschool Program on youths through age 15—a summary.' *In:* Consortium for Longitudinal Studies. *As the Twig is Bent.* Hillsdale, NJ: Lawrence Erlbaum, pp. 71–101.

Seitz, V., Rosenbaum, L.K., Apfel, N.H. (1985) 'Effects of family support intervention: a ten-year follow-up.' *Child Development,* **56,** 376–391.

Simeonsson, R.J., Huntington, G.S., Parse, A. (1980) 'Assessment of children with severe handicaps: multiple problems—multivariate goals.' *Journal of the Association for the Severely Handicapped,* **5,** 55–72.

Swann, W. (1985) 'Is the integration of children with special needs happening: an analysis of recent statistics of pupils in special schools.' *Oxford Review of Education,* **11,** 3–18.

Tobias, P.V. (1975) 'Anthropometry among disadvantaged people.' *In:* Watts, E.S., Johnstone, F., Laske, G. (Eds.) *Biosocial Interventions in Population Adaptation.* The Hague: Mouton, pp. 00–00.

Turnbull, A.P., Winton, P.J. (1984) 'Parent involvement policy and practice: current research and future prospectives.' *In:* Blacher, J. (Ed.) *Severely Handicapped Young Children and their Families: Research in Review.* New York: Academic Press, pp. 377–395.

Warr, P.B. (1980) 'The springs of action.' *In:* Chapman, A.J., Jones, D.M. (Eds.) *Models of Man.* Leicester: British Psychological Society, pp. 289–310.

Zigler, E., Berman, W. (1983) 'Discerning the future of early childhood intervention.' *American Psychologist,* **38,** 894–906.

5
EARLY INTERVENTION IN DEVELOPING COUNTRIES

Roy McConkey

Politics, it is said, is the art of the possible. In September 1990, the largest gathering of world leaders in history assembled at the United Nations to attend the World Summit for Children. They strongly endorsed the Convention on the Rights of the Child, which states in Article 23: 'a mentally or physically disabled child should enjoy a full and decent life, in conditions which ensure dignity, promote self-reliance and facilitate the child's active participation in the community.'

Their resulting Plan of Action was hailed by James Grant, Executive Director of Unicef, as 'an ambitious but feasible agenda for the well-being of children to be achieved by the year 2000.' In particular, it was noted that the necessary knowledge and techniques for reaching most of the goals already exist: 'the provision to families of information and services necessary to protect their children is now within reach in every country and for virtually every community' (Unicef 1990).

For example, 18 years ago Head Start programmes were introduced in the USA with the aim of boosting the developmental progress of preschool children born into socially dis-advantaged homes. The initial optimism soon gave way to controversy but recent empirical research has demonstrated that 'early intervention is a cost-effective method of combating the effects of poverty experienced early in life . . . and it is now viewed as being of value for other high-risk groups, including developmentally disabled children' (Zigler 1990).

This chapter reviews present knowledge about early intervention and the experience of implementing services in developing countries for families with children who are disabled. It draws on the experiences both of projects in industrialized countries (Meisels and Shonkoff 1990, Mitchell and Brown 1990) and of those which have been launched in developing countries (Thorburn and Marfo 1990). Although the future holds promise, a great deal remains to be done before we can be confident that families throughout the world will obtain their share of the knowledge and skills which can prevent a disability from becoming a handicap.

Promoting successful interventions
The aims of early intervention programmes have been summarized by Meisels and Shonkoff (1990) as: 'to enhance child development, minimize potential delays, remediate existing problems, prevent further deterioration, limit the acquisition of additional handicapping conditions and/or promote adaptive family functioning.' However, these goals are easier to state than to realize and have proved deceptively difficult both to attain and to sustain.

Many lessons have been learnt along the way, chief of which is that more therapists or teachers, treating children in specialist centres, is *not* the solution. Instead, interventions are more likely to prove successful when the following conditions are met (McConkey 1994):

• *The focus has to be on the whole child and not just one aspect of her/his development.* Zigler (1990) put it thus: 'the aim of . . . intervention efforts must be to affect positively all aspects of the child's development: social, emotional and physical as well as intellectual . . . all of these aspects are inter-related, one does not function independently of the other.' Particular attention must be paid to the health and nutritional needs of children (Myers 1990).

• *The involvement of the child's family is critical to the success of the intervention.* Bronfenbrenner's (1979) logic is irrefutable: 'the family is the most effective and economical system for fostering and sustaining the development of the child. . . The involvement of parents as partners in the enterprise provides an on-going system which can reinforce the effects of the program while it is in operation and help to sustain them after the program ends.'

• *There will never be a single intervention strategy that will solve all developmental problems.* Despite the claims of their instigators, there is no convincing research evidence that any programmes were more successful than others (Farran 1990). The consequence, as Sameroff and Fiese (1990) suggest, is that 'Cost-effectiveness will not be found in the universality of a treatment but in the individuation of programs that are targeted . . . for a specific child, in a specific family and in a specific social context.'

• *Poverty and the family's social context often render ineffective simple attempts at early intervention.* To quote Zigler (1990) again, 'No amount of counselling, early childhood curricula, or home visits will take the place of jobs that provide decent incomes, affordable housing, appropriate health care, optimal family configurations, or integrated neighbourhoods where children encounter positive role models.'

• *Intervention services must be ongoing throughout childhood.* Children with disabilities cannot be 'inoculated' from handicaps by providing them with an intervention boost during the preschool years. Rather, ongoing support, adapted to their changing needs, is required. In particular, ongoing support of pupils and their teachers is needed in order to maintain placements in ordinary schools (see Chapter 9).

These insights have prompted a redefinition of early intervention services; for example: 'the provision of support to families of infants and young children from members of informal and formal social support networks that impact both directly and indirectly upon parent, family and child functioning' (Dunst 1985). The image has shifted from paid professionals treating preschool children to a network of people—paid and unpaid—helping the parents and child in the family home or neighbourhood. Happily, the latter picture can be realized in developing countries as in the more affluent West, although in both situations support may be found more readily in certain locations, such as rural towns, than in inner-city slums.

Service aims

This 'support' model of early intervention requires a range of responses from service

64

providers. Thorburn (1990) has proposed that the core aims of early intervention services should be:

- the provision of simplified and appropriate technologies at the community level to reduce the disabling effects of impairments. This includes educational and therapeutic advice as well as the provision of aids;
- the training of all levels of people involved—family members, primary level workers, community leaders, etc.;
- the formation of parent groups to provide mutual support and solidarity at a local level but allied to national organizations to advocate for their children's needs;
- the involvement of local people in promoting the participation of people with disabilities in the life of the community;
- the development of public policies and plans to meet the needs of children and their families.

Other tasks could include:

- the primary prevention of disabilities through public health programmes;
- the setting up of playgroups or centres so that families can have a break from caring at least for some of the day;
- supporting pupils with disabilities and their teachers in mainstream nursery and primary schools;
- developing literacy schemes and income-generating projects for families to help alleviate some of their poverty.

Achieving these diverse aims is not easy, even in well-resourced services with years of experience. Among the dilemmas faced by planners of new services with limited resources at their disposal are:

- *Where do you begin?* Do you focus on the child, devising programmes to alleviate her/his disabilities; or do you try to mobilize the families and community to help themselves?
- *How many families do you try to help?* Is it better to bring about even small improvements among a large group than to provide high standards of care for a privileged few?
- *Do you set up a special service?* Should early intervention services be provided solely to families with a child who has an identifiable disability or should they form part of the services which are available to all families in the community?
- *Where should the service be based?* Do you take the service to the family home or base it in a centre, clinic or hospital? As we shall see later, each has its advantages and disadvantages.

To date, we have no objective evidence to prove that any one approach is better than another. Hence the decisions on key issues are based sometimes on the beliefs of the service planners but more often on the policies of the funding agencies, either nationally or internationally. Thus services often begin with what planners can get funding to do, rather than what best suits the needs and wishes of that particular community. This is tolerable provided that the service develops to embrace the range of functions required by the community it serves. As we shall see, that means assessing needs and evaluating the effectiveness of service responses to those needs.

TABLE 5.1
Checklist for home-based early intervention projects

- Strong motivation by people from the local community to start and maintain a project
- Clear statement of service aims and philosophy
- A defined set of clients in a defined geographical area. If none have been identified, a community search will be needed. This can take various forms, from 'door-to-door' surveys to asking health workers and local women's groups
- A planning or management committee, preferably multidisciplinary and well acquainted with existing services
- A project coordinator, preferably a trained and experienced human service professional (from health, education, social work, psychology, etc.) who has dedication, competence and problem solving skills. S/he must be able to coordinate, organize, supervise and advise
- Field workers who are motivated, stable, patient, empathetic, willing to walk! These could be health workers, volunteers, parents, teachers. The number needed will depend on the number of clients—a ratio of 1:15 if the workers are full-time, fewer if part-time
- Methods and tools to be used for identification, assessment, programme planning, teaching and evaluation
- An office to keep records, see clients, have staff meetings. It must be accessible to clients and their families
- A budget for staff stipends, travel and other expenses
- Training for supervisory and field staff
- Community awareness—public relations, public education and involvement of local organizations and leaders
- A register of clients and record systems
- A back-up referral system to refer clients to and from the project for further advice, placement and treatment
- Resource materials—books, test forms, toys, aids, stationery, filing cabinets, training packages, etc.

Adapted by permission from Thorburn (1990).

More problematic are situations where funding policies continue to conflict with the aspirations of service planners and the communities they serve. For example, monies may be available for centre-based services but not for home-visiting services. Possible responses could include searching for alternative sources of funding; engaging in political lobbying to persuade the funders to change their attitude; or finding areas of common ground and focusing efforts on these in future service plans. At present we have neither the accumulated wisdom of experience to guide people on the best strategies to adopt in such situations, nor, worse still, mechanisms for sharing this information across, and often within, countries.

In the coming years hopefully both of these shortcomings will be addressed. Meantime, most service planning and development continues to be based on the judgement of people 'on the ground'. A number of safeguards can be suggested to them:

- *Consult*—find out what families and community need and want as well as seeking out the opinion of professional workers.
- *Clear statement of service aims*—this will make it easy to communicate your intentions to others and serve as a yardstick against which you can measure your effectiveness.
- *Clear statement of beliefs or philosophy on which the service aims are based*—although not easy to do, this is essential in helping others to understand your priorities and approaches.

Developing services
Knowing what needs to be done is but a beginning; making it a reality is another story.

Table 5.1 lists 14 requisites for the establishment and running of early intervention projects, based primarily on experiences in the Caribbean (Thorburn 1990). In this chapter I examine these in more detail, drawing on the experiences of services in various developing countries. The aim is to describe effective and efficient methods which have been used to help children and families in the early years. Of course there are many unresolved issues, and fresh challenges loom. These are noted and possible courses of action are proposed. I shall focus on the following four key issues: (i) nurturing the child's development; (ii) parental beliefs and motivation; (iii) family support; (iv) personnel—selection, training and deployment.

Nurturing children's development
A fundamental premise of all early intervention work is that the disabling effects of impairments can be reduced, thereby enabling children to lead fuller lives. Experiences throughout the world have shown that this can happen.

Nutrition and infection
Health promotion must feature in all early intervention services. Project workers should keep records of the child's weight and immunizations. The family's diet should be reviewed, and primary health personnel could be asked to provide special classes and demonstrations. Specially designed recording scales, child health charts (in six languages), and 'flannel-graphs' (visual aids about nutrition) for use in group teaching are available through TALC (Teaching Aids at Low Cost, P.O. Box 49, St Albans, Herts., AL1 4AX, United Kingdom).

Sensory and physical disabilities
All children should be screened for sensory disabilities—especially hearing loss and visual difficulties—whether or not they have other obvious disabilities (see Chapter 7). Onward referrals should be made for more detailed assessments, for the possible prescription of hearing aids or glasses, and forsurgical interventions. The aim is to minimize the impairment so that adverse effects on a child's development can be reduced. The sooner this happens in the child's life, the better.

Further advice should be sought for children with marked deformities of the limbs, from a physiotherapist or orthopaedic specialist. Amputees may benefit from the fitting of artificial limbs.

Medication can be prescribed to help control fits. Ideally a doctor with specialist knowledge should be consulted. The dosage should be reviewed regularly, especially if there are untoward side-effects such as excessive drowsiness.

Hence, intervention services need to build up a network of supports to whom families can be referred. Issues to do with meeting the cost of aids also need to be tackled. Field workers should accompany the family to appointments whenever possible.

Therapeutic aids
Children who have difficulty in sitting or walking can benefit from a therapeutic aid.

Special chairs or supports will enable children to use their hands for playing with objects or to feed themselves. Likewise, walking frames may enable a child to explore and join in social play. Low-cost aids can be simply and cheaply made from wood or paper technology as described in various publications such as Werner's *Disabled Village Children* (see Table 5.3, p. 79) or those available through TALC (see above). Other aids include those to help with self-feeding (Caston 1985) or simple playthings and toys (Carlile 1988).

It is essential that the family is instructed in the most effective use of any aid which is made for the child and how best to train the child in its use.

Early intervention personnel can be trained in the making of simple aids for their clients. Services have also organized workshops for families and people from the community on producing simple aids. In the Negros region of the Philippines the production of aids is undertaken by adult persons with disabilities as part of their income generation.

Developmental goals

Most children with disabilities can learn to walk, to communicate and to care for their personal needs. However this will be all the harder if the child is left unstimulated. Various publications are available (see Table 5.3) that give ideas for activities which can be used to stimulate a child's development from birth onwards. These guides have a number of features in common:

• Development is split into different areas: gross motor function; fine motor function (use of hands); socialization; communication and language; cognition; self-care; and household tasks. Thus attention is drawn to all aspects of a child's development; key skills are identified and nurtured.

• Within each area, skills are arranged in a progressive sequence from easy to hard. In this way, children can experience success albeit in small steps at a time.

• Activities and teaching techniques are suggested to help children master the skills. Often these include common play activities which families already use, or ones which could be simplified to meet a child's special needs. Wherever possible, play equipment should be made from local materials rather than relying on purchased toys.

• Specific learning targets, appropriate to the child's developmental level and needs, are selected as a focus of teaching over a period of time, *e.g.* two weeks or one month. These targets are updated as the child acquires new competencies.

Although this approach has been very popular in early intervention services for a decade and more, there is surprisingly little objective evidence that it produces significant developmental gains as measured by standard tests (Farran 1990). Gallagher (1992) concluded that: 'the real advantage of . . . intervention programs may, in fact, lie in a new spirit of optimism and encouragement within the family of the affected child.'

Of course this is no mean achievement; families need convincing that their child with disabilities can learn. Key elements are seeing signs of progress and adjusting their expectations to their child's present competencies. Developmental guides can prove valuable in doing this.

Henley and Lansdown (1988) note that 'the well documented progressive decline in cognitive ability with increasing age in Down's Syndrome children can be significantly reduced, or entirely prevented, during the period in which early intervention services are provided.' However, they also conclude from their review of early intervention studies that 'the type of curriculum employed is unrelated to program effectiveness' and that 'there is little evidence to support the view that the earlier intervention is begun, the greater the benefits.'

SERVICE IMPLICATIONS
A developmental curriculum needs to be drawn up to provide a guide to field workers and families (see Table 5.2, p. 78). Particular emphasis needs to be placed on giving workers an understanding of developmental sequences so that they can more accurately match learning targets to a child's present level of competence. Equally, field workers need to be competent in basic teaching techniques such as task analysis, modelling, use of prompting and rewards (McConkey *et al.* 1990, O'Brien and Farrell 1992).

Naturally occurring interactions
Several common shortcomings have been noted of early intervention curricula packages, namely a lack of impact on children's language development, on peer relations and on symbolic thinking. In these areas, children's development is fuelled and channelled by the interactions they experience in their daily lives (Tizard and Hughes 1984).

The active participation of children with disabilities in household routines or ordinary play activities could also be used to stimulate their development. This focus for intervention activities is now attracting greater interest in Western services (McConkey and Price 1986, Harris 1990), and it may be even more appropriate in developing countries. It has several advantages:
• Parents and other family members are already familiar with the activities, thereby reducing the need for training and the feelings of inadequacy which 'professional exercises' often present to families. Families can more easily 'own' and control the interventions, making it more likely that they will continue to use and adapt them (Baker 1989).
• Existing family routines are reinforced or extended, rather than expecting families to adapt to new procedures which may be impractical given home circumstances and responsibilities (McConachie 1986).
• As the activities are drawn from the local culture, the ecological validity of the intervention is assured and the cultural identity of the children may even be strengthened (Ivic 1986).
• For the child with a marked disability, basing interventions around common activities could offer a better opportunity for successfully integrating her/him into the family and the life of the local community.

SERVICE IMPLICATIONS
Field workers when visiting the family home should enquire about and observe the child's play routines with siblings, parents and others. This will enable them to identify examples of good practice and boost the family's confidence. Likewise, family routines need to be examined with a view to involving the child with disabilities in them. Different family members can be identified for certain activities. Field workers must demonstrate how the

activity can be adapted to ensure the child's active participation. The video packages listed in Table 5.4 (p. 79) contain examples.

Monitoring progress

Records need to be kept of the children's progress. This helps to document the service achievements, encourages families who may feel there is little progress, and helps to identify effective interventions as well as areas where new approaches are needed. Among the most commonly used methods are:

- regular diary accounts kept by field workers or coordinators as they visit the family;
- rating scales or questionnaires completed by the family and/or field workers regarding the changes observed over a particular time period, *e.g.* the past six months;
- checklists of skills and attainments which are completed at periodic intervals, say every six months.

The methods chosen should be easy to maintain and amenable to cross-checking by another person, *e.g.* a coordinator. It helps too if the information is in a common format so that it can be easily collated across all the clients.

Evaluations undertaken by external assessors are a favoured way of obtaining less biased accounts of a project's effectiveness. Although still small in number, several evaluations have been published in recent years of home-based projects with encouraging results for the majority of children. For example, two thirds of the children in a Zimbabwean project were deemed to have made either 'good', 'very good' or 'outstanding' progress (Madzima *et al.* 1985). In Mexico and the Philippines, 46 per cent and 53 per cent respectively were rated to have improved 'markedly' or 'modestly' (for fuller details, see O'Toole 1991).

However, the success of a project cannot be measured simply in terms of developmental gains. Changes in parental beliefs, attitudes and interactions with the child can be equally important. An ongoing issue is the appropriateness of measures devised in Western cultures to document changes in children and families from other cultures.

SERVICE IMPLICATIONS

Record systems have to be tailored to the project's aims and resources and should be reviewed as time goes by. It is better to keep simpler records consistently than to strive to maintain overly detailed systems and fail.

Parental beliefs and motivation

'The needs of infants enrolled in intervention programmes can only be fully appreciated and understood within a family context.' This assertion by Shonkoff and Meisels (1990) summarizes current thinking about the crucial influences which all families exert on a child's development.

This section reviews beliefs about the causes of disability and possible cultural influences on child-rearing practices and interactions between parents and children. It explores too the other demands placed on women especially in developing countries and how these can be reconciled with an involvement in intervention programmes.

Cultural perceptions about disability

There appears to be a widespread belief across cultures ancient and modern that the birth of a disabled child is linked to evil spirits and/or parental misconduct (Scheer and Groce 1988). Other cultures may view disabled people as a curse resulting from a sin committed by an ancestor or by the affected person in a previous existence. Such explanations often result in parental feelings of shame or guilt with consequences such as hiding the affected child from neighbours or, in extreme cases, infanticide. Families may seek assistance from traditional healers rather than modern services.

In other families, there may be a fatalistic acceptance of the disability with notions that they have been given a special responsibility. This can result in low expectations of the child and an over-emphasis on physical care and protection.

It must be stressed, however, that these are broad generalizations and that variations in beliefs exist both across cultures and among families within a culture. Also, these beliefs are amenable to change.

SERVICE IMPLICATIONS

Parents need opportunities to share their feelings about disabilities. Giving them the chance to meet and talk with other parents has proved valuable in helping them gain new perspectives.

Families need to be given factual information about the causes of disabilities and how the child might be helped. Seeing examples of children and adults with disabilities involved in everyday activities or gainfully employed has proved effective (see Chapter 11).

The wider family circle, especially grandparents, can exert an important influence on parents; hence opportunities should be sought to keep them informed as well.

Evaluations of the impact of early intervention programmes might usefully try to monitor changes in family and community perceptions of disability and their attitudes to the place of disabled people within communities. This has been little explored to date but is potentially one of the most significant outcomes (see Chapter 15).

Cultural differences in child-rearing practices

Early intervention approaches may also conflict with traditional child-rearing practices. This can result in families 'opting out' of the service. For example: 'Asian parents tend to be more rigid about discipline than Western parents with communication tending to be one-directional (*i.e.* parent to child). Children are not expected to express feelings, wants, likes and dislikes' (Vincent *et al.* 1990). Intervention programmes, by contrast, may emphasize the need for parents to respond to the child's communications and to give praise for compliance with requests rather than accepting it without comment.

Likewise there appears to be widespread variation in the extent to which mothers rely on the face-to-face position for communication (Rogoff *et al.* 1991). Those who commonly hold infants facing away from them become strained and awkward when asked to interact in a face-to-face orientation; a common requirement in many intervention activities.

Ramey and Ramey (1992) have recently posited six 'essential daily ingredients' for early learning and intellectual development based on the accumulated research which has been carried out in Western countries with disadvantaged families. They conclude that parents need to: (1) encourage exploration by the child; (2) celebrate the child's developmental advances, taking family pride in achievements; (3) avoid inappropriate disapproval, teasing or punishment of the child; (4) provide a rich and responsive language environment; (5) emphasize basic cognitive skills of labelling, sorting, sequencing and noting means–end relationships; and (6) encourage the child to practice and extend new skills.

These parenting styles are arguably more necessary when the criterion of success is the child's educational progress in formal schooling. Other parenting styles could be more suited to other cultures, although little research has been undertaken on this topic. However, parenting behaviours as listed above are likely to be found in all cultures, and research suggests that families can be helped to change their style of interactions.

Parents' expectations of the age at which children might acquire basic skills also seem to vary across cultures, with Asian families expecting self-help attainments to be slower than Western parents do (Pomerleau *et al.* 1991). O'Toole (1990) reported that compared to Western norms, mothers in Guyana expected their children to walk and dress themselves at an earlier age, but to talk and be dry during the day at a later age.

Once again, we are dealing in generalizations, but key workers need to be sensitive to cultural and familial differences in making recommendations about interactive activities and when identifying learning targets.

SERVICE IMPLICATIONS

Field workers need to take time to observe families interacting with the child. This offers them opportunities to discover the particular strategies which parents use and enables them to adapt their advice to the parent's preferred style. It is also useful for families to observe other people interact with their child, as this gives them models to follow. Opportunities to talk to and to observe other parents with their child can encourage parents to try new styles of interaction.

Services must beware of imposing Western norms and standards onto the cultures in which they work. A common safeguard is to identify jointly with families their priorities for developmental targets. Also, using workers from the same cultural background as the families helps build a sense of solidarity and trust, a recommendation that is particularly pertinent in providing services to immigrant communities (Tizard *et al.* 1981).

Family roles

'Overwork, poverty, severe social tensions and sheer exhaustion make parental involvement a difficult proposition in developing countries. In such societies, there may be little surplus energy or compassion to spare' (O'Toole 1991). This is a timely reminder that early intervention schemes are more often constrained by what is possible for families to cope with rather than the possibilities envisaged by service workers.

That said, a number of strategies can be followed. Service workers should try to engage the help of all the potential supporters within the family and neighbourhood rather than demanding more of an already overworked mother or grandmother. Older siblings, cousins, aunts and fathers are possibilities. Finding mutually enjoyable activities is a key requirement. Fathers may be more willing to engage in gross motor activities than help with self-care tasks. Moreover, families may cope better with involving the child in their ongoing activities rather than setting up special 'training' sessions.

The family's wider needs may have to be addressed alongside, or even before those of the child with disabilities. For example, women's cooperatives have been set up as a way of generating income alongside crèches for children with disabilities. Further examples are considered in the following section.

A family may not wish to be involved with the service and this wish has to be respected. Ideally alternatives may be offered to them but if this is not possible, renewed invitations can be made at periodic intervals.

Family reactions
Consultations with families can be formalized through the systematic use of questionnaires. In this way, regular feedback can be obtained about the services provided to families and adaptations made in light of their comments.

From published accounts, families appear very supportive of home-based intervention projects. Thorburn (1992) found that three quarters of the 360 families sampled in Jamaica felt that their child had improved as a result of the programme, and nine out of ten would recommend the programme to other parents. Similarly O'Toole (1988) reported that only three out of 56 Guyanan families refused to become involved with the programme, and four out of five mothers claimed that it had not interfered with other responsibilities at home. In the Gaza strip, all but two families reported no problems with the home teachers and everyone rated the relationship as 'very good' or 'excellent' (Johnson and El-Hato 1990).

Changes were also evident in the mothers from Guyana. Before the project, 88 per cent spoke of being sad, depressed or worried about the child's future, whereas six months later they reported being more relaxed (30 per cent) more proud of the child (15 per cent) happier (20 per cent) and more confident (10 per cent) (O'Toole 1988).

These comments have to be balanced against the improvements which parents seek. In all three studies, the most commonly voiced concerns were the establishment of special units or schools for their children and coping with specific difficulties, such as speech and language problems. Similar findings were reported from Sri Lanka (Nikapota 1986) and Zimbabwe (Mariga and McConkey 1987).

Family support
A recurring theme here has been the importance of families in early intervention initiatives. Yet support to them is crucial if they are be sustained in this role. In particular, mothers need a break from caring. The final part of this chapter considers the role of day centres in supporting families, describes strategies for educating and involving the wider community in supporting families, and explore the prospects of integrating early intervention services into broader programmes of child care and community development.

Centre-based services
Early intervention services are often home-based during the child's first three years of life.

Thereafter the issue of centred-based services arises, usually at the request of families. The debate is then presented as a choice between home and centres when in reality both are needed (Henley and Lansdown 1988). However, the balance between these two styles of service provision may need to shift for each family in order to provide them with the optimal help. Having access to only one or the other will not prove suitable to most families.

Problems arise when there are insufficient resources to maintain both types of services and a choice has to made. Each has its own advantages and disadvantages. According to Myers (1990), the points which favour centre-based services are:

• Opportunities will occur for social interactions among the children which may not be available at home. However, this could be managed locally by arranging for the child with disabilities to attend neighbourhood crèches or nurseries.

• Families can have a much needed respite from caring. However, parents may come to depend overly on the centre and may then do less for themselves.

• Centres provide a visibility that is useful politically, both to get programmes going and to sustain them. Yet the danger is that more money may be spent on buildings and equipment than in providing a service to families. Moreover, the building can easily become a segregated resource used only by people with disabilities.

• Centres can facilitate health care and nutritional monitoring, although grouping children can also spread infections.

• Children can have access to special equipment and teaching methods which may not be available at home. However, this can result in a divorcing of family routines and centre practices, with parents made to feel inadequate.

Centre-based services have a number of known disadvantages:

• If there is no through-put of children, the centre may become overcrowded and the staff overworked, and the quality of help on offer will suffer.

• The start-up costs of a centre are usually greater than those of a home-based service.

• Transporting children to and from the centre can pose major problems.

Equally, the advantages and disadvantages of home-based services mirror many of the above points. For example, transport is needed to enable staff to visit homes; could this money be spent on bringing children from home? If both parents are working, then the child may be left unattended during the day.

Hence the need for service planners to strike the right balance between home- and centre-based services for each community for whom the service is being provided. Fortunately a few guidelines have emerged from recent experiences:

• The involvement of parents in the setting up, management and running of the centre is crucial.

• Links should be established with existing schools, and centres should ensure onward referrals. Siblings and neighbourhood children without disabilities could join in some of the centre activities.

• Renting properties, for example houses or halls, gives greater flexibility than opting for purpose-built centres.

• A network of local centres is preferable to one large centre.

• The centres should serve various purposes, *e.g.* a meeting place for families; storing and lending equipment; providing training courses. The centre could be available to other community groups so that it is seen as a community resource.

Community acceptance and engagement
Many parents feel that the attitudes of their local community are a significant barrier to providing a more ordinary life for their child with a disability. Cultural perceptions can be changed using the same approaches described earlier for families. Three strategies in particular have proved effective in educating communities (McConkey 1991). First, people with disabilities, or their families, advocating for themselves and being seen to be productive members of society. Video illustrations can be especially potent in changing perceptions. Second, engaging community leaders in advocating for people with disabilities. This could include village headmen, priests or local politicians. Third, integrating and supporting children with disabilities in ordinary community activities, such as crèches, churches and schools. These local contacts may need to be initiated by service staff and/or parents but it is through such personal contacts that people gain confidence in coping with the person who has special needs.

One of the most practical ways in which neighbours can support families is by child-minding for certain periods of time. In developed countries various schemes have been established in which local people are paid to provide day or night-time care for children with disabilities so that families can have a break. These have reduced the demand from families for their child to be taken into residential care. As yet there are few reports of similar schemes operating in developing countries where they would have to rely on the goodwill of minders.

Much still has to be learnt about effective ways of engaging communities in mutually supportive activities, presuming that it is possible. As O'Toole (1991) noted, 'the vast number of disabled persons live in scattered and rural isolation and in marginalized urban areas . . . to mobilize previously uninvolved populations with no tradition of community participation and with no mechanism for community involvement is a daunting prospect.'

Integrating community initiatives
Myers (1990) bemoans 'the narrow, piece-meal thinking and actions that so dominate the early childhood development field. . . Opportunities should be sought to blend services, to encourage multisectoral collaboration and to fit new components into ongoing programmes whenever it is opportune.' This indictment and challenge is probably even more real for the affluent North than it is for the poorer South.

Early intervention services have common cause with all early childhood health and educational initiatives. First, because some disabilities become apparent only as the child matures. If such children are to be helped from an early age, it has to come within the context of programmes aimed at children without, as well as those with, disabilities. Second, the methods and techniques developed within early intervention services for children with disabilities stand to benefit all the children within a community. In particular, educational packages aimed at informing parents about ways of nurturing a child's development should be available to all families.

Local organizational issues will determine whether early intervention services should be subsumed within wider programmes or retain autonomy while acting in partnership with others. What should not be debated though is the desirability of such programmes working together.

Given the unquestioned link between disability and poverty, early intervention programmes have common cause also with housing and income-generating projects. These can take many different forms such as the formation of local cooperatives and interest-free loans. Once again, imaginative solutions are needed at local level if sectorial boundaries are to be breached and common causes established (see Chapters 11 and 15).

Early intervention personnel

The people providing the service to families are central to its success. Among the questions often asked are what staffing structures are needed, who will you recruit, what training will be given and how will the work of the staff be supervised?

In developed countries, early intervention services are provided by multidisciplinary teams consisting of doctors, psychologists, social workers, therapists and teachers who may see the child and family at home and/or in special clinics or day centres. Few developing countries have the resources to emulate such staffing models, hence it may be some compensation to know that such teams are increasingly criticized; in particular, for their failure to plan for the needs of the 'whole' child within a family context (see Chapter 3). Instead, each discipline claims responsibility for a discrete aspect of the service, defined by traditional professional boundaries (Meisels and Shonkoff 1990). The result is frequently duplication of effort, confused advice to parents and a failure to meet the priority needs of families.

The solution most frequently suggested for building a more coherent service is especially encouraging for service planners in the developing world, namely the concept of having one 'key worker' or 'case manager' for each family who aims to be 'transdisciplinary' in their work. Instead of working to their specialism, key workers are also trained in the basic skills and techniques used by other professionals—therapists, social workers and teachers. Moreover, the key worker should have an understanding of the community where the families live.

In developing countries the most popular staffing model of community-based early intervention services has consisted of project coordinators with a team of field workers (Helander et al. 1989).

Project coordinators

The project coordinators invariably have training and experience in disability services. They have been drawn from a range of human service professions. Their primary role is to train and monitor the field workers rather than to have direct responsibility for families and children. Their job involves regular travelling and contact with a wide range of community and specialist services.

In sum, this post is radically different in style and content to that of hospital-based therapists, for example. Consequently staff who were trained overseas may not be well equipped for this role. Among the common problems for them are: (i) a reluctance to give up the status associated with working in prestige settings and with defined opportunities for career advancement; (ii) a failure to recognize examples of good practice by families and field workers by having too rigid an idea of correct techniques; (iii) a frustration at having to work without the equipment and resources which are necessary for effective rehabilitation; and (iv) the amount of time and energy needed for the itinerant job of service coordinator in rural areas. Similar personnel problems beset services in developed countries as they attempt to move from institutional to community-based services. Unfortunately too, there are few opportunities for coordinators to receive further training for this work, although access to a multidisciplinary group has provided invaluable support.

Field workers
The field workers have primary responsibility for visiting and supporting an assigned number of families. They may have little or no prior experience of disability but they are given specific training for their role. In Zimbabwe, this consists of in-service training spread over two years; resulting in a recognized career post within the health service of Rehabilitation Assistant (House *et al.* 1990).

More commonly though, the training is of shorter duration—around six weeks, or the equivalent if taken part-time (Thorburn 1990). In most projects the field workers are paid, although volunteers from the community have been used successfully (O'Toole 1988).

The personal qualities required for field workers have been well summarized by Thorburn (1990): 'anyone can be selected from any background', but the essential qualities are 'serious intent about work, motivation to assist others in need, an empathetic and respectful (rather than pitying) attitude towards disadvantaged persons, good health, stable family background and literacy.' She notes too that 'persons with too high academic qualifications will tend to drop out because of increased social mobility and work options.'

Jaffer and Jaffer (1990) draw attention to the difficulty which female field workers, especially unmarried ones, could encounter in making home visits in a conservative country such as Pakistan.

Parents of children with disabilities have been successfully deployed as field workers on both a paid and a voluntary basis. Other projects have attempted to use existing personnel such as primary health care workers or nursery teachers. This works best if the individuals volunteer to take on the work or if their existing workloads are light (Thorburn 1990).

Training
The training of field workers is probably the best single determinant of service effectiveness. The better the training, the more effective field workers are likely to be. However the training models used in more affluent countries are *not* well-suited to developing countries. In the first place, they presume that the training is provided in specialist centres or colleges by experienced trainers, neither of which is common in developing countries. And second, the training is often geared toward a professional qualification with preset selection criteria which means that only certain people are accepted for training (McConkey and Bradley 1991).

TABLE 5.2
Suggested topics in the training of field workers

- Service philosophies and goals
- Exploration of one's own attitudes to disability
- Skills in screening and identifying different disabilities
- Referrals to hospitals, schools, etc.
- Listening to and counselling families
- Community attitudes to disability and factors in change
- Assessing resources available in the local community
- Beliefs about, and stages in, child development
- Effects of different disabilities on child development
- Socialization and communication
- Encouraging self-care skills
- Play activities and playthings
- Aids and adaptations
- Physical exercises
- Coping with epilepsy
- Behaviour management
- Designing an individual programme plan
- Observation and recording
- Teaching skills

Rather, a new approach to training has begun to evolve with the following charac-teristics:

• Front-line helpers are the main consumers, *i.e.* untrained service staff, families and com-munity workers. Their levels of literacy are likely to be poor, hence the emphasis needs to be on learning by seeing and doing, rather than from talks and books (Werner and Bower 1982).

• These people need to be given information that is practical and relevant to their needs and to the job they are expected to fulfil. Examples of good practice occurring in their culture and under similar conditions to those which they experience are likely to be the most useful. Hence, indigenously produced materials are necessary (Thorburn and Marfo 1990).

• The training must take place locally and it should be easily repeated for differing groups within the community and over time as new people come along. Trainees have other com-mitments in their homes and community which make it impossible for them to travel even if they could afford to do so. Given the dearth of experienced trainers in most developing countries, some form of distance-learning packages will be required.

• The training must help to develop better services. Too often, training is divorced from service goals by focusing on the acquisition of knowledge and skills, whereas training also needs to embrace methods for changing attitudes, planning service goals and nurturing partnerships within communities (Hope and Timmel 1984).

In summary, many early intervention projects have had to devise their own training programmes for their workers, the families and the local communities. The topics which usually need to be covered are listed in Table 5.2. A number of manuals and books based on experiences in developing countries are now available which tutors and trainees can use

TABLE 5.3
Resource guides used in early intervention projects

Disabled Village Children: a Guide for Community Health Workers, Rehabilitation Workers and Families (1987). Contact: Healthrights, 964 Hamilton Avenue, Palo Alto, CA 94301, USA

Training in the Community for People with Disabilities (1989). Contact: World Health Organization, 1211 Geneva, Switzerland

Portage Guide to Early Education (1976). Contact: NFER Publishing Company, Darville House, 2 Oxford Road East, Windsor SL4 1DF, UK

H.O.P.E. for the Child: Home-based Learning Programme (1985). Contact: Zimcare Trust, P.O. Box BE90, Belvedere, Harare, Zimbabwe

An Early Intervention Programme for Children with Mental Retardation (1991). Contact: Malaysian Care, 21 Jalan Sultan Abdul Samad, Brickfields, 50470 Kuala Lumpur, Malaysia

Special Education for Mentally Handicapped Pupils (1986); *Speech, Language and Communication with the Special Child* (1988); and other publications. Contact: Mental Health Centre, Peshawar, North West Frontier Province, Pakistan

Pictostory leaflets on various topics in early childhood education. Contact: Community Rehabilitation Unit (Speech Therapy), Harare Hospital, P.O. Box ST14, Southerton, Harare, Zimbabwe

Communicating with Children: a Language Training Manual (1991, available in English and Nepali). Contact: Teaching Hospital, Kathmandu, Nepal

Unesco Guides for Special Education. Titles available include: *Guidelines for Partnership between Professionals and Parents*; *Education of Deaf Children and Young People*; *Education of Visually Impaired Pupils in Ordinary Schools.* Contact: Unesco, Special Education Unit, 7 Place de Fontenoy, 75700 Paris, France

TABLE 5.4
Examples of training packages for use in early intervention projects

Living and Learning: Preschoolers and Children with Multiple Handicaps. Produced by: Cheshire Foundation International (1989). Filmed in Malaysia with Malay, Chinese and Indian cultures. Languages—English, Bahasa Malay, Mandarin, Thai. Enquiries to: Cheshire Homes Far Eastern Region, 515Q Jalan Hashim, Tanjong Bungah, Penang, Malaysia

Step-By-Step. Produced by: Guyana Community-based Rehabilitation Programme (1992). Filmed in Guyana. Language—English. Enquiries to: Brian O'Toole, c/o E.C. Commission, P.O. Box 10847, Georgetown, Guyana

Learning Together: a Videocourse for Staff Working with Children Who Have Cerebral Palsy. Produced by: Cheshire Homes International (1992). Filmed in Botswana, Zimbabwe and Zambia. Language—English. Enquiries to: Cheshire Homes International, 26–29 Maunsel Street, London SW1P 2QN, UK

One of the Family. Produced by: National Institute of Education, Maharagama, Sri Lanka (1991). Languages—Sinhala, English and Tamil. Enquiries to: Unesco Special Education Unit, 7 Place de Fontenoy, 75700 Paris, France

Learning Together. Produced by: Ugandan Task Force on Educating Communities about Disability (1991). Language—English. Enquiries to: Unesco Special Education Unit, 7 Place de Fontenoy, 75700 Paris, France

Getting Together. Produced by: The Working Group for Mental Handicap in Malawi (1991). Language—English. Enquiries to: Unesco Special Education Unit, 7 Place de Fontenoy, 75700 Paris, France

during training (Table 5.3), as are a variety of ready-made training packages, based in the main around video programmes (Table 5.4).

The advantages of video can be briefly summarized. It is visual: viewers can see new ideas and approaches in action. A variety of activities can be quickly displayed, and viewers can watch the sequences a number of times to reinforce their learning. Local scenes depict the viewer's reality and emphasize that the messages are appropriate to the culture and that they are already being applied there. It is relatively easy to dub commentaries in local languages onto the video programmes, thereby making training more accessible to everyone.

Video cassettes can be easily taken or sent to any places which have video playback equipment. This is becoming more readily available throughout the world. Recorders and televisions can be battery operated. The programmes can be easily repeated with different groups of parents or community workers.

Our experience has suggested that portraying families and children with disabilities on video can enhance their status within the community as the programmes focus on what the people with disabilities can do for themselves (McConkey 1993).

Finally, a variety of teaching methods are now promoted, especially for adult learners with relatively little education. These include:
• lectures and talks by coordinators, specialist workers, experienced field workers, persons with disabilities and parents who have a child with a disability. These can be followed by question and answer sessions;
• written information—short illustrated leaflets or booklets;
• demonstrations;
• video programmes;
• guided practice;
• group work—sharing ideas and experiences;
• practical assignments.

A number of unresolved issues remain. Who is given responsibility for training? Usually this falls to the project coordinators but the danger is that they are so overwhelmed with other tasks that this function is not properly fulfilled. Allied to this is the lack of opportunity available to trainers to develop their skills and knowledge as teachers of other workers. This need must be addressed at a regional or national level.

What status has this training in terms of nationally recognized qualifications? In Guyana, the training of community-based rehabilitation field workers has been recognized by the University of Guyana as part of the Adult Continuing Education Programme. Local links of this type can prepare the way for new types of qualifications. Particularly pertinent is the dearth of suitable training opportunities for the post of project coordinators and the development of nationally and internationally recognized qualifications for the new type of professional workers in services for people with disabilities.

Training for families
Families often value opportunities to take part in systematic training events. These can comprise a series of evening meetings or one day workshops, and some services have even

organized two week training sessions. Some of the training packages described earlier have been designed for showing to parent groups (see Table 5.4). Such training events can encourage certain parents to become more involved in helping others as a home visitor or worker in a centre on either a voluntary or paid basis.

Conclusion

The past 30 years have witnessed a transformation in thinking about disability and the type of services best suited to the needs of these people. Old notions of illness, doctors and treatments accentuated their differences and encouraged their isolation from society.

After much pressure from people with disabilities and their families, the emphasis now is on their integration into family and community life and working to prevent their disabilities from leading to segregation and social disadvantage. Such attitudes have to be nurtured from birth, hence the crucial role of early intervention services in shaping the future not just of infants with disabilities, but also of their families and communities who will determine whether or not they enjoy a 'full and decent life' as promised by the world leaders in their Convention on the Rights of the Child.

REFERENCES

Baker, B. (1989) *Parent Training and Developmental Disabilities.* Washington: American Association on Mental Retardation.
Bronfenbrenner, U. (1979) *The Ecology of Human Development.* Cambridge: Harvard University Press.
Carlile, J. (1988) *Toys for Fun.* London: TALC.
Caston, D. (1985) *Low Cost Aids.* London: AHRTAG.
Dunst, C. (1985) 'Rethinking early intervention.' *Analysis and Intervention in Developmental Disabilities,* **5**, 165–201.
Farran, D.C. (1990) 'Effects of intervention with disadvantaged and disabled children: a decade review.' *In:* Meisels, S.J. Shonkoff, J.P. (Eds.) *Handbook of Early Childhood Intervention.* Cambridge: Cambridge University Press, pp. 501–539.
Gallagher, J.J. (1992) 'Longitudinal interventions: virtues and limitations.' *In:* Thompson T., Hupp S.C. (Eds.) *Saving Children at Risk: Poverty and Disabilities.* Newbury Park, CA: Sage Publications, pp. 61–70.
Harris, J. (1990) *Early Language Development—Implications for Clinical and Educational Practice.* London: Routledge.
Helander, E., Mendis, P., Nelson, G., Goerdt, A. (1989) *Training Disabled Persons in the Community.* Geneva: World Health Organization.
Henley, S., Lansdown, R. (1988) *Intervention Programs for the Preschool Child: a Survey of the Literature.* Geneva: World Health Organization Division of Maternal and Child Health.
Hope, A, Timmel, S. (1984) *Training for Transformation: a Handbook for Community Workers.* Gweru, Zimbabwe: Mambo Press.
House, H., McAlister, M. Naidoo. C. (1990) *Zimbabwe Steps Ahead: Community Rehabilitation and People with Disabilities.* London: Catholic Insititute for International Relations.
Ivic, I. (1986) 'The play activities of children in different cultures: the universal aspects and the cultural peculiarities.' *In:* Ivic, I., Marjanovic, A. (Eds.) *Traditional Games and Children of Today.* Belgrade: OMEP (World Organization for Early Childhood Education), pp. 83–92.
Jaffer, R., Jaffer, R. (1990) 'The WHO–CBR approach: Programme or Ideology—some reflections from the CBR experience in the Punjab, Pakistan.' *In:* Thorburn, M.J., Marfo, K. (Eds.) *Practical Approaches to Childhood Disability in Developing Countries: Insights from Experience and Research.* St Johns, Newfoundland: Memorial University, Project SEREDEC; Spanish Town, Jamaica: 3D Projects, pp. 277–292.
Johnson, P.R., El-Hato, S. (1990) 'Infant development programs: consumer satisfaction in the Gaza strip.' *British Journal of Mental Subnormality,* **36**, 30–36.

McConachie, H. (1986) *Parents and Young Mentally Handicapped Children: a Review of Research Issues.* London: Croom Helm.

McConkey, R. (1991) *Opening Doors: Educating the Community about Mental Handicap.* Glasgow: Scottish Society for Mental Handicap.

—— (1993) *Training for All: Developing Video-based Training Packages for Parent and Community Education.* Paris: Unesco.

—— (1994) 'Early interventions: planning futures – shaping years.' *Mental Handicap Research,* **7,** 4–15.

—— Bradley, A. (1991) 'Videocourses: a modern solution to an age-old problem.' *In:* Upton, G. (Ed.) *Staff Training and Special Educational Needs.* London: David Fulton, pp. 147–156.

—— Price, P. (1986) *Let's Talk: Learning Language in Everyday Settings.* London: Souvenir Press.

—— Bradley, A., Holloway, S. (1990) *Teaching Skills: a Videocourse.* Penang: Cheshire Homes International.

Madzima, S., Matambo, A.R., Else, J.F. (1985) *Report on the Evaluation of Zimcare Trust's Rural (Home-based) Education Programme.* Harare: Zimcare Trust.

Mariga, L., McConkey, R. (1987) 'Home-based learning programmes for mentally handicapped people in rural areas of Zimbabwe.' *International Journal of Rehabilitation Research,* **10,** 175–183.

Meisels, S.J., Shonkoff, J.P. (1990) *Handbook of Early Childhood Intervention.* Cambridge: Cambridge University Press.

Mitchell, D., Brown, R. (1990) *Early Intervention Studies for Young Children with Special Needs.* London: Chapman & Hall.

Myers, R.G. (1990) *Toward a Fair Start for Children: Programming for Early Childhood Care and Development in the Developing World.* Paris: Unesco.

Nikapota, A.D. (1986) 'Parents' perceptions of needs for care of their mentally retarded children in Sri Lanka.' *In:* Berg J.M. (Ed.) *Science and Service in Mental Retardation.* Baltimore: University Park Press, pp. 396–402.

O'Brien, J., Farrell, P. (1992) *EDY Training Package (Revised Edition).* Manchester: Manchester University Press.

O'Toole, B. (1988) 'A community-based rehabilitation programme for pre-school disabled children in Guyana.' *International Journal of Rehabilitation Research,* **11,** 323–334.

—— (1990) 'Community-based rehabilitation: the Guyana Evaluation Project.' *In:* Thorburn, M.J., Marfo, K. (Eds.) *Practical Approaches to Childhood Disability in Developing Countries: Insights from Experience and Research.* St Johns, Newfoundland: Memorial University, Project SEREDEC; Spanish Town, Jamaica: 3D Projects, pp. 293–316.

—— (1991) *Guide to Community-based Rehabilitation Services.* Paris: Unesco.

Pomerleau, A., Malcuit, G., Sabatier, C. (1991) 'Child-rearing practices and parental beliefs in three cultural groups of Montreal: Quebecois, Vietnamese and Haitian.' *In:* Bornstein, M.H. (Ed.) *Cultural Approaches to Parenting.* Hillsdale, NJ: Lawrence Erlbaum, pp. 45–68.

Ramey, C.T., Ramey S.L. (1992) 'Effective early intervention.' *Mental Retardation,* **30,** 337–345.

Roggoff, B., Mistry, J., Goncu, A., Mosier, C. (1991) 'Cultural variations in the role relations of toddlers and their families.' *In:* Bornstein, M.H. (Ed.) *Cultural Approaches to Parenting.* Hillsdale: Lawrence Erlbaum, pp. 173–184.

Sameroff, A.J., Fiese, B.H. (1990) 'Transactional regulation and early intervention.' *In:* Meisels, S.J., Shonkoff, J.P. (Eds.) *Handbook of Early Childhood Intervention.* Cambridge: Cambridge University Press, pp. 119–149.

Scheer, J., Groce, N. (1988) 'Impairment as a human constant: cross-cultural and historical perspectives on variation.' *Journal of Social Issues,* **44,** 23–37.

Shonkoff, J.P., Meisels, S.J. (1990) 'Early childhood intervention: the evolution of a concept.' *In:* Meisels, S.J., Shonkoff, J.P. (Eds.) *Handbook of Early Childhood Intervention.* Cambridge: Cambridge University Press, pp. 3–30.

Thorburn, M.J. (1990) 'Practical aspects of programme development. 1. Prevention and early intervention at the community level.' *In:* Thorburn, M.J., Marfo, K. (Eds.) *Practical Approaches to Childhood Disability in Developing Countries: Insights from Experience and Research.* St Johns, Newfoundland: Memorial University, Project SEREDEC; Spanish Town, Jamaica: 3D Projects, pp. 31–57.

—— (1992) 'Parent evaluation of community based rehabilitation in Jamaica.' *International Journal of Rehabilitation Research,* **15,** 170–176.

—— Marfo, K. (1990) *Practical Approaches to Childhood Disability in Developing Countries: Insights from Experience and Research.* St Johns, Newfoundland: Memorial University, Project SEREDEC; Spanish Town, Jamaica: 3D Projects.

Tizard, B., Hughes, M. (1984) *Young Children Learning: Talking and Thinking at Home and at School.* London: Fontana.

—— Mortimore, J., Burchell, B. (1981) *Involving Parents in Nursery and Infant Schools.* London: Grant McIntyre.

Unicef (1990) *A First Call for Children.* New York: Unicef.

Vincent, L.J., Salisbury, C.L., Strain, P., McCormick, C., Tessier, A. (1990) 'A behavioral–ecological approach to early intervention: focus on cultural diversity.' *In:* Meisels, S.J., Shonkoff, J.P. (Eds.) *Handbook of Early Childhood Intervention.* Cambridge: Cambridge University Press, pp. 173–195.

Werner, D., Bower, B. (1982) *Helping Health Workers Learn.* Palo Alto, CA: Hesperian Foundation.

Zigler, E. (1990) 'Foreword.' *In:* Meisels, S.J., Shonkoff, J.P. (Eds.) *Handbook of Early Childhood Intervention.* Cambridge: Cambridge University Press, pp. ix–xiv.

6
SURGERY AND DISABLED CHILDREN

David Hall and Kenneth C. Rankin

General and ethical principles

Even the wealthy industrialized nations are unable to afford all that modern medicine can offer. Increasingly, choices have to be made between competing procedures and treatments. In developing countries, the choices may be more painful and the ethical dilemmas more stark than those confronting clinicians in rich countries, but they are not fundamentally different.

The clinician who is contemplating a referral for surgical evaluation of a disabled child will need to consider the following: the benefits and hazards of the procedure; possible alternative courses of action; the surgical expertise and supporting services available, both at the referral centre and in the child's own locality; the implications for the family; and the ways in which the proposed procedure should be explained to the family. In addition, the implications for the community as a whole must be examined.

Benefits

A surgical procedure may successfully improve or repair an impairment, but the improvement will not necessarily result in a reduction of functional disability. For example, some plastic or orthopaedic procedures for limb defects or deformities may improve the appearance of the limb or extremity, but the function may be no better or may even be reduced. It is not enough to ask, 'Is this impairment correctable?'; the clinician must also ask, 'What will the child be able to do as a result of this procedure that s/he cannot do now?'

This does not necessarily mean that one should never contemplate surgery for purely cosmetic purposes. For example, a child who is distressed by an unsightly deformity or birthmark may benefit substantially from surgery in terms of improved self-confidence and self-esteem even though there is no improvement in function. However, if the child is incapable of realizing or understanding the 'stigma' associated with the deformity, for example because of profound intellectual impairment, and the pressure for surgery comes from the parents, the clinician should consider whether it is morally right to operate on the child purely for the satisfaction of parents or of the community as a whole.

An interesting example of this dilemma is posed by the recent development of plastic surgical procedures to normalize the facial appearance of people with Down syndrome. Some parents have argued that society may be more willing to accept people who do not have the typical facial stigmata of the condition and may therefore be more tolerant of their learning problems; but others have pointed out the moral hazards of carrying out surgery on an individual when the real problem is in the attitudes of society.

Another way of assessing the pros and cons of surgical procedures is to ask, 'What will happen if this operation is not done? What will the child's life be like? How much worse will her/his quality of life be?' These questions are particularly relevant when considering the management of a baby with spina bifida. It was thought at one time that if the back was not closed within 48 hours of birth, further neurological deterioration would occur due to progressive damage of the nerve roots; and that if closure was delayed, meningitis would be likely to develop with often fatal results. Although these outcomes can occur, they are actually quite uncommon. Similarly, if hydrocephalus complicates the picture, as it so often does, continued head growth will probably occur and the head may eventually reach a grotesque size. Although untreated hydrocephalus is often eventually fatal, this is not invariably the case.

One is thus faced with the dilemma that to operate and increase the child's chances of survival is likely to result in a child who becomes an adult with many severe impairments; but withholding surgery does not necessarily mean that the child will die and may simply mean that the ultimate level of impairment is even greater. Perhaps the overriding consideration in developing countries is the lack of appropriate follow-up facilities which will militate against embarking on surgery, and in particular against the insertion of a valve and shunt system.

Parents sometimes wonder whether an operation that appears to be necessary and potentially useful needs to be done immediately, or whether it could reasonably be deferred until the child is older or more emotionally mature, or perhaps has overcome some other serious or life-threatening problem. The question arises frequently when correction of deformities in cerebral palsy is under consideration (see below). Many of the other procedures mentioned in this chapter are designed to improve the child's quality of life and can safely be postponed without any reduction of the benefits that can eventually be obtained when the operation is performed.

Costs
Every operation has costs, which can be divided into three kinds: the cost to the child and family in terms of pain, distress, anxiety and disruption of family life; the financial costs to the family; and the cost to the community as a whole. These costs will be incurred no matter what type of health care system a particular country has.

Even the simplest operation involves a degree of discomfort and anxiety. With modern anaesthesia and postoperative pain relief, physiotherapy and equipment, these should not be excessive, but they must not be forgotten in considering the trade-off between costs and benefits. Immobilization, bandages and even sutures can be unexpectedly distressing, particularly to children with severe or profound intellectual impairment. Such children may sometimes produce some baffling and intractable behavioural challenges following an apparently minor procedure—for example, a child may refuse to walk or weight-bear for many weeks following an apparently routine and straightforward Achilles tendon lengthening procedure.

It is important to remember and to remind nursing staff that although children might be unable to describe their pain because they are too young or speak a different language or have severe intellectual or hearing impairment, they still need postoperative pain relief, which must be carefully planned and prescribed before the child returns to the ward from the operation suite.

Financial costs to the family may be important, even when they do not have to pay the costs of medical care. Most operations will involve travel to a large town or city, an often protracted stay there and loss of earnings or productive work during that time. If this results in parents losing their job or neglecting their crops, the health costs to all their children may be greater than the benefits of the operation to the disabled child.

This dilemma is particularly important to appreciate because although most parents will make any sacrifice to make their disabled child 'normal', they do not always appreciate that the aims of an operation are not normality but merely an often very modest improvement in quality of life.

In most countries there will be some families who can afford to travel overseas for medical care. These families often lack a detailed understanding of their child's medical problem and cannot obtain advice which they trust; as a result they undertake very expensive trips, obtaining numerous consultations and investigations, none of which ultimately will significantly improve their child's condition. This wastes not only the family's resources but also precious foreign currency. These families are often particularly difficult for health professionals to advise since they have little faith in local medical expertise and may make this abundantly and even insultingly clear, thus alienating people who could help them.

The surgical team

Some of the surgical procedures described below are straightforward, whereas others require considerable technical skill. There is inevitably a learning curve in the performance of any operation and in the selection of the most suitable patients. There is no doubt that for any given procedure better results will be obtained by surgeons who do that operation frequently. It is important therefore to work closely with a small number of surgeons so that expertise can be gained.

Frequently in developing countries the limiting factor is not the technical skill of the surgeons but the availability of appropriate anaesthetic expertise, theatre facilities and equipment, and postoperative care and rehabilitation. If there is a deficiency in any of these services, the risks and hazards of surgery may well outweigh the benefits.

Counselling of parents

Studies in industrialized countries suggest that parents seldom absorb more than one third of what they are told in a medical consultation. The figure might well be lower if parents are poorly educated or very much in awe of a person perceived to be important, such as a doctor or surgeon. Furthermore, those with a university education usually find it difficult to explain concepts such as anaesthesia or risk to parents who have perhaps had only a few years of primary schooling. The busy doctor or surgeon may be tempted to bypass the time-consuming process of explaining to parents about the treatment that is proposed and instead may adopt the paternalistic view that s/he knows best what is right for this child and family. However, it is unfair, legally risky and probably unethical to exploit parents' ignorance and innocence in this way. It is vital that before committing themselves to the hazards and possible expense of surgery, all parents have a clear understanding of the risks and benefits of the procedure.

The parents may need help in digesting the information given to them and in framing the questions that they ought to ask. For example, a nurse, ward orderly, teacher, or parent whose child has had similar problems and similar treatment might act as a befriender and advocate of the parents, to help them make sure they truly understand and that they can overcome their fears about questioning their doctor. It is also important to work with an appreciation of local traditional and religious explanations of impairment and of healing, rather than to dismiss these.

Perhaps the greatest danger is that parents will expect too much of the operation. For example, an orthopaedic procedure designed solely to improve hip joint stability in a child with cerebral palsy may be misconstrued as an operation designed to make the child walk. It is important also that the children themselves should be involved in the discussion, if they are old enough and intellectually capable of understanding. Even very young children will often have more insight into the conversations they overhear about the proposed surgery than the parents and doctors imagine. They may become very anxious and agitated, unless an effort is made to explain what is proposed and to try to understand their feelings about this.

Impact on the community

Perhaps the most difficult questions for health professionals are the political ones of the proportion of a country's wealth devoted to health care provision, the fair distribution of resources and the priority uses to which these are put. How health care is paid for is an issue in all countries. When only limited resources are available, is it right to use hospital beds, surgical skills and expensive drugs to carry out surgery on a disabled child, when the benefits may be very small?

The dilemma is the more painful because health professionals traditionally do the best for the patient who happens to be consulting them at the time, irrespective of the needs of the rest of the community. But as the gap between economic resources and medical demands gets wider, this traditional attitude is becoming a luxury, and health professionals have to involve themselves in informed discussion about priorities and choices with policy makers and, ideally through a democratic process, with the wider community (cf. the Oregon experiment, see Chapter 3).

When is surgery useful?

Ear, nose and throat (ENT) surgery

In developing countries, suppurative otitis media (OM) is very common, whereas in industrialized nations secretory otitis (also called otitis media with effusion or 'glue ear') is the more usual form of middle ear disease. Suppurative OM may occur in isolation or as an additional problem in children with other impairments. The hearing loss associated with bilateral middle ear disease is of sufficient magnitude to impair language acquisition and classroom learning but, because it is not severe, the child can still respond to loud voices and everyday sounds. As a result, the level of disability is often seriously underestimated in children with middle ear disease, particularly in developing communities where routine audiological checks are not always undertaken. It is particularly important to check children in special schools or centres for the disabled; a child with no other impairment may be able to compensate for the hearing loss to some extent, but the combination of hearing loss with learning difficulties or visual impairment will have severe effects on all areas of development.

It is important to control any active infection with systemic antibiotics and ear drops, together with regular careful cleansing of the ear. If the condition does not resolve with this treatment or if a conductive hearing loss persists, a surgical opinion should be obtained, in order to assess the risk of intracranial complications and the feasibility of reconstructive surgery.

It is particularly important to get the ear dry and clean in children with sensorineural hearing loss, firstly because the additional conductive hearing impairment will make the child's disability even worse, and secondly because the chronic discharge interferes with the wearing of a hearing aid.

The indications for adenotonsillectomy are essentially the same for children with impairment as for the able-bodied population. Particular care should be taken with children who have had a cleft palate, and an expert opinion should be obtained before removing their tonsils or adenoids. Adenoidectomy may be particularly beneficial in children with Down syndrome and craniofacial malformations, because these children frequently have upper airway obstruction which leads to snoring, sleep disturbance and probably an increased risk of middle ear disease.

Drooling is an important problem in children with cerebral palsy and also occurs in many children with severe intellectual impairment. The constant flow of saliva may cause redness and soreness of the chin, neck and upper chest, significant fluid loss and social difficulty. The soreness often responds to a short course of 1% hydrocortisone cream and can largely be prevented by a silicone barrier cream and by regular changes of clothing.

A variety of procedures have been devised to reduce drooling, including behavioural methods and appliances. Surgical procedures involve excision of some salivary gland tissue and transplantation of the salivary ducts. Considerable technical skill is needed. Too limited a procedure is ineffective but excessive dryness of the mouth and accelerated dental decay occur if the procedure is too radical. Behavioural training methods may offer some benefit but need considerable expertise and professional time (Blasco *et al.* 1992).

Dental care and orthodontics
Dentistry and orthodontics for most children with impairments differ from routine dental care only if patient cooperation is more difficult to obtain and the child is less able to indicate the cause and site of pain or discomfort. Good preventive care is important. The possibility of toothache or dental abscess should be considered when a child with impaired communication shows unexplained distress.

Self-mutilating behaviour (biting hands, tongue, etc.) occurs in many children with severe intellectual impairment, whatever the cause, and is not confined to the extremely rare Lesch–Nyhan syndrome, as many people imagine. It can be a response to stress, separation, bereavement or other forms of distress, particularly in children who receive little stimulation or who have minimal ability to communicate by any other means. Changes in the child's routine, identification of possible reasons for distress and the introduction of communication training can sometimes help. If such measures fail or are beyond the resources of the carers, other methods may be needed. A guard can be placed over the teeth by an orthodontist or dental appliance technician. Removal of some or all of the teeth is a drastic step, but occasionally may be the only option available in a deprived community, where orthodontic expertise, expert behavioural therapy and appropriate drugs may not be available.

Reconstructive surgery
Repair of cleft lip and palate is a procedure whose value and benefit are beyond dispute. Although the best results are obtained by a multidisciplinary team including speech therapist, orthodontist, audiologist, counsellor, etc., as well as the plastic surgeon, a straightforward repair without the assistance of these colleagues is still worthwhile. Reconstructive surgery may also be undertaken for a range of other congenital deformities.

Ophthalmology
Rare congenital eye diseases including cataract, buphthalmos and tumours may require early eye surgery of a highly specialized nature. Squint, refractive error and amblyopia are common in all children but their incidence is higher in children with other impairments. Some children, even those with profound and multiple impairments, will make unexpectedly good progress when apparently minor eye defects are corrected.

Neurosurgery
The biggest challenge to the neurosurgeon in developing communities is the combination of spina bifida and hydrocephalus (neural tube defects). Neither the repair of the back lesion nor the insertion of a shunt system for hydrocephalus is particularly difficult from a technical point of view. The problem lies in the ethical dilemma posed by the poor outcome and the multiple complications of surgery in these operations. Shunt systems are subject to malfunction, infection and blockage and may need frequent revisions, often as an emergency. Even with modern imaging techniques it can often be difficult to decide whether and when a shunt needs replacement. Management of a child with a shunt in remote rural areas may present insurmountable problems.

Other neurosurgical procedures, including craniectomy for craniosynostosis, the surgical treatment of epilepsy and combined neurosurgical and plastic reconstruction of craniofacial anomalies, all require facilities and skills that are seldom available except in the most wealthy industrialized nations.

General and urological surgery
Incontinence is among the most distressing of all conditions. Problems of continence occur in children with spina bifida and other spinal lesions. They should of course be distin-

guished from the much more frequent problems of continence that are the direct result of severe learning difficulties or of the immobility and dependence on carers associated with severe cerebral palsy.

The incontinent child is at risk of skin soreness, the smell leads to social isolation, and later in life there is a probability of sexual dysfunction. Urological assessment may be helpful, but only if appropriate drugs and appliances are available to put into action the recommendations of the urodynamic examination and radiological findings. Similarly, care of a stoma (nephrostomy, ureterostomy, colostomy, etc.) may be difficult if suitable bags and other equipment are in short supply.

Feeding difficulties are common in children with severe cerebral palsy. The processes of chewing, bolus formation and swallowing are poorly integrated; choking and aspiration into the lungs are common; and reflux may lead to heartburn, vomiting and even to gastrointestinal bleeding or oesophageal stricture. Various combinations of tube feeding, gastrostomy feeding and drugs such as H2 antagonists (*e.g.* cimetidine) sometimes significantly improve the child's quality of life and at the same time reduce the stress on carers.

Assessment of these cases is difficult and ideally includes a barium study of the oesophagus, an endoscopic examination and a pH monitoring study. These resources are not readily available outside major centres. In the absence of detailed information, it is a major decision to embark on tube feeding in a child with severe impairment, but in some circumstances there may be no alternative.

Orthopaedic surgery
The range of orthopaedic surgery worldwide is now so great that there is hardly any orthopaedic problem which cannot be tackled, though the techniques require varying degrees of sophistication. In developed countries operations are often performed to increase the height of children of small stature due to achondroplasia, or to transport bone from one part of the leg to another; in developing countries, where resources are severely limited, health professionals face considerable dilemmas when confronted with orthopaedic problems. The challenge is to select those children most likely to benefit from the surgery which can realistically be offered in a particular situation.

ADAPTATION TO DISABILITY
In many situations a child can adapt to her/his impairment sufficiently to be able to walk unaided. The commonest example of this is the child with unilateral lower limb poliomyelitis who, with a weak thigh and flail knee, and with a flexion contracture of the hip and equinus contracture of the ankle, is able to walk by stabilizing the knee with the hand. This throws the body weight over the weak hip enabling the sound hip to swing through normally. The resulting effect appears ugly and inefficient to others. However, to improve such a pattern demands extensive surgery, periods in plaster and a subsequent appliance. It is in these circumstances that the expected results of surgery, the appliances required and the profound effect on the whole of the child's gait pattern require to be carefully explained. In many circumstances such children are better left without surgery since they can

walk unaided. This gait pattern can also last for life, since many adults are seen who have walked in that way for decades.

Adaptation to impairment occurs in many orthopaedic conditions. Children with cerebral palsy may walk with flexed hips and knees. If uncorrected before 15 to 18 years of age it may be best to leave well alone. After a period the combination of spasm and contracture is so fixed that any attempt to return the person to the vertical position can result in, at best, a later return to the previous state, at worst, to an inability to walk. It is possible for those with cerebral palsy to walk with 90° flexion contracture of the hips and knees. Their spasm is an important element in locomotion. Removing the flexion contractures can render such children helpless. A study of the child's overall situation, including the way in which they have adapted to their impairment, is necessary before any surgical measures are proposed.

BACKGROUND OF ORTHOPAEDIC CARE IN AFRICA

The examples given below refer to prevailing circumstances in Africa, but are relevant to the situations found in other developing countries.

Given the large amount of orthopaedic impairments in Africa the available resources to manage these are slender. For example, a survey in Malawi recorded 50,000 cases of children with physical impairment (King 1985). In Zambia, a similar survey during the International Year of Disabled Persons (1981) found many children with completely untreated orthopaedic problems.

In other situations, when facilities become available, a large number of disabled people are identified who could benefit from some form of orthopaedic management, from the provision of an orthosis to corrective surgery. It is clear that with the small number of health workers in this field many such patients will not receive adequate assessment and treatment. Where facilities do exist, there may not be trained and skilled staff to treat patients. For some children surgical correction of a deformity is required before rehabilitation can begin. For others an orthosis is required to control malposition. It is necessary to review facilities available and the continuity of care possible before raising the hopes of disabled people. The concept of the 'team approach' may need to be established before embarking on complicated treatment.

SELECTION FOR TREATMENT

The skill of selection for treatment is enhanced by a logical approach to each individual problem. For each child presenting for orthopaedic treatment the following sequence is necessary: diagnosis, assessment and treatment planning.

Making a diagnosis. This will involve history taking, mainly from immediate family members. It is sometimes difficult to obtain an accurate history, since many children come to the clinic accompanied only by their elder brother, aunt or more distant family member. It may be necessary to ask the parents to come. Unfortunately, to compound the problem, histories are often grossly inaccurate and vital information may be forgotten, as in the situation of a haemophiliac boy of 4 years who bled into the leg spontaneously. Only after

91

some days did a family member appear who confirmed a past history of a bleeding tendency. Important in the history is to ask the child what s/he is complaining of. Some less impaired children who are sent for orthopaedic assessment are contented as they are. Direct questioning can be most revealing.

Physical examination forms part of the second stage but will also be important in establishing the diagnosis. A general examination will always assist in working out the problem.

Assessing impairment. In the context of busy clinics in Africa, physical examination needs to be tailored to the condition presented. Although, on occasions, precise diagnosis is difficult, it is often possible to say quite early that the child has had poliomyelitis, cerebral palsy or osteomyelitis. The examination can then concentrate on the most important features of the condition. In poliomyelitis, for example, muscle charting and measuring of contractures are the baselines of management (see below). In cerebral palsy a quite different set of observations is needed, recording balance and reflexes, spasm and muscle tone.

Planning treatment. In Africa this is the most frustrating part of orthopaedics.

First, the treatment plan must be explained to the parents. In many cases it is the father who decides whether operations will be carried out or not. If he is there, well and good; if not the mother or other relative will absorb as much of what the doctor says as possible and return to discuss the situation with the father. They will then return, usually after some weeks, with the answer.

Second, the timing of the procedures or treatment is important. Because much time may be lost in discussions with relatives, the ideal time to start treatment may be delayed. This will have to be accepted. Delay also is inherent in hospital treatment, particularly so in circumstances where non-medical factors intervene, *e.g.* shortage of linen or plaster of Paris.

Third, the sequence of treatment may not be smooth since patients do not return at the times and intervals requested by doctors. This factor must be kept in mind when a sequence of treatment is necessary for success, such as regular changes of plaster for club foot or poliomyelitis.

Fourth, treatment of those conditions for which an appliance is necessary after surgery must be linked to the provision of that appliance. There is little point in carrying out an excellent correction of the knee for poliomyelitis contracture if the knee orthosis required to maintain the corrected position will not be ready for two months (or worse still not at all). During the intervening period the contracture will recur, thus invalidating the previous surgery and demoralizing the patient.

Before surgery it is important to explain to the child in simple terms what the operation involves, and the likely aftercare, *e.g.* whether plaster will be used and for how long. It is a mistake to assume that a child does not appreciate that the treatment will be uncomfortable and involve pain. It is also vital to explain to the parents what the treatment involves, particularly the likely outcome. Most relatives have a very hazy impression of what is being done and what the child will achieve after the treatment. If orthoses will be required this should be explained. It should be emphasized that 'normality' may not be realized. The treatment plan is to make walking easier and to relieve pain.

Although all orthopaedic conditions occur in Africa, those in which correct management can prevent disability will be emphasized here. Examples chosen for description include fractures, bacterial and viral infections (osteomyelitis, septic arthritis, tuberculosis and poliomyelitis), and congenital conditions (club foot).

Fractures. Children's fractures differ from those in adults for the following reasons: (i) growth is taking place, and remodelling will correct many quite marked malpositions; (ii) the younger the child and the nearer the fracture to the growth plate, the more certain it is that remodelling will take place; and (iii) overlap and shortening in the fractured femur is normal and such bones will overgrow within two years.

Fractures in children are increasing. For example, speed of traffic, congestion, lack of awareness and poor driving combine to cause many injuries to children. Fractures require emergency treatment to reduce later morbidity. Because they often appear undramatic, fractures are sometimes relegated to less urgent places on operating lists.

Acute osteomyelitis. Although worldwide much attention is directed toward the eradication of poliomyelitis, there is no doubt that in terms of morbidity the effects of bacterial infection in bone and joint are still profound. The incidence of impairment caused by conditions such as osteomyelitis and septic arthritis can be greatly reduced with correct management.

Surgical intervention in acute osteomyelitis is less important than understanding the bacterial sensitivities of the most common organisms. As in Europe, the commonest infecting organism is *Staphylococcus aureus* and 95 per cent are penicillinase-producing. Because of the widespread indiscriminate use of benzylpenicillin in every African country, penicillinase-producing strains of *S. aureus* are the rule (Afriye and Nana 1983). Therefore, the main thrust of treatment must be with penicillinase-stable antibiotics, given parenterally in high dosage. These are not available in many developing countries, so recourse often has to be made to less effective antibiotics such as trimethoprim or chloramphenicol. Ideally each centre should carry out a survey of bacterial sensitivities, thus being aware of which antibiotics available can be used with greatest effect.

Many cases presenting for treatment already have subcutaneous abscesses which require incision and drainage. Rarely children present in the first 24 to 48 hours and can be given the correct antibiotic. If these children fail to respond by showing persistent elevation of temperature, constant pain and continued tenderness, surgical exploration of the affected metaphysis is required. If in this situation no pus is found under the skin or periosteum then drilling of the metaphysis is necessary.

All patients require to have the limb rested by traction or plaster, and to have pain relieved by analgesics, and may also require intravenous fluids and occasionally blood transfusion.

Patients whose osteomyelitis is not completely cured on first admission may have the following problems:

(1) Progress to chronic osteomyelitis. This involves the patient having chronic discharging sinuses, and recurrent bouts of pain and fever associated with the presence of dead bone surrounded by the new bone formed by the raised periosteum.

(2) The infective process causes death of the cortex (outer part of the bone), forming a sequestrum. This is the focus of bacterial infection and the basis of continuing problems.

(3) Pathological fracture. The bone weakened by infection is not strong until new bone (involucrum) grows around the dead bone. During this stage there is risk of fracture and the bone must be protected against this for at least three months.

(4) Growth abnormalities. Severe infection can damage the growth plate, although the normal epiphysis resists damage in most cases. This will result in deformities ranging from loss of length to all varieties of angulation. Occasionally the damage is so severe that the entire growth plate is lost with consequent marked limb shortening.

Septic arthritis. Since the basic causation is the same as osteomyelitis, the earlier remarks regarding antibiotic treatment apply also in septic arthritis. Where the two conditions differ is in the need for and urgency of operation. In septic arthritis pus forms within the joint, and the harmful effects on the articular cartilage and the other structures are so severe and rapid that unless drainage of the joint is carried out surgically at the earliest possible moment permanent damage will result.

Septic arthritis can occur at all ages from the neonatal period on, reaching a maximum between 5 and 15 years. Accurate diagnosis is most difficult in the neonatal period since the baby may show signs only of systemic infection, and careful examination is necessary to elucidate the painful, swollen and tender joint. Neonates with septic arthritis can have a normal temperature.

There is little place for aspiration of joints in this condition. The problem arises when aspiration is attempted and fails; frequently this is taken to mean that infection is not present in the joint and no further action is taken. However, aspiration may fail for a variety of reasons: as infection advances, the pus thickens and fibrin clots form; also, aspiration is more difficult to achieve in some joints such as the hip. If the joint is then not opened surgically the harmful effects of the infection will continue (despite antibiotics) with eventual complete destruction of the joint. The surest policy is to open by arthrotomy every joint in which septic arthritis is diagnosed. In this way no infected joint will be put at risk and no false assumptions made that the joint is not infected.

Arthrotomy is a simple procedure and requires no special skill. After drainage the skin should be closed, the joint capsule remaining open. Immobilization is required for three weeks with the joint in a functional position.

Septic arthritis is commonest in the hip and knee and these joints pose particular problems. The intracapsular epiphysis of the hip is vulnerable in severe infection. The combination of pressure inside the joint and toxic damage to both the articular cartilage and the blood supply leads to two major complications. The most serious problem is dislocation, if diagnosis is not made early. This is an irreversible event and will result in lifelong impairment. It is not possible to reduce the hip after a septic dislocation, and the limb will be short and unstable with a pseudoarthrosis developing. Damage to the blood supply of the upper femoral epiphysis is also common and will cause permanent impairment due to avascular necrosis.

The knee must be splinted in extension during the acute phase of the infection so that a flexion contracture will not develop. Knees treated without splintage frequently develop contractures of 30–40° which are very difficult to correct.

Tuberculosis of bone and joint. Tuberculosis is still one of the main causes of morbidity and mortality in Africa. If the diagnosis is made early the outlook for recovery to a normal joint is excellent. However, making a diagnosis early is precisely the difficulty in this situation. The onset of pain, swelling and stiffness is insidious. The child may not complain for some time and even then the joint does not look very abnormal. The signs once the child is brought to hospital are non-specific and unimpressive. Mild swelling, slight warmth and modest restriction of movement are found. There may be tenderness on palpation and pain on movement. There are no diagnostic blood findings (the erythrocyte sedimentation rate may be slightly raised and there is a relative lymphocytosis), and radiology in the early stages may not confirm the diagnosis. The only way to make a positive diagnosis is through a biopsy, which is difficult particularly when the large numbers of children presenting with these vague and non-specific symptoms and signs are considered.

When the condition progresses without treatment, pain is more persistent, the swelling more profound and the joint becomes contracted. By this stage the X-ray shows diagnostic signs of definite joint narrowing, diffuse osteoporosis and areas of bone destruction, particularly next to the cartilage at the edge of the joint.

In areas where large numbers of patients are seen and there are no facilities for histology, the only reasonable course of action is to give anti-tuberculous treatment for six weeks initially and to assess the response. Resting the affected joint is also required, *i.e.* plaster of Paris cylinder for the knee or traction for the hip. It is clear that by employing this method, some patients who do not have tuberculosis of the joint will be treated as such. But in those who do, the joint will be saved from destruction. Once the joint has improved on anti-tuberculous drugs these can then be continued for the full course. When the joint is pain-free and the swelling has settled, movements can be restarted and the child allowed to walk. In clinical terms the knee requires six weeks of immobilization and the hip three months.

Spinal tuberculosis. The need to use a clinical trial of treatment as a diagnostic measure is very important in spinal tuberculosis. Early lesions in quite young children are seen. Since complaints of pain may again be vague and imprecise, particular attention must be paid to any back pain. The only clinical sign may be a very slight prominence of one spinous process, with the suggestion of angulation. This area may be tender to palpation. Unless the condition has progressed far there will be no neurological signs in the lower limbs. The only confirmation of diagnosis is by X-ray. Even that is only corroborative. The narrowing of any intervertebral disc space must be taken very seriously and, if combined with the

95

above signs, tuberculosis must be assumed and treatment started. Delay without treatment can risk the progression to paraplegia if follow-up is poor.

Some children will present with much more advanced signs, making diagnosis easier. An angular kyphus (prominence) of the spine is virtually diagnostic of tuberculosis. X-ray changes of disc space narrowing together with destruction of the adjacent vertebral bodies confirms the diagnosis. There remains the problem of differentiating tuberculous infection from that caused by other bacteria. However, tuberculosis of the spine is much more frequent. A child who presents with high fever and acute illness with symptoms and signs in the spine must be considered as having a vertebral pyogenic osteomyelitis. In contrast to those with tuberculosis these patients will have abnormal blood investigations (a high white cell count with a polymorphonuclear leucocytosis and a raised erythrocyte sedimentation rate).

Poliomyelitis. The combinations of deformity in poliomyelitis are legion. Since times past this condition has given rise to all known orthopaedic problems to such a degree that it was axiomatic that to know poliomyelitis was to know orthopaedics. Severe degrees of widespread poliovirus infection in one patient may still be seen. Such patients have scoliosis, weak arms and legs, contractures of a major degree and are unable to sit or stand. Where possible all attempts should be made to maintain a sitting posture which will allow children to have the mobility of a wheelchair.

Lesser degrees of paralysis involving mainly the lower limbs are common. Many poliomyelitis patients have deformities which influence function and look unsightly. The difficulty from an orthopaedic viewpoint is to decide which patients require surgery and which should be left alone.

The clinical history should include details of when the attack took place, how mobile the patient was before the attack and how development took place thereafter. In practice much of the detail will not be available; the mother may know only that the child started to walk, then had a febrile illness after which s/he could not walk.

If old enough the child must also be questioned, particularly when the poliomyelitis deformity affects only one (usually lower) limb. They should be asked how the impairment affects normal life, walking and other activities. Some children come to be seen not because they themselves were conscious of a problem but because someone else thought they should.

The child should be fully examined with a view to obtaining four types of information: (i) the general state of the child including presence or absence of scoliosis; (ii) the degree of contractures, by accurate measurement of the most commonly affected joints, *e.g.* hips, knee, ankle and foot; (iii) the extent of muscle paralysis, involving muscle charting according to the MRC grading system (Medical Research Council 1943); (iv) the mobility status of the child, whether walking, crawling or unable to move about independently.

Certain aspects of each child will be immediately obvious. Those with extensive severe paralysis are brought into the clinic on a wheelchair or carried by attendants. Children who are unable to walk but can crawl are often carried by parents.

The decision on whether to offer treatment in this group can be particularly difficult. The decision should be taken after discussion with caregivers and the clinic team if one exists. The first objective is to talk in realistic terms, usually to bring expectations down to earth.

Children with poliomyelitis can be grouped according to disability as follows:

(1) Children with widespread paralysis, extensive contractures and unable to walk. These children can rarely be helped by orthopaedic surgery, certainly as it is available in much of Africa. A child before skeletal maturity with a significant scoliosis can be made comfortable for sitting by spinal correction and fusion. If seen early enough, prevention of contractures would be the most useful single factor. Such children rarely have sufficient muscle power to walk even if correction is carried out.

(2) Crawling children under the age of 15 years. These children usually have strong arms but severe contractures of the hips and knees. They have sufficient gluteal muscle power and pelvic control to crawl using their contracted limbs. It is possible with extensive surgery to correct the contractures. However, the surgery is long and painful and the limb contractures prone to recurrence. Only with rigorous discipline do such children remain in the corrected position and learn to walk, requiring long leg calipers and crutches. Although all children want to walk, unless they are assisted through the adolescent phase they will quickly return to the contracted state and to crawling. Consideration must therefore be given to leaving the child crawling. In many countries there will be no other alternative. Crawling gives such children mobility. They can move quickly, get on and off chairs, and transfer from a chair to a bed or to washing facilities. In short they are independent. Many such children have the full use of their upper limbs and therefore can work. The worst result for this group is to undergo surgery which fails. They are then left unable to crawl and dependent on others for many routine activities which they used to do alone. Often the problem with crawling children (and adults) is that they are an offence to others. However, the decision to treat such children should be made clearly in the interests of the child and not to satisfy inherent desires to make them look normal.

(3) Older crawling children. As children with poliomyelitis grow up it is progressively more difficult to correct deformities. From what has been said in relation to younger children it must be clear that there is even less justification to attempt correction of contractures in young adults. Since bodily images change around puberty it is natural that requests for corrective surgery increase in this age group. All young adults wish to walk, and the pressure from the patient is extreme. Most orthopaedic clinics in Africa have a large number of crawling poliomyelitis victims who believe that the doctor can straighten their limbs and make them walk. The risks of surgery in this group are even higher, since failure to completely straighten the limb is common and the risk of complications much greater. The benefits of mobility in the crawling position can be more easily explained to young adults and this must be the main function of the orthopaedic service.

Unilateral lower limb involvement is the commonest type seen and consists of a flexion contracture of the hip, flexion contracture of the knee and equinus of the ankle and foot. Some of these deformities may not be present and the child may only have one, *e.g.* equinus of the ankle. In other children the hip and/or knee contractures are so bad that the foot cannot reach the ground. In extreme cases the limb is thin and atrophic but the child or parents want the leg straightened.

Consider what is required for correction in these cases: the hip must be fully corrected to neutral; the knee must be completely corrected to full extension; the ankle must be corrected to neutral; the leg length discrepancy must be made up. Since the leg is flail and there is no stability in the knee, it follows that a knee orthosis is required. To control the ankle, an ankle–foot orthosis with plantar flexion resistance is needed. The length must be made up by a raise to the shoe. All this is to be applied to a leg which has no muscle power. The effect is to produce an encumbrance of major dimensions which the child may not use since s/he still has to rely on the one good leg and crutches. Only if the limb in question can be corrected in such a way that the child's mobility is improved should these procedures be undertaken.

The more severe the deformities the lesser are the chances of satisfactory correction. Bilateral lower limb involvement will mean greater motivation required by the child. With both lower limbs in calipers most of the energy required for walking comes from the upper limbs. The energy use is very great, and heavy children may not be able to sustain this for long.

Congenital abnormalities: club foot. This—the commonest congenital abnormality—has a high incidence in Africa. It is more common in boys and has a genetic factor. Completely uncorrected club foot is seen often, and these children can walk well if supplied with special boots. Thus if no treatment is offered because the combination of skills is not available, all is not lost.

Consider what is necessary to achieve good results in treating club feet:
(1) Diagnosis must be made at birth.
(2) Treatment must be started as soon after birth as possible.
(3) Neonatal treatment begins with manipulation and strapping of the feet, at first daily. Later, depending upon choice, plaster of Paris needs to be applied.
(4) The baby must be seen frequently in the early stages; weekly is a minimum in the first month.
(5) If correction is not achieved by 3–4 months, operation is indicated.
(6) Operative treatment requires an experienced orthopaedic surgeon and an anaesthetist competent with children of 3–4 months.
(7) Staff are required who can supervise the aftercare.
(8) Postoperative care is vital to the success of the operation and must continue until the child is 5 years old, hopefully walking with a plantigrade foot and able to sustain self-correction.

All of the above are not absolutely necessary but most are. Thus, if treatment is not started at birth it can still start later but a good result cannot be expected. The skilled surgeon and physiotherapist or rehabilitation assistant *are* necessary. There will be poor results from inadequate surgery and incomplete follow-up. Even with all of the above carried out, recurrences are common and difficulties arise. The situation in Africa is that almost none of the above criteria can be fulfilled, even in major cities with teaching hospitals.

TABLE 6.1
Club foot surgery in different age groups in childhood: a summary

Age	Operation	Continuing care	Possible result
Birth to 3 months	Nil	Manipulation and strapping. Regular plaster change	Correction or incomplete correction requiring surgery
3–6 months	Postero-medial soft tissue release	Ten days in backslab. Full plaster for three months, changed monthly. Protection of position until walking	Correction or relapse
6 months to 2 years	Postero-medial soft tissue release	As above	Complete correction unlikely; relapse probable
2–6 years	Postero-medial soft tissue release	As above	Partial correction
6–8 years	Calcaneo-cuboid wedge	Plaster for 3 months	Partial correction
8–13 years	Nil		
13–15 years	Triple arthrodesis	Plaster for 3 months	Complete correction

Treatment is doomed to failure if embarked upon in circumstances in which defects in continuity are likely. Mothers of children with club feet are very aware of what is being done. If they see progress and consistency in the treatment they will tend to keep coming back, even in difficult circumstances of travel and expense. If they experience gaps in care, incomplete treatment and no progress in the management of the foot they tend to default. Thus before starting the programme of management all factors must be taken into account. The list above defines the ideal conditions for a good result. However, children are brought at all ages and stages of club foot having had no previous treatment. The treatment possible at various stages can be defined but it must be emphasized that over the age of 6 months, and particularly over 2 years, treatment is essentially unsatisfactory, operations are difficult to carry out and aftercare even more exacting.

The key to success in the 3–6 months age group is a radical postero-medial soft tissue release. This operation, which involves elongation of all long flexor tendons and the Achilles tendon, must include capsulotomy of the subtalar joint from posteriorly to the talo-navicular region and the posterior half of the deltoid ligament. Only by completely releasing the medial structures in this way can a possible complete correction be achieved. Over-correction is almost never seen in Africa. Lesser procedures will always be accompanied by recurrence.

It has been commonly assumed in the past that when club foot treatment fails, the last resort of triple arthrodesis can be carried out between 13 and 15 years. This has been taken to imply that even in the presence of a previously untreated club foot a triple arthrodesis can be carried out. This has led to many poor results due to surgical operations trying to correct very severe degrees of deformity. Therefore any surgery over the age of 10 years must be considered against the background of possible function if the child is left alone (Table 6.1).

SUMMARY

The scope for orthopaedic surgery in developing countries is very wide. All known conditions occur including those now rare in the Western world. All parents have expectations for the future growth and development of their children, and will accept major surgery if this is necessary and can be carried out.

A major limiting factor for orthopaedic practice stems from late presentation of all conditions. Severe deformity may not be correctable. In addition, restrictions of treatment may be dictated by inadequate facilities. Postoperative nursing is usually good and allows operative treatment in safety where the surgeon has experience, understanding and is competent. Physiotherapy may be available and is essential to many treatment programmes, *e.g.* club foot. Rehabilitation assistants or similar health workers may form the largest group of care givers required for orthopaedic surgery.

Where treatment is being started for the first time in a new locality it is important to start slowly and be sure of success in the early months. Confidence once built up in the community will be an important factor in being able to develop services in the long term. The reputation of a hospital, health team or surgeon is widely known in any locality. If progression to more complicated procedures is possible this must be after the initial process of recruitment and training of a good team, and establishing a high standard for the simpler procedures.

Selection for surgery is the most difficult part of the treatment programme. Keeping expectations within reasonable limits is vital, particularly where the child can function despite the impairment. The advantages and disadvantages of not intervening surgically must be carefully discussed with the parents and, where possible, with the child. Continuity is important; once a programme has started, all concerned look to regularity of treatment for a good outcome.

It will be many years before orthopaedic services reach even half of the population in developing countries. The effort required to start even a modest programme is great but will mark an important beginning in addressing the problems of children with physical impairment.

REFERENCES

Afriye, K., Nana, Y. (1983) 'Acute osteomyelitis at Mpilo Central Hospital.' *Proceedings of the Association of Surgery of East Africa*, **6**, 77–79.
Blasco, P.A., Allaire, J.H., and Participants of the Consortium on Drooling (1992) 'Drooling in the developmentally disabled: management practices and recommendations.' *Developmental Medicine and Child Neurology*, **34**, 849–862.
King, M. (1985) 'Malawi against polio.' *Proceedings of the Association of Surgery of East Africa*, **8**, 170–171.
Medical Research Council (1943) *War Memorandum No. 7, Revised 2nd Edn.* London: HMSO.

7
EARLY IDENTIFICATION OF IMPAIRMENTS IN CHILDREN

Stuart Logan

'Between 10% and 20% of children in Britain still reach school age with defects, often treatable ones, that have gone undetected. . . the only certain remedy is to examine all children several times during the preschool years.' (*Lancet* 1975)

This 1975 *Lancet* editorial on 'developmental screening' reflects a view still widely held. In the USA, the Committee on Children With Disabilities (1986) postulated three reasons for supporting programmes for the early identification of problems in development and functioning: (1) to identify the barriers to children's participation in the educational process; (2) to assist these children and their families in finding medical, educational or other appropriate services; (3) to overcome or mitigate the adverse effects of the disability. The committee argued that this early identification was best achieved by the universal and regular use of screening tests for developmental problems, suggesting that 'Simple instruments that identify developmental problems are readily available.'

Although some have begun to question the need for universal screening of apparently healthy children for developmental disorders (Hall 1991), most developed countries have in place preschool surveillance systems which attempt to identify children with a wide variety of impairments. These surveillance systems often have other broader functions but these are beyond the scope of this discussion.

The process of identification of a child with an impairment includes two stages: the selection of those children who *may* have an impairment and then a diagnostic assessment. The purpose of identification should be to intervene effectively. The process of assessment is dealt with in Chapter 8; this chapter will focus on how children are selected for assessment. This selection may depend on concern being expressed by parents or teachers or may include formal screening.

The first question that must be addressed in discussion of early identification is whether it actually conveys significant benefits to affected children and their carers. The answer will be specific for each type and level of impairment. Furthermore, evaluation of potential effects of a programme must include consideration of how not just the child is affected, but also the family (WHO 1979). Even in the absence of effective therapeutic interventions for the child, there is evidence that early diagnosis may facilitate family adaptation, if appropriate counselling is available (Cunningham *et al.* 1984, Quine and Pahl 1987, McConachie *et al.* 1988). In addition, early identification may allow parents to make better informed decisions about family planning. Finally, even if intervention has been shown to improve outcome, the appropriate assessment and therapeutic facilities must be available locally at an acceptable cost. The efficacy and appropriateness of specific early intervention programmes are considered in other chapters (*e.g.* Chapters 3 and 5).

In most less developed countries, services for disabled children are relatively sparse. The availability of service will often be related to the ability of parents to pay. In these countries, the identification of children with impairments usually depends on recognition of problems by the parents or teachers. It has been suggested that programmes for early identification should become part of routine maternal and child health services even in poor countries, although others have suggested caution (Hall *et al.* 1991).

In this chapter I will examine screening and other possible approaches to the early identification of impairments in children, particularly in the context of countries where resources are severely limited.

Screening

Child health surveillance programmes became widespread in the UK and other developed countries in the 1960s and early '70s (*Lancet* 1986, Köhler and Jakobsson 1987, Hutchison and Nicoll 1988). Surveillance is an unfortunate term which has been used to cover a number of different activities (Butler 1989), but one element of such programmes has generally been screening for a variety of medical and developmental conditions. These programmes have not been widely evaluated but the evidence does not suggest that they are particularly effective, although this may in part be due to the nature of the evaluations. Most programmes developed for historical reasons, but once started are difficult to stop, even where evidence of efficacy is lacking.

In clinical practice the patient approaches the professional with a problem, but in screening programmes the professionals approach the population, claiming to offer something of benefit. This, it is argued, means that the moral context in which screening must be judged is different from that in which we evaluate clinical practice. Professionals must not simply be certain that their service is doing as well as possible within the constraints of knowledge and resources but must actually be certain that the programme does more good than harm.

The criteria against which a potential screening programme should be examined in order to fulfil this requirement are well established. They were first proposed by Wilson and Jungner in 1968 and have been much amended since (Table 7.1) The criteria can be divided into three sections, referring to the condition, the tests and the programme.

Condition criteria
(1) The natural history of the condition must be known. This implies the need to know not only the pattern of development of the condition and its outcome with and without treatment but also its prevalence in the population.
(2) There must be a clear case definition and consensus about the management of borderline cases.
(3) The relative benefits provided by early rather than late treatment must be known.
(4) The condition must have a stage at which it is not likely to be recognized without screening.

TABLE 7.1
Principles of screening

1. The condition for which screening is undertaken should be an important health problem
2. There should be an acceptable treatment for cases identified
3. Facilities for diagnosis and treatment should be available
4. There should be a recognizable latent or early symptomatic stage
5. There should be a suitable test or examination
6. The test should be acceptable to the population
7. The natural history of the condition should be understood
8. There should be an agreed policy on whom to treat as patients
9. The cost of case finding should be non-wastefully balanced in relationship to expenditure on medical care as a whole
10. Case finding should be a continuing process and not a once and for all event

Reproduced by permission from Calman (1994).

These demands may seem unremarkable but are often not met by conditions for which screening is carried out.

We have limited knowledge about the natural history of disorders affecting childhood development. The central difficulty is often that of case definition. Most clinicians can agree about whether or not a child has quadriplegia; there is much less agreement about so-called 'clumsy children' or about what constitutes speech delay. There are actually few conditions apart from single gene disorders in which there is a clear dividing line between those with and those without the condition; it is usually more a matter of asking how much of a condition someone has, rather than whether or not they have it (Illingworth 1987). Where conditions are defined in terms of skills, these usually have a continuous, if skewed, distribution in the population and the cut-off points chosen are arbitrary. Children with severe impairments are relatively easy to identify, and therefore screening programmes are most often proposed for the detection of the mild impairments which are most difficult to define satisfactorily. These problems of definition have bedevilled attempts to determine the natural history of impairments in childhood and often confuse discussion about the relative effectiveness of interventions.

The assessment of the effects of early intervention for disabled children is hampered by a lack of clear evidence. The 'gold standard' for the evaluation of any intervention is a randomized controlled trial but these are seldom feasible in the field of disability. It may be ethically difficult to withhold potentially useful interventions once an impairment has been identified, although it might be argued that for some intrusive interventions there is an ethical problem in their use without adequate evaluation. The goals of intervention are often long-term, which causes practical difficulties in the organization of trials, and there are few established measures of outcome. The conditions which underlie childhood impairments are heterogeneous and variable in prognosis. The evidence for the efficacy of early rather than late management is therefore largely based on case studies and is difficult to translate into a quantitative form suitable for the formal assessment of the benefits of screening.

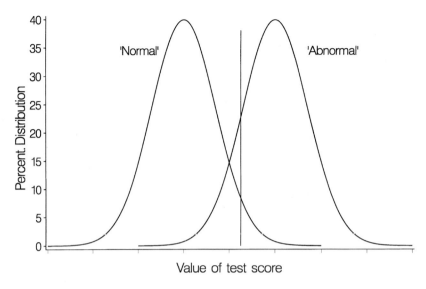

Fig. 7.1. Diagrammatic representation of population distribution of hypothetical screening test scores in 'normal' and 'abnormal' children. The vertical line is the 'decision rule', moved left or right to determine the cut-off point for intervention.

Test criteria

(1) The screening and diagnostic tests must be repeatable and valid (*i.e.* they must measure what they purport to measure).

(2) The sensitivity and specificity of the tests must be high.

(3) The screening tests must be relatively simple and inexpensive.

(4) It must be possible to train large numbers of potential screeners to a high level of reliability.

(5) They must be acceptable to both public and professionals.

The function of a screening test is not to diagnose who has a condition but to separate the population into those at high risk of having it from those at low risk. The high risk group are then offered diagnostic assessment.

Although screening tests must be relatively simple and inexpensive they must produce low rates of false positives and false negatives. There are very few tests where there is not an overlap in the results achieved by children with and without the condition of interest. There is usually a trade-off between sensitivity, the proportion of true positives correctly identified by the test, and specificity, the proportion of true negatives correctly labelled. With many tests it is possible to move the point at which someone is labelled positive, the so-called decision rule, in order to change the sensitivity and specificity of the test. Figure 7.1 illustrates the situation graphically. The two normal distributions represent the scores achieved on some hypothetical test by children who are actually 'normal' and those who are actually 'abnormal'. The vertical line represents the 'decision rule', the cut-off used to determine who is classified as 'abnormal' on the test. Because the distributions of scores in the two groups overlap, wherever the cut-off is placed some children will be mis-classified. If the decision rule is moved to the left, fewer 'abnormal' children will be missed by the test but at the cost of more 'normal' children being classified as 'abnormal'. Conversely, moving the cut-off to the right will decrease the sensitivity but increase the specificity. Deciding where to place the cut-off depends on balancing the consequences for false positives and false negatives. For instance, if we consider language development in childhood, it is generally believed that there is a group of children with language delay who would benefit from speech therapy intervention but there is also a group of children whose expressive speech falls into the lowest part of the population distribution but for whom speech therapy is probably unnecessary. If we used a screening test in 2-year-olds trying to pick out the children with a problem we might set the cut-off as having fewer than 20 single words or as not making two-word sentences. The second option would obviously lead to many more children having unnecessary diagnostic tests but would also probably miss fewer children who actually have significant language problems.

It is important to accept that there are virtually no perfect tests available for screening; all have some false positives and false negatives. Tests are usually developed in popula-tions which have a high prevalence of abnormality, which may give a falsely optimistic impression of their suitability for screening in the general population. There are particular problems with many of the tests used for screening for developmental delay. The use of tests such as the Denver or Bayley scales is often treated as unproblematic, but it has been pointed out that they were in fact designed as tools for assessment and not as screening instruments (Dworkin 1989).

The measures which are most important in determining how a screening programme will function in a population are the positive and negative predictive values of the tests. The 'positive predictive value' is the likelihood that an individual labelled 'abnormal' by the screening test actually has the condition. The 'negative predictive value' is the likelihood that an individual screened negative actually does not have the condition. Unlike sensitivity and specificity, which are properties of a test, these measures are greatly influenced by the prevalence of the condition in the screened population. Table 7.2 shows the effect of applying a test with a sensitivity of 95 per cent and a specificity of 98 per cent to two different populations, one where the prevalence of the condition is 1 in 10 and the other where it is 1 in 1000. Obviously the implications of having a positive screening test are very different in the two populations. In the first, the positive predictive value of the test, that is the chance that someone with a positive screening result actually has the condition, is 84 per cent. When the prevalence is 1/1000, however, the positive predictive value of the same test is only 32 per cent. In very low prevalence conditions the positive predictive value of even very good tests is usually very low.

Obviously most screening programmes will generate large numbers of false positives for each true positive detected. Neonatal screening for congenital hypothyroidism, gener-ally regarded as worthwhile in countries where the appropriate infrastructure is available, has a positive predictive value of around 4 per cent, *i.e.* for each true case detected, 25 children will be positive on the screening test and require diagnostic assessment (Layde 1984). This is important because these false positives can easily swamp the diagnostic

TABLE 7.2

Effects of prevalence on performance of screening tests*

(a) Hypothetical population of 100,000; true prevalence of cases 1/10.

		Truth		
		'Abnormal'	*'Normal'*	*Total*
Screen	+	9,500	1,800	11,300
	–	500	88,200	88,700
Total		10,000	90,000	100,000

Thus, the chance that an individual who is positive on the screening test actually has the condition (positive predictive value) is 84%.

(b) Hypothetical population of 100,000; true prevalence of cases 1/1000.

		Truth		
		'Abnormal'	*'Normal'*	*Total*
Screen	+	950	1,980	2,930
	–	50	97,020	97,070
Total		1,000	99,000	100,000

Thus the chance that an individual who is positive on the screening test actually has the condition (positive predictive value) is 32%.

*Example based on a test with 95% sensitivity and 98% specificity.

facilities leading to delays in making the correct diagnoses. In addition, there are costs to families in their child being labelled as 'abnormal' on screening tests even if they are later told that the child does not have the condition (Marteau 1990). Parents may find it difficult to accept completely the truth of a negative diagnostic test after a positive screening test. These doubts and anxieties may have long-term implications for the way the parents react to their child.

If the decision rule for the screening test is set in such a way as to minimize the number of false positives, this may be at the cost of missing a large number of true cases. The reassurance that their families, and professionals who see them later, are given by the negative result may well lead to diagnosis being delayed further than if no screening programme was in existence.

Diagnostic assessments are also imperfect, although, as they are applied to a population which has been selected as being at high risk of the condition, they appear to perform better. Nonetheless, some individuals will be incorrectly labelled at this stage. This may well result in considerable costs to the child and must be taken into account when evaluating potential screening programmes. For instance, many clinicians will have experience of children who have been incorrectly diagnosed as having sensorineural hearing loss. The spread of neonatal screening for this condition, using tests which are not highly specific, makes it likely that a small number of children with normal hearing will be fitted with hearing aids leading to potentially severe developmental consequences.

Similarly, screening for neuromotor problems will lead to a few unaffected children being diagnosed as having mild cerebral palsy which will inevitably affect the way they are treated by their parents.

Screening tests which are costly or time-consuming or which parents perceive as intrusive are likely to lead to low uptake of screening. If screening is to be used on whole populations in less developed countries they must be simple enough to be applied by workers with limited training. The tests must also be quick to perform so that they can form part of the routine maternal and child health visits.

Programme criteria
(1) The achievement of high rates of coverage must be possible.
(2) Appropriate facilities for diagnosis, assessment and intervention must be available.
(3) Overall, the benefit derived from the screening programme must outweigh the costs.
(4) The cost–benefit analysis must take account of opportunity costs.
Even where a condition fulfils the criteria and the appropriate tests are available, a cost–benefit analysis must be carried out to determine whether the programme is worthwhile. Without achieving high rates of coverage any screening programme is likely to be of limited benefit. Ill health tends to concentrate in the least privileged members of a community and they are usually those least likely to be reached by health services including screening programmes (Tudor Hart 1971). Much of the experience of 'developmental screening' in Europe suggests that after the first year of life attendance drops rapidly, particularly among the poorer members of the community. The result is that those most likely to have the conditions of interest are those least likely to attend for screening. This increases the cost per case detected and decreases the yield of the programme.

One of the effects of instituting a screening programme may be to reveal a large pool of unmet need. Unless this results in a political commitment to the allocation of resources for assessment and management, the individual children identified may receive little benefit. In Czechoslovakia under the communist government, a comprehensive developmental screening programme involving repeated medical examinations was offered to all children. This large investment in screening services was, however, not matched by investment in facilities for the ongoing management of children with problems, many of whom were cared for in unsuitable institutions (Struk, personal communication 1988). Similarly, many districts in Britain screen children for moderate speech and language problems, but the shortage of speech and language therapists means that few children can be offered more than token assistance.

Long delays between screening and diagnostic assessments tend to reduce the attendance rates for diagnosis, which will also reduce the yield of the programme. Mabott (personal communication, 1990) reported that in one British screening programme for sensorineural hearing loss, the mean waiting time between an infant failing a screening test and a diagnostic appointment was ten weeks. In this programme at least 10 per cent of parents did not bring their children for diagnostic assessment after failing two or more screening tests.

Even if a proposed screening programme meets all of the above criteria, it is still important to try to demonstrate that this is a better way to spend the resources than on other competing programmes. The cost and benefits must be weighed against alternative methods of identifying and managing children with impairments and against use of the resources in other parts of the service.

Parental identification of impairment

Studies in developed countries have shown that most impairments in children are identified by parents rather than by professionals (Johnson 1984, Hall 1991). Parents of disabled children frequently report having been reassured repeatedly that their worries were groundless before a professional finally acknowledged the child's impairment. This has led to suggestions that identification can best be left to parents.

For parents to successfully identify impairments in their children at an early stage and to take them to the appropriate services, requires that a number of conditions be met. Firstly, the parents must be able to distinguish between 'normal' and 'abnormal' development. Secondly, they must acknowledge their anxieties and not be deterred by denial or by fears of social stigma. Thirdly, they must believe that intervention is available that will improve the quality of the children's lives. Finally, appropriate services must be available.

Inevitably these conditions are often not fulfilled. In settled communities in less developed countries there may well be a fund of knowledge about child development that helps parents toward the recognition of impairments in their children. However, increasing numbers of people in these countries now live in extremely adverse conditions in shanties or informal settlements. Many will be isolated from informal care networks which might have served as sources of advice. In addition, when meeting the requirements for daily life is a constant struggle, an appropriate response may well be to give child developmental problems a low priority.

The major block to the early identification of impairments in children in less developed countries is, however, the paucity and expense of services. Parents may well have concerns about their children's development but unless adequate assessment and intervention are available at a reasonable cost they cannot pursue these concerns.

Conclusions

Programmes for early identification contain many pitfalls, even where services are well resourced. Screening programmes are particularly problematic as few conditions fulfil the standard screening criteria. In countries with inadequate resources, few screening programmes for childhood impairments can be justified. Many authors now recommend that programmes should emphasize the facilitation of identification by parents rather than formal screening. This does, however, imply the need to ensure that channels are available for parents to act on their concerns.

It is important to take account of opportunity costs when considering priorities in health care. There are conditions where screening might be of benefit but where a public health approach may actually offer greater potential benefits for the same cost. For instance, deficiencies of micronutrients such as iodine and vitamin A have been associated respectively with intellectual impairment and blindness, but screening and treatment of those at high risk is likely to offer less overall benefit than population nutrition programmes.

In less developed countries the priority is to develop services for assessment and management of children who have impairments. Until accessible services are in place, attempts to facilitate early identification are likely to be of little benefit. The availability of services will, in itself, tend to encourage early identification, particularly if accompanied by appropriate publicity. Finally, in setting priorities it is important to remember that the primary needs of disabled children are the same as the needs of all children (see Chapter 2). Unless basic needs are met, there is no point in distinguishing between disabled and non-disabled children.

REFERENCES

Butler, J. (1989) *Child Health Surveillance in Primary Care.* London: HMSO.

Calman, K. (1994) 'Developing screening in the NHS.' *Journal of Medical Screening*, **1**, 101–105.

Committee on Children With Disabilities (1986) 'Screening for developmental disability.' *Pediatrics*, **78**, 526–528.

Cunningham, C.C., Morgan, P.A., McGucken, R.B. (1984) 'Down's syndrome: is dissatisfaction with disclosure of diagnosis inevitable?' *Developmental Medicine and Child Neurology*, **26**, 33–39.

Dworkin, P.H. (1989) 'Developmental screening—expecting the impossible?' *Pediatrics*, **83**, 619–622.

Hall, D.M.B. (Ed.) (1991) *Health for All Children. 2nd Edn.* Oxford: Oxford Medical.

—— Moosa, A, Familusi, J.B. (1991) 'Disorders of the central nervous system.' *In:* Hendrickse, R.G., Barr, D.G.D., Matthews, T.S. (Eds.) *Paediatrics in the Tropics.* Oxford: Blackwell Scientific, pp. 470–520.

Hutchison, T., Nicoll, A. (1988) 'Developmental screening and surveillance.' *British Journal of Hospital Medicine*, **39**, 22–29.

Illingworth, R.S. (1987) 'Pitfalls in developmental diagnosis.' *Archives of Disease in Childhood*, **62**, 860–865.

Köhler, L., Jakobsson, G. (1987) *Children's Health and Well-being in the Nordic Countries. Clinics in Developmental Medicine No. 98.* London: Mac Keith Press.

Johnson, A.M. (1984) 'Visual problems in children: detection and referral.' *Journal of the Royal College of General Practitioners*, **34**, 32–35.

Lancet (1975) 'Developmental screening.' *Lancet*, **1**, 784–786. *(Editorial.)*

—— (1986) 'Developmental surveillance.' *Lancet*, **1**, 950–951. *(Editorial.)*

Layde, P.M. (1984) 'Congenital hypothyroidism.' *In:* Wald, N.J. (Ed.) *Antenatal and Neonatal Screening.* Oxford: Oxford University Press, pp. 239–257.

Marteau, T.M. (1990) 'Reducing the psychological costs.' *British Medical Journal*, **301**, 26–28.

McConachie, H., Lingam, S., Stiff, B., Holt, K.S. (1988) 'Giving assessment reports to parents.' *Archives of Disease in Childhood*, **63**, 209–210.

Quine, L., Pahl, J. (1987) 'First diagnosis of severe handicap: a study of parental reactions.' *Developmental Medicine and Child Neurology*, **29**, 232–242.

Tudor Hart, J. (1971) 'The inverse care law.' *Lancet*, **1**, 405–412.

WHO (1979) *Early Detection of Handicap in Children. Report on a WHO Working Group. EURO Reports and Studies 30.* Copenhagen: World Health Organization Regional Office for Europe.

Wilson, J.M.G., Jungner, G. (1968) *Principles and Practice of Screening for Disease.* Geneva: World Health Organization.

8
CRITIQUE OF CURRENT PRACTICES IN ASSESSMENT OF CHILDREN

Helen McConachie

Assessment should be an integral part of enquiring into how best to support a child's adaptation and progress through her/his everyday social experiences. However, assessment of children identified as having an impairment is bedevilled by inappropriate conceptual frameworks. Medical models look for classification of 'abnormality' as part of diagnosis; educational models may describe a child's current skills but not what might account for the child's 'failures'. How a child functions arises from the interaction between genetic inheritance, impairments and environment (including interactions and expectations). Assessment models are required which reflect the child's potential for resilience and adaptability, and which illuminate a profile of strengths as well as weaknesses. Assessment may be undertaken for a variety of reasons, for instance:

- to find out whether the child is developing 'normally' or 'abnormally';
- to predict the child's future developmental progress;
- to understand how the child learns;
- to establish learning objectives;
- to find out how the child reacts to environmental events;
- to determine environmental factors that influence the child's behaviour;
- to identify teaching strategies;
- to evaluate a programme of education or treatment.

This chapter reviews the purposes of assessment, the approaches usually adopted to meet those purposes, and the underlying assumptions which may invalidate their use with children who have impairments or children in developing countries with or without impairments. The emphasis in discussion will be on young children with severe intellectual impairment, and who may or may not have additional sensory or physical impairment. I begin with traditional psychometric testing of development and intelligence.

Standardized assessment

The first two reasons for assessment given above rest on the assumptions that any particular ability or attribute can be defined, measured and summed, and that it develops according to processes more influenced by organic impairment and/or maturation than by environment. This model is a medical/physical one and applies well to simple measures such as of children's height; it is also relatively easy to apply to measures of sensory or motor functions (such as degree of visual acuity, or age of first walking). However, there is much greater controversy over the measurement of intellectual functioning.

Firstly, there is the problem of *definition*: most approaches to the assessment of intelligence are not based on any clear theory about the nature of intelligence. Western tests concentrate on the dimensions of reasoning, communication and physical coordination. However, cross-cultural conceptions of 'intelligence' show some striking differences, particularly the inclusion of characteristics of social responsibility, cooperation and obedience (*e.g.* in Africa and in Latin America). Thus, assessments based on a Western conception, which undervalue dimensions such as social cooperation and self-help skills, will not be measuring the characteristics of children which the community perceives as constituting intelligence (Berry 1984, Serpell 1988, Lynch and Hanson 1992).

Secondly, there are a multiplicity of problems in *measurement* of intelligence or intellectual disability. Tests of intelligence are standardized, *i.e.* they employ particular pieces of equipment or verbal procedures, presented in the same way to every child, and have results tables (norms) for comparison derived from large samples of children stratified for age, sex and area of the country of origin of the test. Items are chosen and retained in the test which are thought to be relatively unaffected by specific teaching (which some children may not have experienced) and which show a capacity to differentiate a range of high and low scores. By definition, items are not chosen because of their importance or relationship to useful everyday functions, nor are they chosen to give a basis for planning a teaching programme (*e.g.* items will include stacking small blocks, or counting backwards) (Neisworth and Bagnato 1992). Abilities such as creativity or sense of humour, for which measurement would require individualized presentation of opportunities, can therefore not be assessed within standardized test procedure. The standardization samples of children almost always specifically exclude children with a known impairment, and so items are usually chosen without any regard to the level of sensory or physical functioning demanded of the child. Paradoxically, the children for whom the tests are most used (to 'diagnose' intellectual impairment) are not the children for whom the tests were designed. Constructional tests are timed, so penalizing children with physical difficulties; children with motor speech difficulties may be asked to imitate number sequences to test short-term memory; children with visual impairment are asked to manipulate tiny miniature dolls; and so on.

Leaving these problems aside, there remains an aura that tests of early development or intelligence measure something relatively precisely and 'scientifically'. If that were the case, then comparable tests should give comparable results. Two widely used scales of infant development are the Bayley (1969) and Griffiths (1954); where these have been compared, they tend to give substantially different results (*e.g.* in one study of 50 high-risk infants—Ramsay and Fitzhardinge 1977). Furthermore, the published test–retest reliability may not apply to children with impairments. Wishart (1991) has demonstrated that children with Down syndrome tend to have very different patterns of pass/fail from testing sessions only one week apart, thus giving two very different summary results.

In the history of the assessment of intelligence, most criticism has been directed at the 'IQ score', the *summary* measure. Indeed, Binet, the founder of intelligence testing, explicitly rejected the idea that intelligence should be regarded as a single, scalable entity. He was concerned that an IQ figure would be used to deny children education (as indeed it

111

has been), when his original task and intention was to identify those children who needed extra teaching (see Binet and Simon 1916). The norms generated from the standardization sample of children employ a statistical model in which points are arbitrarily defined as discriminating 'normal' from 'abnormal' levels of IQ. Particularly in the case of children with impairments, total scores can be reached in very different ways (*e.g.* motor skills compensating for poor language scores, or conversely low performance on motor and language tasks masking relatively intact cognitive abilities). A preferable approach may be to report profiles from subscales of a test (though these often have poor internal reliability and cannot be shown to measure statistically different entities). Recent discussion of profiles of cognitive strengths/weaknesses associated with particular genetic conditions may, however, prove to have some utility in the design of appropriate educational strategies (*e.g.* the relative strength of simultaneous versus sequential processing in individuals with fragile X syndrome) (Hodapp and Dykens 1991, Wishart 1991).

Finally, there is the question of what processes are implied to underpin development. The historical basis of developmental assessment of very young children is a *maturation* model, where milestones are noted and arbitrary cut-off points used to define a child's motor development or expressive language as 'delayed'. Gaussen (1984) has described developmental milestones as 'conceptual millstones', instead exploring the implications of newer research on child development. The emphasis is on children developing competence in interaction with their social environment (*e.g.* Schaffer 1977). Children with disordered early development are even more sensitive to and dependent on their environment; furthermore, their own 'differentness' and hard-to-interpret responses may affect caregivers, thus altering further (and not necessarily in helpful directions) their interaction experiences (Sameroff and Chandler 1975) (see Chapter 3).

Consideration of this model of child development has two immediate implications for interpreting assessment. First, the interdependence of child and environment calls into question the evaluation of developmental progress in apparently distinct areas of development. Particularly in the case of severely and/or multiply impaired children, impairment in one area (*e.g.* motor disorder) can have important consequences for other areas (*e.g.* language comprehension). For example, a child who does not reach out to touch her mother's coffee mug does not experience 'No, that's hot!', and so has reduced learning opportunities. Therefore, for our approaches to assessment to be appropriate they should reflect how the child interacts with her/his own environments, and also the interrelationship between different areas of functioning.

Second, the maturation model suggests that intelligence is quantifiable and essentially fixed. Development should be linear (allowing for errors of measurement) and predictable through childhood given no extreme adversity such as head injury. However, the reality is very different: research with young children who have impairments indicates that the course of early development is discontinuous and marked by plateaux, regressions and accelerations (Dunst *et al.* 1981, Wishart 1991). Even in children with no impairments, the picture is frequently of discontinuity. Test results on children between 13 and 18 months of age account for only 25 per cent of the variance in results at 3–4 years, and 9 per cent at ages 8–18 years (McCall 1981). Generally assessments before the age of 2 years have little predictive validity for later intelligence assessments. And this is a statement about groups; when the course of development of intelligence is followed for individuals, large amounts of variability can be found. Moffit *et al.* (1993) tested and retested New Zealand main-stream school children at ages 7, 9, 11 and 13; 13 per cent of the children had highly variable IQ profiles, including substantial movement back and forth across the 'normal/abnormal' divide, not explained consistently by adverse experiences. However, a very long-term study of children who had attended classes for slow learners did suggest that adversity (*e.g.* parental divorce or alcoholism, being taken into care, etc.) can affect 'intelligence'. By 31 years of age, the 'slow learners' had generally increased in measured IQ, and to a greater extent (average 16 IQ points) where they had experienced two or more types of adversity (Svendsen 1983). It is usually accepted that children identified early as having severe intellectual impairment are likely to remain so (DuBose 1977, Goodman and Cameron 1978). However, Fagan and Singer (1983) reviewed the evidence of multiple studies of young children with severe impairments tested first at 1 year and found even lower predictive validity than for non-impaired children.

In summary, traditional testing which compares children on the basis of developmental milestones, or to a standardization sample, has the following conceptual problems as an approach with children who have impairments:
• early 'intelligence' is not definable in an agreed way, and means different things at different ages;
• measurement is inexact, with tests usually designed as if sensory and physical impairments can be separated out from more cognitively loaded skills;
• summary scores give a false impression of precision, and have low predictive validity especially from early childhood.

There are additional practical problems with this approach to assessment. There is evidence that young children who have impairments show test scores that are more seriously reduced when they have been tested by an unfamiliar adult than is the case for children without impairments (Fuchs *et al.* 1985). Severely visually impaired children are frequently 'tactile defensive', that is, they avoid manipulating new objects or toys. These and other reactions are compounded by difficulties encountered in applying traditional tests in developing countries. Cross-cultural research has shown the importance of interactional factors in determining how children respond to tests. In many cultures children seldom engage in intensive, structured, one-to-one play and dialogue with an adult, and are not encouraged to show off individual competence to strangers. They may lack experience in verbal labelling and dealing with words outside the practical contexts in which they are customarily used. In addition, there are many differences in familiarity with the materials and items used in tests, such as pencil and paper, developed in the West (Mittler and Serpell 1985, Baine 1990).

Adaptations?

Can any usefulness be salvaged from the traditional approach to assessment? Newer standardized tests such as the Kaufman Assessment Battery for Children (K.ABC—Kaufman and Kaufman 1983) have been derived from a stronger theoretical and research base than the older IQ tests. The K.ABC gives a description of a child's functioning in the areas of sequential and simultaneous processing and achievements/skills, with the expectation that scores will change if and as the child's environment changes. There is some flexibility over administration of the subtests to serve the needs of children with various impairments, and 'teaching' items are included to explain the nature of the tasks. There are some other tests available which have been designed specifically for children who have impairments. For example, the Columbia Mental Maturity Scale (Burgemeister *et al.* 1972) and the Leiter International Performance Scale (Leiter 1969) can be accomplished with a simple eye-point response; the Hiskey–Nebraska Test of Learning Aptitude (Hiskey 1966) and the Snijders–Oomen Non-verbal Intelligence Scale (Snijders and Snijders-Oomen 1976) have norms for young deaf children; and the Reynell–Zinkin Scales (Reynell 1979) have age-equivalents for severely visually impaired children.

Nevertheless, the problems of definition of what is being measured, spurious precision, reduced responding and especially lack of predictive validity remain. With children who have severe impairments, standardized tests can be used at best as a screening procedure, and as such may have a positive role at times in demonstrating a more sophisticated age-equivalent level of functioning in a child than had previously been thought by teachers and others, masked by severe sensory or physical impairment.

Psychologists and others in developing countries have considered many approaches to cultural adaptation of standardized assessment. The two primary approaches have been: (a) review of the content of Western tests followed by restandardization on local samples of children; and (b) development of new tests using concepts and material derived from the local culture (Serpell 1988, Baine 1990). The steps required in revising and restandardizing a test have been outlined by Lansdown and Graham (1992) and include translation and then retranslation into the language of origin to check preservation of meaning, replacement of culturally unfamiliar materials, pilot testing, item analysis, and administration to a large representative sample. Serpell (1988) notes for developing countries that 'uneven access to schooling makes it difficult to conceive of a unitary, standardized test that could serve as a valid measure of intelligence for all sections of the national population.' If a certain group in the population is contending with and successfully adapting to a systematically different set of demands from the majority, then tests for assessing adaptability must be devised which are relevant to those demands.

Thus, the development of new tests seems necessary, a daunting undertaking. One example is the Independent Behaviour Assessment Scale (IBAS) (Munir 1992) used in the validation of the 'Ten Questions' screening assessment (Zaman *et al.* 1990) (see Chapter 1). This scale was designed specifically for use with children who have some degree of intellectual impairment, and is normed on a large non-impaired urban and rural sample. The item choice was informed by conducting an 'ecological inventory' (further described under Criterion-referenced Assessment below) so that tasks observed to be culturally and age-appropriate in Bangladesh were selected. The scale has 188 items developmentally sequenced within four domains: motor, socialization, communication and daily living skills. A more limited approach is represented by the development of the Hand Positions Test and Panga Munthu Test (Ezeilo 1978, Serpell 1989). In the former the child is required to mimic a series of positions of the tester's hands; in the latter, the child makes a model of a person out of plasticine which is then scored for detail and proportionality. Both tests show an increase in scores with age in samples of non-impaired children. One difficulty is to know precisely what cognitive dimensions are being tested and whether they do tap what is suggested to constitute 'intelligence'. The latter test showed limited correlation with children's school marks, and no relationship with teachers' judgement of children's 'intelligence' (or the apparently equivalent concepts in the local language) (Ezeilo 1978).

These assessments overcome some of the problems of standardized testing outlined above. Nevertheless they retain others such as being inappropriate for children with severe sensory or physical impairment, and being respectively too superficial or non-functional to inform the planning of relevant educational programmes.

It is hard to resist the conclusion that current approaches to standardized assessment have little role in services for children with severe impairments. Standardized test results have some role in research evaluating a programme of education or treatment, where individual change scores rather than IQ equivalents are computed (*e.g.* O'Toole 1990); or, as mentioned above, in some initial screening as an imperfect description of current status. However, the two purposes of assessment addressed originally (to discover 'abnormality' and to predict future progress) are fundamentally flawed. Let us consider some more useful purposes and approaches.

The process approach
A variety of strategies for adapting assessment methods have been proposed which might overcome children's difficulties in responding or compensate for previous culturally determined differences in experience. These include setting out fewer test items at a time; giving pre-training on items; and introducing different, more motivating materials or activities. These and other measures usually invalidate the requirements for standardized testing; however, such adaptations are legitimate, indeed highly desirable, when one is exploring the circumstances under which a given child can do certain tasks and perform at her/his highest level of understanding. As Robinson and Fieber (1988) put it:

'. . our task in assessment and intervention with infants and toddlers with significant motoric impairment is to identify situations or tasks that permit adequate insight into such children's underlying competence, and also to appreciate more fully the limitations that significant motoric impairments place on the acquisition of the information and schemes that underlie the successful performance of cognitive tasks.'

The second half of this quotation emphasizes the interdependence in development between different areas of ability and in child–environment interaction. Impairment will be likely to alter experience. Thus the rate of, and routes taken in, development by a child with impairments should be looked at individually and not compared with an inappropriate conception of 'normal' (Davidson and Simmons 1992).

A process-oriented approach to assessment is based on viewing the child as active in creating her/his own developmental path and as discovering ways of learning which can be measured. Thus it can begin to answer another purpose of assessment listed in the introduction to understand how a child learns. The fundamental strategies involved in this approach to assessment include adapting tasks so that the child can best respond, and observing responses to stimuli over several trials and sessions.

There are a number of key considerations in establishing the appropriate assessment materials and methods. The first is *motivation*: some children may find their own toys more motivating than new objects (*e.g.* hiding a child's own toy or drinking cup may be more likely to produce searching). Many children with impairments tire easily and need frequent rests during an assessment session. Other children have a habit of throwing, and so will need the assessor to sit next to them, to anticipate and inhibit throwing, rather than the usual face-to-face position. Assessment of a child's use of gestures to make requests may be best established by singing together two or three nursery action songs (*e.g.* in Britain these might be 'Row, row, row the boat', 'Pat-a-cake', and 'Round and round the garden'); the assessor then provides opportunities for the child to request using a gesture (rowing, clapping or palm-extension respectively). The second is *materials*: materials may be modified to facilitate responding. For example, pictures may be spaced out and tilted up on a rack; usual-size, everyday objects are preferable with severely visually impaired children (Fraiberg 1977); good contrast between materials and the surface they are presented on is important. The third is *positioning*: the child must be in a suitable position to respond, so that none of her/his attention needs to be used up in maintaining head or body control. This may require some adaptability, for example, even necessitating the assessor and child to adopt a side-lying position on the floor! The fourth is *mode of response*: eye-pointing is the most usual alternative response to speech or movement. However, it is important to establish the child's preferred position and distance for presentation of materials. In addition, many young children like to attempt to manipulate materials despite severe motor disorder, so should not be prevented from so doing; fortunately, they usually glance before reaching. Additional points are summarized by Fewell (1983), Langley (1986) and Robinson and Fieber (1988).

Such considerations have also begun to influence strategies for standardized assessment, such as computer-based presentation of stimuli with various switch-access options (*e.g.* Special Needs Assessment Software—Douglas 1990), and preferential looking to video presentation of alternative action sequences to assess verbal comprehension (Cauley *et al.* 1989). However, most of the conceptual problems of standardized assessment remain.

The discussion of motivation leads into consideration of the second fundamental strategy. If a child's experiences have been severely limited by impairments, then rapid learning of a new level of task complexity within the assessment session may be an indication of the child's capacity. For example, a severely motor impaired child may never have pulled on a string to retrieve an object. If the child quickly learns to do so, with the string wrapped around her/his wrist, then basic understanding of how to achieve a goal by indirect means may be inferred. Test–teach–retest has an honourable history as an assessment strategy (*e.g.* Haeussermann 1958), and has obvious relevance to establishing appropriate teaching goals. Finally, assessment of the child also requires observation of social interactional variables; it will be important to see how the child reacts to comparable stimuli in different situations. The most obvious is to compare responses when tasks are presented by one of the child's parents versus the probably unfamiliar assessor; playfulness and vocalization/speech may especially be increased with the parent.

The evaluative framework and chosen tasks used in process-oriented assessment are based on two main approaches in psychology for exploring early cognition—the Piagetian approach, and the information processing model. Piaget's detailed observational research of how infants learn through experimenting with new experiences led him to describe the development of early intellectual processes under various domains (Piaget 1953). These were refined into seven scales by Uzgiris and Hunt (1975): (1) the development of visual pursuit and the permanence of objects; (2) means for obtaining desired environmental events; (3) vocal imitation; (4) gestural imitation; (5) operational causality; (6) construction of object relations in space; (7) schemes for relating to objects. Examples from the first scale would include 'noticing the disappearance of a slowly moving object', 'finding an object which is completely covered' and 'finding an object following a series of invisible displacements'. Any type of cover and any object can be used, including very motivating substances such as food items. The child's level of sophistication of processing is noted, using the six developmental stages within the sensorimotor period described by Piaget, and achieved usually by 2 years of age. Rough age-equivalents can be given for each stage, but generally this approach to assessment is more concerned with description of the sequences within a child's developing understanding. Various authors have developed further the assessment outlines suggested by Uzgiris and Hunt, specifying in more detail suitable objects and directions for administration, in order to achieve reliability between different assessors (*e.g.* Dunst 1980). Coupe and Levy (1985) have developed the Object Related Scheme Assessment Procedure (an elaboration of the seventh scale mentioned above) for use specifically with children who have severe intellectual impairment and who may have additional physical or sensory impairment. Jeffree (1986) in a Unesco publication has further simplified the approach, using a visual presentation to make it useful in a wide variety of circumstances and linking it to later stages of development through observation of play sequences.

Links across areas of behavioural development have been demonstrated by many pieces of research. Sensorimotor understanding stages have been shown to be related to adaptive behaviour achievements, such as skills on the way to independent drinking from a cup (Woodward and Stern 1963), and self-feeding with a spoon in visually impaired children (Kitzinger 1980). For example, until children understand relationships between objects such that they discover how to retrieve an object out of a container, they are unlikely to pick up pieces of food from a bowl to feed themselves. Similar links are noted between stages reached in spoken words and in means–end understanding (*e.g.* Bates *et al.* 1979). Whether these links are in some way causal (*e.g.* whether cognitive processing is prerequisite for language) has been a matter for continuing debate. Certainly development in one area can be seen without necessary accompaniment in the other; blind children often first use words long before they understand how to search for objects (Bigelow 1990). In addition, links have been shown across time; assessed levels of vocal and gestural imitation, and understanding of object permanence, have been shown to predict

117

levels achieved four years later by severely intellectually impaired children on measures of language and socialization (Kahn 1992).

There are of course some limitations with this approach to assessment. Firstly, Piaget's theoretical approach was derived from his own cultural background, and focused on the child as an individual mini-scientist, without reference to influences on development arising from interaction with familiar adults and other children. Therefore, it would also be important to note children's developing skills in social interaction and early vocal and non-vocal communication in addition to their actions on objects (Coupe and Goldbart 1988). An assessment scheme combining these areas for children with dual sensory impairment has been developed by Stillman and Battle (1983, 1986). Secondly, observations on developing movement skills would need to be added (*e.g.* Touwen 1976). A very comprehensive framework for considering early development in children who are profoundly and multiply impaired is provided by Hogg and Sebba (1986), and one for less severely impaired children by Linder (1990). Thirdly, the assumption that development proceeds in a continuous linear fashion in intellectually impaired children is contested by Wishart's (1991) findings that children with Down syndrome tended to show a learning style characterized by acquiring and then losing certain competencies, necessitating later re-learning.

Finally, this approach to assessment, which concentrates on sensorimotor development, is of questionable validity for children with severe motor impairment. Piaget's theoretical position was that children learn through active engagement with their environment. However, it has become clear from later research that learning about spatial and object relations can proceed independently of active movement experience (Zelazo 1982). This has allowed development of assessment procedures which measure young children's attention and habituation to visually and auditorily interesting sequences, requiring little or no active response. Instead a cluster of responses may be noted including visual fixation, cardiac deceleration and smiling. The child is seated in front of a puppet theatre or video monitor and watches, for example, a hand moving a lever down whereupon three lights come on. This is repeated a number of times, and habituation sets in—the child starts to lose interest. Then a novel event is introduced (*e.g.* the lights fail to come on). Measures of looking time can be shown to predict later assessed levels of intelligence better than traditional testing of young children (Slater *et al.* 1989). Also, a number of studies with groups of children with impairments have suggested the applicability of the technique to assessment of cognitive ability (*e.g.* Lewis and Brooks-Gunn 1984). However, as yet, in practice the approach is limited to research settings.

In conclusion, process-oriented assessment offers some strategies for estimating levels of cognitive processing in children with severe levels of impairment, attempting to work with rather than against their idiosyncratic ways of functioning. However, it is conceptually important to note that, because it focuses on the child, it also has limited predictive validity. Current levels of functioning are just one element in a child's 'potential for development'. The whole picture requires consideration of the child's current and future environments and learning opportunities.

There is a second problem for the process-oriented approach in common with standardized assessment. Because the child is central in the approach, any developmental or learning problems identified are implied as belonging to the child. The effect of this upon administrative decisions such as admission to school may be contrary to practitioners' good intentions (Wolff 1989). The assessment approaches which need to be adopted should be wider, and include consideration of the important environments of a child with impairments in order to guide planning of the most appropriate intervention strategies.

Let us take a particular example. In a book describing community-based rehabilitation in Zimbabwe, House *et al.* (1990) put emphasis on attitudes as being of more immediate concern to parents bringing their children to rehabilitation centres than the children's impaired skills. Social stigma, feelings of isolation and emotional pain are some of the problems reported in their own and others' attitudes. Parents may not expect that the child can change and develop. The authors stress that assessment should immediately relate to aspects which constitute the parents' greatest difficulty with the child (*e.g.* self-help skills) and which will change most quickly the attitudes of others (*e.g.* behaviour, concentration). If assessment starts by looking at what the child cannot do, then it reinforces the child's 'differentness' and does not allay fear. Thus, psychologists, teachers, therapists and others who assess children may have a profound influence on how families perceive their child and what they can expect for their child and themselves (Ballard 1991).

This brings us back again to the purposes of assessment. It is not simply a matter of measurement; for long enough it has been said that assessment must lead to intervention. But it becomes clearer that appropriate intervention must also inform the assessment strategy adopted. In the remainder of this chapter, we will consider a number of other assessment approaches applicable to children with impairments, of use in developing countries and with direct bearing on intervention. These have greater or lesser analysis of the child's environment implied within them. We start with criterion-referenced assessment, and touch on its relationship with the teaching curriculum.

Criterion-referenced assessment
This rather awkward title refers to forms of assessment presented as checklists of behaviours which an individual child may or may not be able to do (*i.e.* meet the criterion). Essentially this approach to assessment is not concerned with comparing individual children to others, but instead with looking at skills across a number of areas of development in order to plan educational objectives. In practice, many checklists used with children who have impairments are based on a model of 'normal' developmental progressions, and provide rough age-guides for items or groups of items. The appropriateness of this can be questioned (see above, p. 112).

Criterion-referenced assessment gained in popularity in light of the WHO definition of 'mental retardation' (WHO 1985). This has two elements: 'intellectual functioning that is significantly below average'; and 'marked impairment in the ability of the individual to adapt to the daily demands of the social environment'. The latter is of particular importance when one considers that more than half of young people who have been in special schooling in Western countries and classed as having mild to moderate learning difficulties 'disappear' from the registers of service users after school, having quite sufficient adaptive skills to run a home, raise a family, and hold down a job (should employment levels allow). The greater diversity of roles for adults in society allows young people with intellectual impairments to choose situations in which they are able to meet the expectations of the social environment (Richardson *et al.* 1984). Criterion-referenced assessments of adaptive behaviour include the Adaptive Behavior Scale (ABS) (Nihira *et al.* 1974) which has been widely applied outside the USA where it originated (*e.g.* in India). It is important in evaluating such scales to note the original WHO definition, as many can be criticized for interpreting adaptive behaviour primarily as daily living skills, and relatively ignoring the dimension of social competence (Greenspan and Granfield 1992).

Examples of criterion-references assessments used with children would include the Portage checklist from the Guide to Early Education (Bluma *et al.* 1976), the Parental Involvement Project Developmental Charts (Jeffree and McConkey 1976), and the Vineland Adaptive Behavior Scale (Sparrow *et al.* 1984). These differ in scope and age-range, but essentially cover most of the easily observable aspects of development including play. Only the Vineland includes maladaptive behaviours. The checklists are usually filled in through collaboration between a professional helper and someone who knows the child very thoroughly. Direct observation or testing may be needed for some items (*e.g.* going up steps using one foot at a time). Issues of reliability and validity have been little addressed in criterion-referenced assessment (Bricker 1989). A common problem is misinterpretation of items, which are briefly expressed (*e.g.* how many steps? holding on to a rail or a person, or not holding on?). Children may also behave differently in different settings or with different people, and different observers may give more or less help to the child. However, in many cases the resolution of disagreements will lead to more careful observation and consequently more accurate goal-setting for intervention.

The Portage checklist (but not the other two mentioned above) is linked to a curriculum. That is, there are teaching suggestions specified for each checklist item and a curriculum delivery system. Curriculum-based assessment like this has many advocates (*e.g.* see Bricker 1989, Notari *et al.* 1991) but requires very careful linkage if the curriculum for the individual child is to be functional, to be generalizable across environments, to address the behaviours which block progress, etc. Children's uniqueness tends to render this ideal unrealizable. Certainly, any curriculum-based assessment would require massive adaptation for use in other cultures. The Portage system has been widely adopted (Sturmey 1990), but problems encountered shed light on the assumptions embodied in the curriculum. It was originally developed for use by home visitors with mothers of mildly impaired children in a rural part of the USA. Other cultures hold differing assumptions about children's development and independence, about parents as teachers, about impairment, and so on (Syed 1986). A home visitor from a different area and class may not be well accepted as an adviser, and slow progress may cause parents quickly to lose interest (Balasundaram and Woods 1990) (see Chapter 11).

If the linkage with a curriculum is problematic, what about the criterion-referenced assessments themselves? The Parental Involvement Project charts are relatively brief; the other two are lengthy and may be rather daunting for parents. They all have few items at the early stages of development and so are of limited usefulness with more severely or multiply impaired children. The separation into areas of development obscures linkages between areas (*e.g.* language and play). Language assessment is based on rather dated models, and does not adequately tap the child's spontaneous use of language, or other modes of communication such as gesture or signing, to get adults' attention, make requests or ask questions. To be usable in developing countries, the language checklists in particular would need considerable adaptation, as the course of development will differ in a non-European language. In addition, the relative ages at which certain behaviours are typically expected may vary widely across cultures. Self-reliance may be emphasized less in some Asian families than in British or American ones; children with no developmental problems may continue to be bathed or dressed by parents for longer (Syed 1986). In other circumstances, children may more quickly learn self-reliance or be given independence in moving about in the community.

These considerations lead to the necessity of conducting an 'ecological inventory' in developing or adapting a test for a new situation. The steps suggested by Baine (1986) are to:

(1) pick a target group of children by age, level of impairment, and location;
(2) survey the environments of those children;
(3) identify sub-environments (*e.g.* field, river, well, temple, kitchen) where the children currently go, and potentially may go to in the future with other children of the same age who have no impairments (*e.g.* school, public bus);
(4) list the tasks in each sub-environment which are performed by children (*e.g.* carry food home safely, look after goats);
(5) analyse the tasks into sequences of steps and skills, which can be used in assessment and teaching.

One final consideration for criterion-referenced assessment is examination of the sensory and physical impairments which may accompany intellectual impairment. For several reasons, standard testing may be hard to carry out, and a preferable approach is the development of non-technical checklists to structure the observations made by teachers, parents and other carers during the child's ordinary daily life. Assessment of physical development, hearing and vision in severely intellectually impaired children has been very usefully summarized by Sebba (1987).

Given a criterion-referenced assessment instrument with developmentally and logically sequenced skills, organized into sub-environments appropriate to local cultural expectations for children, and with items specified clearly to avoid misinterpretation, how is the information to be used in planning teaching? A full answer is beyond the scope of this chapter (but see Kiernan 1981, Baine 1986, Jeffree 1986). However, there are some priorities which can be set. The first is to consider blocks to learning, which may be highly individual. One example would be repetitive hand-biting; if this is being prevented by having the child wear thick gloves, it will make practical skills very difficult to learn. As a second example: for parents, a child's poor self-help skills may be a block to having varied interaction experiences, as a great deal of time has to be spent in dressing, feeding, toileting and washing. Programmes aimed at overcoming such blocks will be a priority (Kiernan 1977). A second priority is socialization: if the child is to develop successfully, s/he must accept and interact with other people. A third priority is communication. A basic ability to communicate is essential, even simply to express needs and preferences, and ways need to be found through gesture, sign, eye-pointing, choice-making, etc. for a child to communicate, in order to avoid behaviour problems arising from frustration and to increase children's enjoyment of interaction with others.

Direct observation

The above discussion of setting priorities in teaching clearly implies the need for direct observation of the child, reacting to events in various environments (see back to the purposes of assessment). There are two broad approaches used in this form of assessment: functional analysis of events surrounding particular child behaviours, and rating scales.

Functional analysis can in principle be applied either to desirable responses (*e.g.* vocalization, playing cooperatively) or to undesirable ones (*e.g.* self-mutilation, hitting other children). The observer notes instances of the specified behaviour and records what happened just before and just after (*i.e.* the antecedents, the behaviour, and the consequences—the 'ABC'). Over a period of repeated observations, patterns emerge which lead to ideas on intervention strategy, often through changing the antecedents or the consequences. This approach to assessment has brought about consideration of undesirable behaviour in children with severe impairments in terms of its possible communicative functions (*e.g.* Baumgart *et al.* 1990). Some children may show undesirable behaviour to get adult attention; others may do so because they feel overstimulated and anxious. The intervention strategies will likewise need to differ.

Direct observation can also be used to look at patterns of parent–child interaction. For example, McCollum (1984) describes an intervention study with a 2-year-old child who had cerebral palsy and whose mother found interaction with him confusing and disappointing. Using videotape, the professional worker and the mother noted positive child behaviours (*e.g.* vocalizing) and analysed two mother behaviours which tended to increase the frequency of vocalization (*i.e.* an antecedent—the mother moving her face closer to the child playfully; and a consequence—imitating the vocalization). Thus, the mother found ways to increase her child's responsiveness, making interaction more predictable and mutually more pleasurable. In Nigeria, Nwanze has followed a similar approach with mothers whose children had delayed language development (see Serpell and Nabuzoka 1991). A second example comes from a book written by a parent involved in a Portage service (Lloyd 1986). When her child (who has Down syndrome) started to attend playgroup she was concerned that he showed more immature social behaviours than he did at home with his younger brother and sister. The home visitor and she stopped working on individual teaching, and instead observed the child at playgroup using the Target Child Coding scheme of Sylva *et al.* (1980). They analysed what social skills he lacked in that setting, and how to change the environment to elicit more from him.

Rating scales take a more global and qualitative approach to observation. For problem behaviours, examples would include the Childhood Autism Rating Scale (Schopler *et al.* 1985), and adaptations of the Behaviour Screening Questionnaire (Richman *et al.* 1982) which give greater emphasis to disruptive habitual behaviours not frequently seen in children without impairments (Cunningham 1987). For parent–child interaction, one example is the Parent/Caregiver Involvement Scale (Farran *et al.* 1986) developed for use with children having a variety of types and levels of impairment. It rates 11 aspects of the parent's interactive behaviour, including 'physical involvement', 'responsiveness', and 'play interaction', for amount, quality and appropriateness.

Direct observation does pose some problems as an assessment approach. One is time, as repeated observations are needed in order to begin to see the pattern of how the child reacts to various events. Secondly, the presence of an observer tends to alter behaviour patterns. However, the nature of the alteration is not easy to predict; experimentally, both parents and teachers have been shown to be able to make their child 'look good' or 'look bad' if requested to do so. On balance, observational data probably do usually reflect real patterns (Murphy 1987). As long as there is clarity in defining the behaviour(s) to be observed, direct observation is likely to be more reliable (*i.e.* greater inter-observer agreement) than interview data or rating scale formats which simply ask for adults' opinions on the child's behaviour.

Direct observation can thus provide a baseline assessment from which to plan educational programmes that are individually appropriate to the child. It also gives measures which can be repeated to evaluate the effectiveness of the programme. Nevertheless, the focus is still narrow: increasingly, research into the determinants of disabled children's developing social and cognitive competence emphasizes factors beyond the child and her/his immediate interactions (Dunst and Trivette 1988).

Assessment of environments
The term 'environments' encompasses the total context of children's behaviour, not only the physical characteristics of the environment but also the roles of other individuals, social rules, parent and teacher expectations, and so on. All of these have an impact on children's development and learning, and so should potentially be included in a process of assessment for intervention. A number of measures of environmental variables have been developed for research purposes and have then begun to be utilized in practical services. In this section some family and educational measures will be briefly considered.

Socio-cultural factors determine the quality of life and opportunity available to children who have biologically based impairments. A number of adverse factors may interact with intellectual impairment, including poverty, malnutrition, short spacing between births, physical overcrowding, physical or mental illness of one or both parents, and growing up in poorly managed orphanages or other child care institutions (WHO 1985). Several of these conditions coincide for families living in poor circumstances in developing countries. Sen (1992) describes vividly the possible effects of overcrowding in India, where large families often live in cramped housing. In the first year of life this may not be disabling for a child with impairments; indeed it may offer constant stimulation. But soon the child's variety of experience is limited, with few objects to touch. As the child starts to move around, s/he gets in the way of adults who may be ill-tempered and frustrated as a result of their own limited space. The child's activities are curtailed, and little stimulation is directed to the child or notice taken of her/his interests. Parents preoccupied with survival are unlikely to ask the child questions, and the child is expected to conform. There has been considerable interest in developing countries in measuring the educational potential of a child's home circumstances. Sometimes an adaptation of the HOME Inventory (Caldwell and Bradley 1984) has been created for a particular culture. In Tanzania, this required the addition of questions about roles of other children in caregiving, and of other adults in the extended family; also the instrument was first used with urban families where some Western aspects of lifestyle are more likely to have been adopted (Mbise and Kysela 1990). It will later be tried with rural families. The Inventory measures aspects of the family environment such as stimulation through toys, games and reading materials, pride, affection and warmth, language stimulation, and variety in stimulation, through a mixture of interview and observation. Similar instruments are described by Sen (1992) and Serpell and Nabuzoka (1991). The latter, the Home Environment Potential Assessment, is intended also to identify key people in the home environment who may be willing to take responsibility for intervention activities.

The degree of social support felt by parents has been shown in research to be a powerful determinant of parental well-being (see Chapter 3). Feeling supported has also been shown to increase with appropriate intervention involving counselling and problem solving (the Parent Adviser Scheme, with English-speaking and Bangladeshi families in Britain), leading also to significant positive effects upon children's developmental progress (Davis and Rushton 1991). Measures such as the Family Support Scale (Dunst *et al.* 1984) are administered by interview, and require parents to rate how helpful 18 different sources of informal and formal support have been in the past three months. Adaptations for other cultures might include adding traditional healers, herbalists, voodoo priests, 'espiritistas', etc. to the list of sources (Lynch and Hanson 1992).

Many other measures of parental distress or well-being, parental attitudes to the child, coping strategies, and style of family functioning have been developed (McConachie 1991). However, perhaps more important in assessment appropriate to intervention is a measure of parents' perceptions of their needs. Seligman and Darling (1989) describe the Parent Needs Survey, which is used directly in drawing up a broad intervention plan. The 26 items fall under six headings: information, treatment, formal support, informal support, material support and competing needs. Similar instruments could be developed for brothers, sisters and grandparents.

Where children are living in large residential settings away from home, measures such as the Child Management Scale (King *et al.* 1971) can be used to document care practices along a dimension from child-oriented to institution-oriented (*e.g.* whether children have a choice about when they have a bath, how their birthdays are recognized, etc.).

In educational settings it is important to document the key skills which will make a difference to how children 'fit in'. These might include compliance with instruction, attention control, and social interaction with other children. In planning integration of children with intellectual impairment into mainstream school in a developed country, Rietveld (1983) observed that a key skill required in that setting was independently selecting an activity. She therefore taught children how to make choices, before they started in school. More structured approaches to assessment include the Instructional Environment Scale (Ysseldyke and Christenson 1987) which measures such aspects as teacher expectation, motivational strategies, informed feedback and adaptive instruction.

These approaches to assessment of the child's environment have yet to prove their usefulness and generalizability in assessment for intervention. Given the many aspects which could be assessed, the combination of measures most pertinent and acceptable to families has to be found. However, it does seem as if these are the right kinds of questions to be included in appropriate assessment.

Evaluation

As mentioned in concluding the section on standardized assessment, test results may have a role in evaluation of the effectiveness of a service. Desirable outcomes could include accelerated child progress, reduced problem behaviours, or increased parent responsiveness to the child in interaction. McConkey (1990) has described a range of simple approaches to record keeping and to measuring consumer satisfaction, child progress and changes in caregivers, which those individuals and agencies providing services in developing countries may adopt to assess the effectiveness of their work with some objectivity.

However, assessment of outcomes is only part of the story. Equally important is process evaluation, that is, how an intervention works, not just whether it does. Any intervention consists of a complex package of elements evolving over time. Therefore, assessment needs to include qualitative as well as quantitative measures, and to involve parents (and also perhaps children). Possible negative effects must be looked for, as well as benefits. The goals of the service need to be specified clearly: are they simply focused on child progress in skills, or are community integration and family adaptation central goals? (see Chapter 15). Mitchell (1991) has described a scale for evaluating early intervention programmes which has been applied in Canada, New Zealand and the Gaza strip. A total of 51 criteria have been set following wide consultation, and programmes are rated for the extent to which these are met. For example, 'Where the programme is staffed by several professionals, one team member is assigned primary liaison responsibilities for each young child with special needs and his or her family.' The process evaluation allows parents and staff to reconsider aspects of the service which fall short of the criteria in order to improve them. The scale complies with the features required of a good criterion-referenced assessment, having explicit bases in theory, clearly specified items, and instructions on appropriate activities required to score an item. It offers an objective framework for what can otherwise be rather imprecise value judgements.

Conclusions

I conclude this chapter by reviewing some of the fundamental requirements suggested for appropriate assessment of young children who have impairments (Ballard 1991). First, assessment should focus on children's behaviour in real and interesting activities, and include as priorities communication and social skills. Second, assessment should involve observing the child on several occasions, in various settings. Third, assessment materials and methods should be culturally appropriate. Fourth, assessment should include the demands made upon the child by the environment, both in interaction patterns with others and in terms of expectations of appropriate behaviour. Fifth, assessment and teaching should be interlinked. The child's active processing of new experiences and information is a focus for assessment, not simply the tally of 'failed' items. Sixth, parents and teachers should be meaningfully involved in assessment. Assessment is the first stage in developing a relationship between service providers and parents, and so needs to be attuned to their perspectives and priorities.

Finally, and most importantly, the results of assessment should help to create the conditions for provision of effective intervention for the child. The key resources in the child's environment, the family's and community's attitudes, and the aspects of the child's behaviour found most difficult, all dictate the form and goals of intervention and therefore must be part of the design of appropriate assessment.

REFERENCES

Baine, D. (1986) *Testing and Teaching Handicapped Children and Youth in Developing Countries. Guides for Special Education No. 3.* Paris: Unesco.
—— (1990) 'Guide to the development, evaluation, and/or adoption and modification of tests for early childhood education in developing countries.' *In:* Thorburn, M.J., Marfo, K. (Eds.) *Practical Approaches to Childhood Disability in Developing Countries: Insights from Experience and Research.* St Johns, Newfoundland: Memorial University, Project SEREDEC; Spanish Town, Jamaica: 3D Projects, pp. 199–224.
Balasundaram, P., Woods, P.A. (1990) 'A home–based system of service delivery: some difficulties and lessons learned.' *Paper presented to CAMHADD/UNICEF Workshop, Male, Maldives.*
Ballard, K. (1991) 'Assessment for early intervention: evaluating child development and learning in context.' *In:* Mitchell, D., Brown, R.I. (Eds.) *Early Intervention Studies for Young Children with Special Needs.* London: Chapman & Hall, pp. 127–159.
Bates, E., Benigni, L., Bretherton, I., Camaioni, L., Volterra, V. (1979) *The Emergence of Symbols: Cognition and Communication in Infancy.* London: Academic Press.
Baumgart, D., Johnson, J., Helmstetter, E. (1990) *Augmentative and Alternative Communication Systems for Persons with Moderate and Severe Disabilities.* Baltimore: Paul H. Brookes.
Bayley, N. (1969) *Manual for the Bayley Scales of Infant Development.* New York: Psychological Corporation.
Berry, J.W. (1984) 'Towards a universal psychology of cognitive competence.' *International Journal of Psychology,* **19,** 335–361.
Bigelow, A. (1990) 'Relationship between the development of language and thought in young blind children.' *Journal of Visual Impairment and Blindness,* **84,** 414–419.
Binet, A., Simon, Th. (1916) *The Development of Intelligence in Children.* (Translated from articles in *L'Année Psychologique* from 1905, 1908 and 1911, by E.S. Kite.) Baltimore: Williams & Wilkins.
Bluma, S., Shearer, A., Frohman, A., Hilliard, J. (1976) *Portage Guide to Early Education.* Portage, Wisconsin: CESA; Windsor: NFER—Nelson.
Bricker, D.D. (1989) *Early Intervention for At-risk and Handicapped Infants, Toddlers, and Pre-school Children.* Palo Alto, CA: Vort.
Burgemeister, B.B., Blum, L.H., Lorge, I. (1972) *Columbia Mental Maturity Scale, 3rd Edn.* Sidcup, Kent: Harcourt Brace Jovanovich.
Caldwell, B.M., Bradley, R.H. (1984) *Home Observation for Measurement of the Environment (HOME). Revised Edition.* Little Rock: University of Arkansas.
Cauley, K.M., Golinkoff, R.M., Hirsh-Pasek, K., Gordon, L. (1989) 'Revealing hidden competencies: a new method for studying language comprehension in children with motor impairments.' *American Journal on Mental Retardation,* **94,** 53–63.
Coupe, J., Goldbart, J. (1988) *Communication Before Speech.* Beckenham: Croom Helm.
—— Levy, D. (1985) 'The Object Related Scheme assessment procedure: a cognitive assessment for developmentally young children who may have additional physical or sensory handicaps.' *Mental Handicap,* **13,** 22–24.
Cunningham, C.C. (1987) *The Effects of Early Intervention on the Occurrence and Nature of Behaviour Problems in Children with Down's Syndrome. Final Research Report.* Manchester: Hester Adrian Research Centre.

126

Davidson, I.F.W.K., Simmons, J.N. (1992) 'Young blind children: towards assessment for rehabilitation.' *International Journal of Rehabilitation Research*, **15**, 219–226.

Davis, H., Rushton, R. (1991) 'Counselling and supporting parents of children with developmental delay: a research evaluation.' *Journal of Mental Deficiency Research*, **35**, 89–112.

Douglas, J. (1990) *Special Needs Assessment Software*. Windsor: NFER–Nelson.

DuBose, R.F. (1977) 'Predictive value of infant intelligence scales with multiply handicapped children.' *American Journal of Mental Deficiency*, **81**, 388–390.

Dunst, C.J. (1980) *Clinical and Educational Manual for Use with the Uzgiris and Hunt Scales of Infant Psychological Development*. Austin, TX: PRO-ED.

—— Trivette, C.M. (1988) 'Determinants of parent and child interactive behavior.' *In:* Marfo, K. (Ed.) *Parent–Child Interaction and Developmental Disabilities: Theory, Research and Intervention*. New York: Praeger, pp. 3–31.

—— Brassell, W.R., Rheingrover, R.M. (1981) 'Structural and organisational features of sensorimotor intelligence among retarded infants and toddlers.' *British Journal of Educational Psychology*, **51**, 133–143.

—— Jenkins, V., Trivette, C.M. (1984) 'The Family Support Scale: reliability and validity.' *Journal of Individual, Family and Community Wellness*, **1**, 45–52.

Ezeilo, B. (1978) 'Validating Panga Munthu Test and Porteus Maze Test (wooden form) in Zambia.' *International Journal of Psychology*, **13**, 333–342.

Fagan, J.F., Singer, L.T. (1983) 'Infant recognition memory as a measure of intelligence.' *In:* Lipsett, L.P. (Ed.) *Advances in Infant Research, Vol 2*. Norwood, NJ: Ablex, pp. 31–78.

Farran, D.C., Kasari, C., Comfort, M., Jay, S. (1986) *Parent/Caregiver Interaction Scale Training Manual*. Chapel Hill: Frank Porter Graham Child Development Center, University of North Carolina.

Fewell, R.R. (1983) 'Assessing handicapped infants.' *In:* S G Garwood, S.G., Fewell, R.R. (Eds.) *Educating Handicapped Infants: Issues in Development and Intervention*. Rockville, MD: Aspen Systems, pp. 257–297.

Fraiberg, S. (1977) *Insights From the Blind*. London: Souvenir Press.

Fuchs, D., Fuchs, L.S., Power, M.H., Dailey, A.M. (1985) 'Bias in the assessment of handicapped children.' *American Educational Research Journal*, **22**, 185–198.

Gaussen, T. (1984) 'Developmental milestones or conceptual millstones? Some practical and theoretical limitations in infant assessment procedures.' *Child: Care, Health and Development*, **10**, 99–115.

Goodman, J.F., Cameron, J. (1978) 'The meaning of IQ constancy in young retarded children.' *Journal of Genetic Psychology*, **132**, 109–119.

Greenspan, S., Granfield, J.M. (1992) 'Reconsidering the construct of mental retardation: implications of a model of social competence.' *American Journal on Mental Retardation*, **96**, 442–453.

Griffiths, R. (1954) *The Abilities of Babies: a Study in Mental Measurement*. London: University of London Press.

Haeussermann, E. (1958) *Developmental Potential of Preschool Children*. New York: Grune & Stratton.

Hiskey, M.S. (1966) *Hiskey–Nebraska Test of Learning Aptitude*. Lincoln, NE: Union College Press.

Hodapp, R.M., Dykens, E.M. (1991) 'Toward an etiology-specific strategy of early intervention with handicapped children.' *In:* Marfo, K. (Ed.) *Early Intervention in Transition—Current Perspectives on Programs for Handicapped Children*. New York: Praeger, pp. 41–60.

Hogg, J., Sebba, J. (1986) *Profound Retardation and Multiple Impairment, Vol. 1: Development and Learning*. London: Croom Helm.

House, H., McAlister, M., Naidoo, C. (1990) *Zimbabwe Steps Ahead: Community Rehabilitation and People with Disabilities*. London: Catholic Institute for International Relations.

Jeffree, D.M. (1986) *The Education of Children and Young People Who are Mentally Handicapped. Guides for Special Education No. 1*. Paris: UNESCO.

—— McConkey, R. (1976) *Parental Involvement Project Developmental Charts*. Sevenoaks: Hodder & Stoughton.

Kahn, J.V. (1992) 'Predicting adaptive behaviour of severely and profoundly mentally retarded children with early cognitive measures.' *Journal of Intellectual Disability Research*, **36**, 101–114.

Kaufman, A.S., Kaufman, N.L. (1983) *Kaufman Assessment Battery for Children*. Circle Pines, MN: American Guidance Service.

Kiernan, C.C. (1977) 'Toward a curriculum for the profoundly retarded, multiply handicapped child.' *Child: Care, Health and Development*, **3**, 229–239.

—— (1981) *Analysis of Programmes for Teaching*. Basingstoke: Globe Education.

King, R.D., Raynes, N.V., Tizard, J. (1971) *Patterns of Residential Care*. London: Routledge & Kegan Paul.

Kitzinger, M. (1980) 'Planning management of feeding in the visually handicapped child.' *Child: Care, Health and Development*, **6**, 291–299.

Langley, M.B. (1986) 'Psychoeducational assessment of visually impaired students with additional handicaps.' *In:* Ellis, D. (Ed.) *Sensory Impairments in Mentally Handicapped People.* London: Croom Helm, pp. 253–296.

Lansdown, R., Graham, P. (1992) 'The uses and abuses of psychological tests in childhood.' *In: Assessment of People with Mental Retardation.* Geneva: World Health Organization, pp. 42–52.

Leiter, R.G. (1969) *Leiter International Performance Scale Battery for Children.* Chicago: Stoelting.

Lewis, M., Brooks-Gunn, J. (1984) 'Age and handicapped group differences in infants' visual attention.' *Child Development*, **55**, 858–868.

Linder, T.W. (1990) *Transdisciplinary Play-based Assessment: a Functional Approach to Working with Young Children.* Baltimore: Paul H. Brookes.

Lloyd, J.M. (1986) *Jacob's Ladder: a Parent's View of Portage.* Tunbridge Wells: Costello.

Lynch, E.W., Hanson, M.J. (1992) *Developing Cross-cultural Competence: a Guide for Working with Young Children and Their Families.* Baltimore: Paul H. Brookes.

Mbise, A.S., Kysela, G.M. (1990) 'Developing appropriate screening and assessment instruments: the case of Tanzania.' *In:* Thorburn, M.J., Marfo, K. (Eds.) *Practical Approaches to Childhood Disability in Developing Countries: Insights from Experience and Research.* St Johns, Newfoundland: Memorial University, Project SEREDEC; Spanish Town, Jamaica: 3D Projects, pp. 225–243.

McCall, R.B. (1981) 'Predicting developmental outcome: résumé and redirection.' *In:* Brown, C.C. (Ed.) *Infants at Risk: Assessment and Intervention.* Palm Beach, FL: Johnson & Johnson, pp. 57–69.

McCollum, J.A. (1984) 'Social interaction between parents and babies: validation of an intervention procedure.' *Child: Care, Health and Development*, **10**, 301–315.

McConachie, H. (1991) 'Families and professionals: prospects for partnership.' *In:* Segal, S.S., Varma, V.P. (Eds.) *Prospects for People with Learning Difficulties.* London: David Fulton, pp. 85–101.

McConkey, R. (1990) 'Evaluating the impact of programmes.' *In:* Thorburn, M.J., Marfo, K. (Eds.) *Practical Approaches to Childhood Disability in Developing Countries: Insights from Experience and Research.* St Johns, Newfoundland: Memorial University, Project SEREDEC; Spanish Town, Jamaica: 3D Projects, pp. 157–176.

Mitchell, D. (1991) 'Designing and evaluating early intervention programmes.' *In:* Mitchell, D., Brown, R.I. (Eds.) *Early Intervention Studies for Young Children with Special Needs.* London: Chapman & Hall, pp. 297–326.

Mittler, P., Serpell, R. (1985) 'Services: an international perspective.' *In:* Clarke, A.M., Clarke, A.D.B., Berg, J.M. (Eds.) *Mental Deficiency: the Changing Outlook. 4th Edn.* London: Methuen, pp. 715–787.

Moffitt, T.E., Caspi, A., Harkness, A.R., Silva, P.A. (1993) 'The natural history of change in intellectual performance. Who changes? How much? Is it meaningful?' *Journal of Child Psychology and Psychiatry*, **34**, 455–506.

Munir, S.Z. (1992) 'Development of the Independent Behaviour Assessment Scale (IBAS) and construction of norms for use in Bangladesh.' *Paper presented at the 9th IASSMD Congress, Gold Coast, Australia, August 1992.*

Murphy, G. (1987) 'Direct observation as an assessment tool in functional analysis and treatment.' *In:* Hogg, J., Raynes, N.V. (Eds.) *Assessment in Mental Handicap: a Guide to Assessment Practices, Tests and Checklists.* London: Croom Helm, pp. 190–238.

Neisworth, J.T., Bagnato, S.J. (1992) 'The case against intelligence testing in early intervention.' *Topics in Early Childhood Special Education*, **12**, 1–20.

Nihira, K., Foster, R., Shellhaas, M., Leland, H. (1974) *American Association on Mental Deficiency Adaptive Behavior Scale.* Washington, DC: AAMD.

Notari, A., Slentz, K., Bricker, D.D. (1991) 'Assessment–curriculum systems for early childhood/special education.' *In:* Mitchell, D., Brown, R.I. (Eds.) *Early Intervention Studies for Young Children with Special Needs.* London: Chapman & Hall, pp. 160–205.

O'Toole, B. (1990) 'Community-based rehabilitation: the Guyana evaluation project.' *In:* Thorburn, M.J., Marfo, K. (Eds.) *Practical Approaches to Childhood Disability in Developing Countries: Insights from Experience and Research.* St Johns, Newfoundland: Memorial University, Project SEREDEC; Spanish Town, Jamaica: 3D Projects, pp. 293–316.

Piaget, J. (1953) *The Origins of Intelligence in Children.* London: Routledge & Kegan Paul.

Ramsay, M., Fitzhardinge, P.M. (1977) 'A comparative study of two developmental scales: the Bayley and the Griffiths.' *Early Human Development*, **1**, 151–157.

128

Reynell, J. (1979) *Manual for the Reynell–Zinkin Scales for Young Visually Handicapped Children.* Windsor: NFER–Nelson.

Richardson, S.A., Koller, H., Katz, M., McClaren, J. (1984) 'Career paths through mental retardation services: an epidemiological perspective.' *Applied Research in Mental Retardation,* **5,** 53–67.

Richman, N., Stevenson, J., Graham, P.J. (1982) *Pre-school to School: a Behavioural Study.* London: Academic Press.

Rietveld, C.M. (1983) 'The training of choice behaviours in Down's syndrome and non-retarded preschool children.' *Australia and New Zealand Journal of Developmental Disabilities,* **9,** 75–83.

Robinson, C., Fieber, N. (1988) 'Cognitive assessment of motorically impaired infants and preschoolers.' *In:* Wachs, T.D., Sheehan, R. (Eds.) *Assessment of Young Developmentally Disabled Children.* New York: Plenum Press, pp. 127–161.

Sameroff, A.J., Chandler, M. (1975) 'Reproductive risk and the continuum of caretaking casualty.' *In:* Horowitz, F.,Hetherington, M., Sigel, S. (Eds.) *Review of Child Development Research, Vol. 4.* Chicago: Society for Research in Child Development, pp. 187–244.

Schaffer, H.R. (1977) *Studies in Mother–Infant Interaction.* London: Academic Press.

Schopler, E., Reichler, R.J., Renner, B.R. (1985) *Childhood Autism Rating Scale (CARS).* New York: Irvington.

Sebba, J. (1987) 'Assessments of physical development, hearing and vision that can be used by educational and care staff.' *In:* Hogg, J., Raynes, N.V. (Eds.) *Assessment in Mental Handicap: a Guide to Assessment Practices, Tests and Checklists.* London: Croom Helm, pp. 129–157.

Seligman, M., Darling, R.B. (1989) *Ordinary Families, Special Children: a Systems Approach to Childhood Disability.* New York: Guilford Press.

Sen, A. (1992) *Mental Handicap Among Rural Indian Children.* New Delhi: Sage.

Serpell, R. (1988) 'Childhood disability in the sociocultural context: assessment and information needs for effective services.' *In:* Dasen, P.R., Berry, J.W., Sartorius, N. (Eds.) *Health and Cross-cultural Psychology: Toward Applications.* Newbury Park, CA: Sage, pp. 256–280.

—— (1989) 'Psychological assessment as a guide to early intervention: reflections on the Zambian context of intellectual disability.' *In:* Serpell, R., Nabuzoka, D., Lesi, F.E.A. (Eds.) *Early Intervention, Developmental Disability and Mental Handicap in Africa.* Lusaka: University of Zambia, pp. 145–159.

—— Nabuzoka, D. (1991) 'Early intervention in Third World countries.' *In:* Mitchell, D., Brown, R.I. (Eds.) *Early Intervention Studies for Young Children with Special Needs.* London: Chapman & Hall, pp. 93–126.

Slater, A., Cooper, R., Rose, D., Morison, V. (1989) 'Prediction of cognitive performance from infancy to early childhood.' *Human Development,* **32,** 137–147.

Snijders, J.Th., Snijders-Oomen, N. (1976) *Snijders–Oomen Non-verbal Intelligence Scale (S.O.N. 2 1/2 – 7).* Harlem, The Netherlands: H.D. Tjeenk Willink Groningen.

Sparrow, S.S., Balla, D.A., Cicchetti, D.V. (1984) *Vineland Adaptive Behavior Scale.* Circle Pines, MN: American Guidance Services.

Stillman, R.D., Battle, C.W. (1983) *Callier–Azusa Scale – H: Cognition and Communication.* Dallas: University of Texas.

—— —— (1986) 'Developmental assessment of communicative abilities in the deaf–blind.' *In:* Ellis, D. (Ed.) *Sensory Impairments in Mentally Handicapped People.* London: Croom Helm, pp. 319–335.

Sturmey, P. (1990) 'Portage Guide to Early Education: partnership with parents and cross-cultural aspects.' *In:* Evans, P.L.C., Clarke, A.D.B. (Eds.) *Combatting Mental Handicap: Social and Environmental Factors in the Prevention and Amelioration of Mental Handicap.* Bicester, Oxfordshire: AB Academic, pp. 145–159.

Svendsen, D. (1983) 'Factors related to changes in IQ: a follow-up study of former slow learners.' *Journal of Child Psychology and Psychiatry,* **24,** 405–413.

Syed, R (1986) 'A question of cultural differences: Portage and Asian families.' *Paper presented at the 10th National Portage Conference, Winchester, UK, September 1986.*

Sylva, K., Roy, C., Painter, M. (1980) *Childwatching at Playgroup and Nursery School.* London: Grant McIntyre.

Touwen, B.C.L. (1976) *Neurological Development in Infancy. Clinics in Developmental Medicine No. 58.* London: Spastics International Medical Publications.

Uzgiris, I., Hunt, J.M. (1975) *Assessment in Infancy: Ordinal Scales of Psychological Development.* Urbana, IL: University of Illinois Press.

WHO (1985) *Mental Retardation: Meeting the Challenge.* Geneva: World Health Organization. (Offset Publication No. 86.)

Wishart, J.G. (1991) 'Learning difficulties in infants with Down's syndrome.' *International Journal of Rehabilitation Research,* **14,** 251–255.

Wolff, P. (1989) 'The concept of development: how does it constrain assessment and therapy?' *In:* Zelazo, P.R., Barr, R.G. (Eds.) *Challenges to Developmental Paradigms: Implications for Theory, Assessment and Treatment.* Hillsdale, NJ : Lawrence Erlbaum, pp. 13–28.

Woodward, M.W., Stern, D.J. (1963) 'Developmental patterns of severely subnormal children.' *British Journal of Educational Psychology*, **33**, 10–21.

Ysseldyke, J.E., Christenson, S.L. (1987) 'Evaluating students' instructional environments.' *Remedial and Special Education*, **8**, 17–24.

Zaman, S.S., Khan, N.Z., Islam, S., Banu, S., Dixit, S., Shrout, P., Durkin, M. (1990) 'Validity of the 'Ten Questions' for screening serious childhood disability: results from urban Bangladesh.' *International Journal of Epidemiology*, **19**, 613–620.

Zelazo, P.R. (1982) 'Alternative assessment procedures for handicapped infants and toddlers: theoretical and practical issues.' *In:* Bricker, D.D. (Ed.) *Intervention with At-risk and Handicapped Infants: from Research to Application.* Baltimore: University Park Press, pp. 107–128.

9
EDUCATION: RESPONDING TO SPECIAL NEEDS THROUGH TEACHER DEVELOPMENT

Mel Ainscow, N.K. Jangira and Anupam Ahuja

It is beyond doubt that across the world many children do not receive adequate education, including large numbers who have disabilities. This is so despite the fact that it is now more than 40 years since the nations of the world, speaking through the Universal Declaration of Human Rights, asserted that 'everyone has a right to education'.

The text of the 1990 World Conference on Education for All (Unesco 1993), held in Thailand, pointed out that the following realities persist:
- More than 100 million children, including at least 60 million girls, have no access to primary schooling.
- More than 960 million adults, two thirds of whom are women, are illiterate, and functional illiteracy is a significant problem in all countries, industrialized and developing.
- More than one third of the world's adults have no access to the printed knowledge, new skills or technologies that could improve the quality of their lives and help them shape, and adapt to, social and cultural change.
- More than 100 million children and countless adults fail to complete basic education programmes; millions more satisfy the attendance requirements but do not acquire essential knowledge and skills.

Alongside this horrific set of statistics we also know that over 140 million children have significant disabilities (Mittler 1993).

In this chapter we consider the development of educational responses to children with special needs internationally, with particular reference to the situation in developing countries. This review leads us to the conclusion that relatively small changes in schooling, supported by better teacher preparation, can facilitate the education of many children with disabilities and make better arrangements for many others who experience difficulties in learning. To illustrate this argument we describe the work of a Unesco teacher education project that is being used to support teachers in responding to diversity in their classrooms.

The international scene

Probably the most helpful source of data with respect to special educational provision internationally arises out of a survey of 58 countries conducted in 1986–87 (Unesco 1988*b*). The information provided by this survey illustrates the discrepancies in the level of progress among the various regions and countries. It was found, for example, that 34 of the countries had fewer than 1 per cent of pupils enrolled in special educational programmes; ten of these countries had special education provision available for fewer than 0.1 per cent of pupils.

Precise figures for developing countries are particularly difficult to establish, but the studies that are available confirm the disturbing scale of the problem. For example, Ross (1988) summarized data gathered from 13 countries in eastern and southern Africa indicating that virtually all these countries had special education enrolments for only approximately 0.1 per cent or fewer of the school population. Such data led Hegarty (1990) to conclude that, 'The stark reality underlying these figures is that the great majority of children and young people with disabilities do not receive an appropriate education—if indeed they are offered any education.'

It is possible to detect certain patterns in the historical development of special education across different countries. The pace of these developments varies, of course, from country to country. It is also important to note that the field of special education is of relatively recent origin. In its early stages the emphasis is usually on provision for children with distinct disabilities, but with the expansion of public education in many countries, broader forms of special education may be introduced.

As with ordinary education, education for children with disabilities in many countries began with individual and charitable enterprise. There followed in time the intervention of government, first to support voluntary efforts, and finally to create a national framework in which public and voluntary agencies could act in partnership to see that all children receive a suitable education. In many developing countries, however, such a national framework has still to be established (Unesco 1988a).

Many of the current practices of special education have developed since the early 1960s. This period has been marked by significant shifts in beliefs within the field, and, indeed, the process of change is still apparent in many parts of the world.

During the early part of the period there was a marked emphasis on making provision for children with particular impairments. In many countries provision of special education depended on a process of assessment leading to a child being categorized with respect to a perceived impairment. Thus, over the years, special education came to see itself, and to be seen by others, as a separate world catering for that small population of the child population perceived as being disabled. Those involved in special education had relatively little contact with mainstream schools. This tendency to isolation was reinforced in some countries by the fact that many of the providers of special education were voluntary organizations and that some special schools were located in places distant from the community.

The late 1960s and early '70s began to see considerable changes in emphasis. A concern with equal opportunities in a number of Western countries heightened awareness of children in ordinary schools who were perceived as making unsatisfactory progress. Consequently there was a substantial growth in various forms of remedial education, including the establishment of special classes within or attached to mainstream schools. This pattern of development can also be witnessed in developing countries.

Evidence of new legislation internationally is provided by a recent survey (Unesco 1988b). Two thirds of the respondents in the survey (i.e. 38 out of 58 countries) made reference to new legislation under discussion or being introduced. This ranged from loosely formulated discussions of the need for various legislative developments to definite plans to introduce regulations governing specific aspects of educational provision.

The issue of integration

Evidence from the Unesco (1988*b*) survey indicates that the predominant form of provision for special education in many parts of the world is in separate special schools. However, such schools often serve very limited numbers of children, leaving many children with disabilities with little or no education. These observations led the participants in Unesco's consultation in Special Education (1988*a*) to state: 'Given the size of the demand and the limited resources available, the education and training needs of the majority of disabled persons cannot be met by special schools and centres.'

Consequently, a way forward requires changes in both special and mainstream schools. Mainstream schools have to develop forms of organization and teaching that cater for greater pupil diversity, while those special schools that do exist must develop an outward looking stance and take on significantly new roles (Hegarty 1990).

There is considerable evidence that in many countries throughout the world integration is a central element in planning of special education (*e.g.* Unesco 1988*b*, Ainscow 1990, Pijl and Meijer 1991). Such an emphasis seems sensible for developing countries, given the extent of the need and the inevitable limitations of available resources. It is also important to note that in many developing countries there is substantial 'casual' integration of children with disabilities in ordinary schools (Miles 1989).

Developed countries are experiencing their own difficulties in establishing effective policies for integration. The existence of well-established separate provision in special schools and classes creates complex policy dilemmas, leading many countries to operate what Pijl and Meijer (1991) refer to as 'two tracks.' In other words, these countries have parallel, but separate, segregation and integration policies.

In some countries integration represents an aspiration for the future. In Germany, for example, while some pilot initiatives based on the idea of integration are underway, students who are declared eligible for special education must be placed in a special school; statistics for 1986 showed that 4.2 per cent of all students between 6 and 16 years of age were in separate schools for special education. On the other hand, some countries (including Denmark, Norway and Spain) have shown considerable progress in implementing the integration principle universally. Here the local community school is often seen as the normal setting for pupils with special needs.

Discrepancies between stated policy and actual practice are evident in many countries. For example, Pijl and Meijer (1991) note that despite the fact that special schools were abolished in Italy in 1977 most of the so-called integrated pupils are 'integrated outside the classroom'. Often this means that they are taught by support teachers in separate classrooms. It is reported that the reasons for these problems in implementing a policy of integration are that regular school teachers still do not regard the teaching of pupils with special needs as their responsibility and are often not equipped (by training or materials) to do so.

A problem reported from a number of industrialized countries is that despite national policies emphasizing integration there is evidence of a significant increase in the proportions of pupils being categorized in order that their schools can earn additional resources (Ainscow 1991). As a result of her analysis of policies in Australia, England and Scandinavia, and the USA, Fulcher (1989) has suggested that the increased bureaucracy that is often associated with special education and the inevitable struggles that go on for additional resources have the effect of escalating the proportion of schoolchildren labelled as disabled.

International activities

Since the International Year of Disabled Persons (1981) there has been considerable international collaboration with respect to the development of special education policies and programmes. Agencies such as Unesco, Unicef and OECD have acted to encourage collaborative developments, and many national agencies have invested resources to give them support. The World Declaration on Education for All that arose as a result of the 1990 conference in Jomtein, Thailand, gives further impetus to these efforts. Specifically, in Article 3.5, it states: 'The learning needs of the disabled demand special attention. Steps need to be taken to provide equal access to education to every category of disabled persons as an integral part of the education system.' This challenge is enormous, particularly in developing countries.

Preferred ways of conducting international efforts remain a matter of debate. For example, Miles (1989) is doubtful of the value of introducing Western models of special education into countries such as Pakistan and India. He suggests that the reasons that they often do not seem to work are complex but include what he refers to as 'conceptual blockage'. He notes that Western special education is constructed on views of children and schooling that may be largely alien to much of the population of the Indian subcontinent. Furthermore, he is critical of the work of advisers visiting Third World countries as part of what he characterizes as a 'Western conceptual crusade' which seems to ignore the realities of Third World situations.

At the International Consultation on Special Education (Unesco 1988a) participants reviewed and assessed international developments related to special education over the previous decade. They also made suggestions concerning the focus of actions to be taken. Conscious of the magnitude of the problems, and stemming from a commitment to the principles of normalization, integration and participation, they recommended that the complementary approaches of *community-based rehabilitation* and *integrated education* represent the most effective ways forward.

Community-based rehabilitation (CBR) is being used by an increasing number of developing countries as a strategy to eliminate the constraints of institution-based rehabilitation. Its implementation in a particular context will depend to a large degree on a country's strategies for socio-economic development. Often countries start by setting up a CBR project in a selected district, which provides the basis for gaining national experience and expertise. This is followed later by the launching of a wider programme, possibly as part of a national plan. Werner (1987) provides an impressive manual of suggestions for setting up such initiatives in rural communities, including examples of Child-to-Child activities. These are intended to encourage school-aged children to help their disabled peers (see Chapter 11). It is interesting to note that these approaches which have been developed for use in developing countries mirror some of the techniques now being used to create inclusive schools in the West (*e.g.* Lipsky and Gartner 1989). In particular, both emphasize collaboration, including cooperative learning approaches, as a means of utilizing existing resources for the purposes of problem solving in educational contexts.

The Unesco (1988*b*) survey presents a gloomy picture with respect to the international scene in teacher preparation. Only a minority of the 58 countries reported coverage of disability issues in pre-service training programmes for all teachers. In-service training opportunities for teachers in regular schools were similarly limited. A wide range of training opportunities were reported for teachers specializing in special education—a five year course in a teachers college at one extreme, to on-the-job instruction offered on an *ad hoc* basis at the other.

While it is difficult to generalize across widely diverse countries, it seems clear that the main thrust of training at present is directed at specialists who will work in segregated special schools. However, it can be argued that the vast majority of children with disabilities, and many others who experience difficulties, could be helped in mainstream schools by relatively minor adjustments to the teaching that is provided (Hegarty 1990). Thus an investment in the pre-service preparation of teachers with respect to strategies for accommodating pupil diversity, and some attention to in-service activities, could bring about major improvements in the special education provision offered by schools.

Problems and issues

From this summary of international developments with respect to the education of children and youth said to have special needs, it is possible to draw out a number of important problems and issues that require urgent attention. While in its relatively short existence the field of special education has made much progress, an analysis of the current scene around the world presents a disturbing picture. Hegarty (1990) sums up the situation when he states: 'Those with disabilities, who ironically have the greatest need of education, are the least likely to receive it. This is true of developed and developing countries alike.'

In developed countries many pupils with disabilities, and others who fail to achieve satisfactory progress in school learning, are formally excluded from the mainstream education system or receive less favourable treatment within it than other children. On the other hand, in many developing countries the continuing struggle to achieve compulsory education for a majority of children takes precedence over meeting the needs of those with disabilities.

The International Consultation on Special Education (Unesco 1988*a*) outlined a number of general obstacles to improvement. These are:

- Inadequacy of perceptions and thus in policy formation which is very much linked to attitudes, whether they be cultural, religious, political, or ideological.
- Rigidity in legislative and administrative provision, especially as related to rigid characterization of disability and categorical allocation of resources often not matched to individual needs.

- The discrepancy between what exists and our present knowledge of what should exist due to poor dissemination of knowledge.
- Special education in some countries is still perceived as a charitable venture—a welfare programme. Responsibility for special education does not always rest with educational authorities.
- The administrative and professional separation that continues to divide the educational community into 'special' and 'regular' components isolated from each other.

As the field of special education internationally continues to seek an appropriate way forward, there has recently emerged from within its own ranks a new set of voices arguing for further reform. Once again these voices reflect developments in different parts of the world. While inevitably they are not in full agreement with respect to their analysis and recommendations, they all adopt a critical perspective, seeking to question the field's theories and assumptions. Examples of writers sharing this perspective include in England, Tomlinson (1982); in Papua New Guinea, Carrier (1983); in Australia, Fulcher (1989); in New Zealand, Ballard (1990); and in the United States, Skrtic (1991). They all draw on theories from fields outside of special education, such as sociology, politics, philosophy and organizational analysis. Their work, and that of others adopting similar stances, offers a more radical analysis of the policy and practice of special education, pointing to new possibilities for reform.

One of their concerns is with the way in which pupils within schools come to be designated as having special needs. They see this as a social process that needs to be continually challenged. More specifically they argue that the continued emphasis on explaining educational difficulties in terms of child-centred characteristics has the effect of preventing progress in the field. The argument is summed up by Dyson (1990) who states: 'The fact remains that the education system as a whole, and the vast majority of institutions and teachers within it, are approaching the twenty-first century with a view of special needs the same as that with which their counterparts approached the present century. That view, for all its avowed concern for the individual child, promotes injustice on a massive scale. It demands to be changed.'

This radical perspective leads to a reconceptualization of the special needs task (Ainscow 1991). This suggests that progress in the field depends on a general recognition that difficulties experienced by pupils come about as a result of the way schools are organized and the forms of teaching that are provided. In other words, as Skrtic (1991) puts it, students with special needs are artefacts of the traditional curriculum.

This new perspective on the special needs task is the one that has been adopted and developed in the Unesco teacher education project *Special Needs in the Classroom*. It is based on the view that the way forward must be to reform schools in ways that will make them respond positively to pupil diversity, seeing individual differences as something to be nurtured and celebrated. Within such a conceptualization, a consideration of difficulties experienced by pupils and teachers can provide an agenda for reform and, indeed, insights as to how this might be accomplished.

However, this kind of approach is only possible in schools where there exists a respect for individuality and a culture of collaboration that encourages and supports problem solving. Such cultures are likely to facilitate the learning of *all* pupils and, alongside them, the professional learning of all teachers. Ultimately, therefore, this line of argument makes the case that increasing equity is the key to improvements in schooling for all.

The origins of the Unesco project

The initiative for the Unesco project grew out of its continuing work in encouraging member countries to develop strategies for responding to children's special needs in ordinary schools. A survey of 14 countries, commissioned by Unesco and carried out by a research team from the University of London (Bowman 1986), identified three major priorities for policy development. These were: (i) the provision of compulsory education for all children in the population; (ii) the integration of pupils with disabilities into ordinary schools; and (iii) the upgrading of teacher training as a means of achieving the first two priorities.

The findings of this survey were used as the basis of a series of regional workshops. An outcome of these events was that Unesco was urged to assist in the dissemination of teacher training materials that could be used to facilitate improvements with respect to meeting special needs in ordinary schools. It was also recommended that in carrying out this work, the following points should be kept in mind:

(1) The need to develop national policies for teacher education that progress in a continuous fashion from the pre-service stage through to the in-service stage.

(2) The importance of supervised practical experience as a major element of teacher education programmes.

(3) The importance of taking account of what has been referred to as the 'hidden population' of pupils with special needs. These are children who do not have significant disabilities but who nevertheless experience difficulties in learning. (The original survey, for example, indicated that up to 45 per cent of pupils repeated one or more grades in some countries, for a variety of reasons.)

(4) A necessity to increase flexibility of curriculum practice and teaching methods in mainstream classrooms in order to be more responsive to the needs of individual children.

(5) The principle of self-help, brought about by encouraging teachers to develop skills of self-evaluation.

(6) The importance of recognizing the value of collaboration among groups of teachers within a school.

(7) The need to help and encourage teachers to make better use of three sources of nonprofessional help in the classroom: the pupils themselves; the parents, relatives and others in the community; and paid ancillary help or teachers' aides.

The regional workshops also generated some more specific recommendations regarding the possible content of teacher education programmes.

Consequently in 1988 one of the present authors (M.A.) was invited to direct a project to be called *Special Needs in the Classroom*, which would aim to develop and disseminate a Resource Pack of education materials.

Clearly the design of suitable teacher education materials represented an enormous challenge. In particular there was the issue of how to produce a pack that could take account of such a wide range of national contexts, especially those in developing countries. This being the case a number of measures were taken during the formulation of the materials in an attempt to achieve a level of flexibility that could take account of diverse settings. These were as follows.

(1) Advisory teams consisting of teacher educators and teachers were created in different parts of the world. These teams provided comment on draft materials and contributed materials and ideas of their own for inclusion in the pack.

(2) A number of special educators and others involved in teacher development around the world read and commented upon draft materials.

(3) A pilot workshop for teachers and teacher educators from various African countries was held in Nairobi, Kenya in April 1989. This allowed various materials and approaches to be evaluated.

(4) Further trials were carried out in Turkey during September 1989.

(5) An international resource team was created to field-test and evaluate pilot materials. This team is now involved in the dissemination of the project materials.

The initial dissemination was, therefore, carried out in order to field-test a pilot version of the Resource Pack consisting of four modules of working materials, and, in so doing, to develop an international resource team which can be used to support the widening of the work of the project.

In April 1990 two coordinators from each of eight countries (Canada, Chile, India, Jordan, Kenya, Malta, Spain and Zimbabwe) took part in a two week workshop/seminar at the University of Zimbabwe. The group included university lecturers, educational administrators, teachers and one headteacher. The first week took the form of a demonstration workshop during which materials from the Resource Pack were used to conduct a series of course sessions for the coordinators and a further group of local teachers and student teachers. In the second week, the demonstrated workshop was evaluated during a seminar in which the international coordinators planned together the ways in which they would field-test the Resource Pack in their own countries.

The field-testing was completed by March 1991, and each team of coordinators prepared an evaluation report about their work. The main aim of the field-testing was to gather information which could be used to inform the further development of the Resource Pack and to plan its future dissemination. In this way, it was possible to develop the 16 coordinators into an international resource team who are now collaborating in the design and promotion of the overall project. Currently, dissemination initiatives are underway in a number of countries, including major national projects in China, India and Thailand.

In terms of evaluation, the central question was, 'How can the Resource Pack be developed and disseminated in a way that will be appropriate for teachers in different countries?' With this in mind, the evaluation was based on a multi-site case study approach (Miles and Huberman 1984) in which individual reports attempted to explain what happened as the resource materials were used in a particular context. Reports included interpretations of these events from the points of view of *all* participants. A particular interest, of course, was the ways in which the materials and ideas related to the social, cultural and educational tradition of each participating country (Miles 1989).

The evaluation data indicate that in all of the field-testing sites the materials were used as intended and that course leaders worked in ways which were largely consistent with the rationale of the project. The reports reflect a sense of acceptance and optimism about the approaches that were used. This was apparent even when coordinators were working in very difficult and stressful conditions, not least in Jordan where the field-testing took place during the period just prior to the outbreak of war.

Particular contextual factors created difficulties in certain places. For example, a number of coordinators reported hostility from certain of their colleagues who, it seems, were unhappy with the emphasis on group work used in the project. Some of the student teachers experienced negative reactions from experienced teachers when they attempted to reorganize classrooms in order to move away from more traditional organizational formats. Difficulties sometimes arose when the materials were used as part of school-based staff development programmes. Once again, negative reactions seemed to occur when approaches were introduced which appeared to challenge existing patterns of working.

It is also worth noting a significant trend that emerged with respect to the reactions of those teachers who had previously been exposed to specialized training in special education. There is some evidence in the evaluation data that members of this group experienced greater difficulty in accepting the value of the approaches used in the Resource Pack (Ainscow 1993a,b). It may well be that the dominant individualized focus within the special education community acts as a barrier to a consideration of broader, contextual responses.

Overall, however, the evidence supports the view that the content of the materials in the Resource Pack is appropriate for teachers in each of these national contexts, focusing on issues that they find meaningful and relevant. Furthermore it seems that the activities and processes used are successful in helping teacher educators and, in turn, teachers, to develop their thinking and practice (Ainscow 1993a,b).

As a result of this research the Resource Pack was rewritten. It now contains the following elements.

- *Study materials.* These include an extensive range of readings, stimulus sheets and classroom activities for use during course or workshop sessions.
- *Course Leaders' Guide.* This provides detailed guidance as to how to organize courses and facilitate sessions based on the study materials. A series of case studies describing projects that have been carried out in a number of countries is also included.
- *Training videos.* These include examples of the various recommended approaches in use during courses and film of follow-up activities in schools.

It is important to understand that the materials and activities in the pack encourage course leaders to model at the adult level strategies for teaching which take account of and, indeed, make positive use of student diversity. In this way the features of the pack that are seen as facilitating adult learning within course sessions are intended to be used as a basis for working with classes of children in schools.

The content of the materials emphasizes two main strategies for helping teachers to consider alternative perspectives to educational difficulty as a means of improving classroom practice. These are as follows.

(1) *Reflective enquiry.* Influenced by the writings of Donald Schon (1983, 1987), this is an approach to professional development that encourages practitioners to question taken-for-granted knowledge that is implicit in their actions.

(2) *Collaboration.* Here teachers are encouraged to use the resources of others around them (including colleagues and pupils) to support them as they reflect upon difficulties that arise in their classrooms.

Our attempts to introduce teacher educators and teachers to these two strategies are based upon five sets of approaches that have been developed and refined within the project (Ainscow 1993*a,b*). These are:

(1) *Active learning*: approaches that encourage participants to engage with opportunities for learning.

(2) *Negotiation of objectives*: approaches that enable teacher development activities to take account of the concerns and interests of individual participants.

(3) *Demonstration, practice and feedback*: approaches that model examples of practice, encourage their use in the classroom and incorporate opportunities for supportive feedback.

(4) Continuous evaluation: approaches that encourage enquiry and reflection as ways of reviewing learning.

(5) *Support*: approaches that help individuals to take risks.

Teams in over 30 countries have now used the Unesco Resource Pack as part of their teacher education activities. As they do so they are involved in further research that will contribute to the refinement and expansion of the ideas included in the materials.* In the next section we provide, as an example, an account of the developments currently going on in India.

The project in India

The use of the Resource Pack in India has to be seen alongside earlier initiatives. In particular, Project Integrated Education for the Disabled (PIED), begun in 1986, had included a teacher education element. This initiative, organized by the National Council of Education Research and Training (NCERT), had encouraged the enrolment of children with special needs in ordinary schools.

Although PIED was seen as a significant breakthrough in encouraging the participation of children with special needs, it had several limitations. First of all, despite the emphasis on integration, there was evidence that categorization and labelling continued. Associated with this was a tendency to withdraw children with special needs from certain activities. Second, while the enrolment of children with special needs in mainstream schools did increase, there was also evidence of a marked increase in the numbers of children already in school who were designated as having special needs. Third, despite efforts to make the teacher education component of PIED learner-centred, it continued to have a didactic emphasis. Finally, the design of the project meant that it seemed costly given the vast number of schools and teachers to be influenced.

*Readers wishing to have more information about the Unesco project *Special Needs in the Classroom* should contact Lena Saleh, Special Education Programme, Unesco, 7 Place de Fontenoy, 75700 Paris, France.

Following the involvement of NCERT in the field-testing of the Unesco Resource Pack, it was decided that the materials should be disseminated nationally through teacher education institutions. The first phase of this initiative is a multi-site action research project called *Effective Schools for All* which started in November 1991.

The project began with a training workshop held in Mysore in Southern India. 33 co-ordinators from 22 institutions (nine District Institutes of Education and Training (DIETs), eight Colleges of Education, three Schools and two non-government organizations) from different parts of the country attended the workshop. It was a mixed group of six heads of institutions, three teachers and 23 teacher educators. The selection of participants was done in such a way that two persons from each institution were invited for the training. This was done in order to promote mutual support and collaboration. It also helped in providing procedural and resource support. Some teams consisted of the head of the institution and a teacher educator or teacher, while others were represented by two teachers or teacher educators. In the case of the latter, care was taken to see that the head of the institution was informed about the policy of the Resource Pack material to ensure full support.

The training was based on the adaptation of the Unesco Resource Pack material carried out as a result of the feedback from the earlier international workshops and the learning experiences gathered from the pilot testing of the Resource Pack in pre- and in-service training in India (Jangira and Ahuja 1992). Four days were devoted to training the participants in the use of the Resource Pack strategies. This was followed by a day devoted to workshop debriefing. An opportunity for participants to practice with feedback followed. The last two days were devoted to planning and finalization of the action research projects to be carried out in each institution.

The training sessions helped participants reflect upon their own thinking and practice with respect to ways in which they respond to pupils' special educational needs. They also helped participants determine their own learning objectives within the general aim of the course and think about themselves as learners. In addition the sessions helped them to consider the integration of children with special needs and its influencing factors. Some sessions allowed rich discussions based on sharing different experiences on ways of effective teaching and meeting individual needs in the classroom. The participants were also encouraged to reflect on the nature of the support that is available in their settings and how they could develop a supporting network. In particular, they were asked to keep a learning journal in which they could record their experiences during this project.

Action research projects for the participating institutions were designed with a view to developing capabilities in teacher educators and institutions to encourage implementation of the innovative material and strategies, and to provide research evidence. The assumption was that these innovations, spread over a year and a half, would become a part of institutional practice. It was also hoped that the participants would evolve into 'change agents' to reform the teacher development process, thus making it responsive to how teaching can take account of *all* children in the classroom. Further, these institutions can be used to provide resource support to others in order to facilitate similar initiatives.

The action research followed a pre-test/post-test single group research design. School children and teachers were selected randomly. For trustworthiness of the research the importance of learning together and seeking collaboration were stressed. Participants were also asked to describe their methods and the context of the research. Caution was to be exercised before making conclusions. Data were to be reported with examples. The need to take into account different types of data from interviews, attitude scales, evaluation of proceedings, photographs, and audio and video tapes was emphasized. It was also stressed that there was a need to keep colleagues informed, design a short-term pilot, seek collaboration, be open to reactions, be self-critical, and have fun!

For the evaluation of the organization and management of the training workshop, participants used a daily evaluation sheet, participant questionnaire, group reports, course leader and participants' learning journals, and observations. Course leaders were also asked to note specific reactions to sessions using structured methods such as 'stance taking' and 'rounds', as recommended in the Resource Pack.

For evaluating the effectiveness of the workshop, measures were adopted to observe changes in the teaching behaviour of teachers, and in children's feelings about learning and teaching in the classroom. This was done using the following specially designed measures: (1) Attitude towards Teaching and Learning; (2) Pupil Participation in Learning Teaching Inventory; (3) Classroom Drawings (teachers and children); (4) Learning Preference Questionnaire.

Teachers were also asked to observe and note changes in their instructional behaviour, and the attendance, achievement and attention span of children after the follow-up exercises carried out in classrooms.

Progress so far

A three day project review meeting was organized in November 1992 to help participating teams share their experiences regarding planning, implementation and problems encountered. This also helped participants in considering pre-testing experiences, evaluation procedures, follow-up measures and a report writing format.

Then, in March 1993, a final evaluation conference took place. By that time almost all the institutions involved had finished their action research projects. Their work involved a total of 338 experienced teachers, 248 pre-service teachers, 9896 children and 115 schools.

In a few cases, rural areas had been included in the project. Some institutions had involved state government and local education department officials. School-based follow-up exercises had been planned and implemented. Some institutions obtained particularly encouraging results in teaching mathematics and science using the approach. The Resource Pack materials had been translated into a variety of languages. Photographs had been taken, and some project sites are planning video programmes. All had actively maintained learning and course journals in order to record their experiences.

The whole school approach used in two schools was particularly effective. In these two schools, teachers and heads were actively engaged in the action research activities. Recently one of them has been able to smoothly integrate blind children into its mainstream. A significant innovation while using the whole school approach has been the use of the Resource Pack materials without an external change agent. Here we have found that staff have been involved collaboratively without any intervention.

Comments from members of the project team engaged in training in- and pre-service teachers and in planning follow-up work with children in classrooms include the following:

'Initially pre-service teachers were unsure about planning a lesson. However, as they used the approach, planning became effective and enjoyable.' (DIET Wayanad Kerala)

'Most subjects can be taught using this approach.' (Amar Jyoti School, Delhi)

'The approach was found effective in teaching English. The method helped in generating a rich discussion. It resulted in intermingling of boys and girls in the class.' (DIET Rajinder Nagar, Delhi)

'Economical to teach with this approach. It reduces teachers' work load and results in better time management.' (Navjug School, Delhi)

'In situations where it was difficult to organize group work (fixed or heavy furniture), conducting sessions outside the classroom worked well.' (Seva-in-Action, Bangalore)

'This approach helps to make learning more enjoyable.' (DIET Sonitpur, Assam)

'For orientating the teacher training institute staff about the approach using the student teachers as models proved useful.' (Regional College of Education, Bhubaneshwar)

'Clearing administrative hurdles in stages helps to make the project a success.' (DIET Tirur, Tamil Nadu)

'When this approach is followed, initially there is a resistance from the students. However, over a period of time they accepted it.' (DIET Sonitpur, Assam)

A whole school approach

Our experience in many countries has been that the most effective use of the Unesco Resource Pack is as part of a whole school, staff development programme. To illustrate this argument we will describe as an example the work carried out by one school in India.

Navjug is a municipal primary school in New Delhi. It caters in the main for children of poor families, including some from slum dwellings. Over the last nine years the head-teacher, Mrs Uma Tomar, has developed it from a small school with nine staff to the present organization which has 27 teachers and caters for 640 pupils with an age range of 5–13 years. Class sizes are usually just over 40.

The school follows the NCERT syllabus, based on national policy (1986), but is unusual in that it has established a policy of flexible teaching approaches. Standards in the school are high with many pupils going on to secondary education, some gaining scholarships.

During the last 18 months or so Mrs Tomar and her staff have used the Unesco pack as the basis of a school-wide staff development initiative. All staff have participated in workshop sessions using materials from the pack, and have carried out follow-up exercises in their own classrooms. This project has been given considerable status, and large amounts of time have been allocated in order to support activities.

Visiting the school, it is clear to see the impact of these staff development activities. All the classrooms emphasize active learning approaches, with cooperative group work much in evidence. Pupils are frequently involved in role play and peer tutoring. Recently, particular emphasis has been placed on the idea of pupil involvement in assessment.

Specifically, pupils have been asked to take a much more active role in assessing one another's progress during formal examinations. This is remarkable given the rather rigid format of the examination papers. It has also led at times to some uncertain reactions from local education authority representatives.

Displayed around the main courtyard of the school are large, colourful posters, rather reminiscent of Chinese wall newspapers. These illustrate the work carried out by staff and, sometimes, pupils as a result of activities based on the Unesco Resource Pack. These posters take a variety of forms. All tend to use wording taken from the pack (*e.g.* active learning, parents as partners), and many include pieces of writing produced by individual teachers. Some are accounts of classroom activities carried out and case studies of work with particular pupils.

Talking with staff, one is struck by the impact of the many staff development experiences they have shared. Enthusiasm is evident for the ideas they have explored, and they talk with obvious delight of the reforms they have made in their own classroom practices. A particular area of enthusiasm is for the idea of collaboration. The teachers explain how they have learned to work in teams as a result of exercises using the Resource Pack. These teams plan together, teach together and help one another in problem solving. Staff recall that at the outset they found collaboration difficult and that they needed strong leadership. Now, however, this is not necessary, and as one teacher noted, 'at the end we were *all* leaders.'

Good use has been made of the idea of partnership teaching (*i.e.* two teachers working in one classroom) in order that colleagues can assist one another in developing aspects of their practice. To make this happen, of course, organizational sacrifices have to be made. So, for example, the headteacher will herself provide cover by taking classes in order to release teachers. Sometimes classes will be taught together. Staff also make similar arrangements in order to release one another to attend courses and workshops.

A further area of collaboration in the school involves non-teaching personnel (*e.g.* general helpers, drivers). All of these colleagues are seen as making a contribution to the creation of flexible conditions that will enable all pupils to succeed in their learning. Indeed, they are seen as being essential members of the overall staff team.

The impact of all these developments on pupils' outcomes is clearly evident. Academic standards are high, and the social atmosphere is warm and relaxed. A strong emphasis is placed on nurturing and celebrating individuality. With this in mind, attempts are made to provide a broad curriculum within which different forms of achievement can be recognized. Within this diverse environment some children with significant disabilities are fully included.

The evidence of this school indicates that the Unesco Resource Pack can make a significant contribution to wider school improvement initiatives. Clearly the emphasis on team work that the pack encourages has been turned to significant advantage at Navjug School. However, it has to be recognized that other organizational variables, such as effective management, are also at work. Indeed, Navjug seems to illustrate all of the features noted in the research on effective schools (*e.g.* Stoll 1991). In this respect it demonstrates that a school that caters for individuality is, in fact, an effective school for all.

Lessons learnt

On the whole it seems that teachers and student teachers have few reservations in meeting special needs, if they are provided with appropriate training and support. The materials and the process encourage them to be more reflective and better problem solvers, not only for meeting the special needs of all children but also for professional tasks relating to teaching and school organization in general. It has also activated and motivated teachers and pupils to learn and take responsibility for their own learning. Writing a learning journal, reflecting on it and sharing with others seems to make teachers professionally alive. This develops reflection and the problem solving capabilities of teachers, thus improving their effectiveness. Teachers also learn the utility of collaborative work in teaching and organization of schools.

We have also found that the same spirit of collaboration is passed on to the pupils. Encouraging independence in learning in students and teachers develops initiative in both. Teachers also realize that even within the rigidity of the Indian school system, reasonable autonomy in curriculum transaction can exist.

The multi-site action research project is turning out to be a good reflective and innovative approach to teacher development. As such it is leading us to new insights. It is also developing the insights of the participating teachers and teacher educators. In the process, a dozen resource persons who can provide effective training using the Resource Pack strategies, and design and implementation of similar action research projects, have been identified. The institutions involved have been used as resource centres for further work in about 200 DIETs during 1993–94. Rich material well adapted to a variety of contexts in the country is being developed. New material applied to the teaching of school and teacher training syllabuses is a significant contribution.

It is expected that gradually this approach will be applied in all 400 DIETs in order to make these an integral component of teacher development in nationally and internationally funded education for all projects.

Concluding remarks

In this chapter we have explored the international situation with respect to the education of children with special needs. While noting that the situation in many countries in both the developed and developing countries is a cause for considerable concern, we have also argued that relatively small changes in the practice of ordinary schools can make a significant impact. In this respect we believe that some reforms of pre-service and in-service teacher education could be a major contribution to such developments. As we have noted, however, such reforms do challenge existing arrangements and practices.

REFERENCES

Ainscow, M. (1990) 'Special Needs in the Classroom: the development of a teacher education resource pack.' *International Journal of Special Education*, **5**, 13–20.
—— (Ed.) (1991) *Effective Schools for All.* London: Fulton; Baltimore: Paul H. Brookes.
—— (1993a) 'Teacher education as a strategy for developing inclusive schools.' *In:* Slee, R. (Ed.) *The Politics of Integration.* London: Falmer, pp. 201–218.
—— (1993b) 'Teacher development and special needs: some lessons from the Unesco project "Special Needs

in the Classroom".' *In*: Mittler, P., Brouillette, R., Harris, D. (Eds.) *World Yearbook of Education 1993: Special Needs Education.* London: Kogan Page, pp. 238–251.

Ballard, K.D. (1990) 'Special education in New Zealand: disability, politics and empowerment.' *International Journal of Disability, Development and Education*, **37**, 109–124.

Bowman, I. (1986) 'Teacher training and the integration of handicapped pupils: some findings from a fourteen nation Unesco study.' *European Journal of Special Needs Education*, **1**, 29–38.

Carrier, J.G. (1983) 'Masking the social in educational knowledge: the case of learning disability theory.' *American Journal of Sociology*, **88**, 948–974.

Dyson, A. (1990) 'Special educational needs and the concept of change.' *Oxford Review of Education*, **16**, 55–66.

Fulcher, S. (1989) *Disabling Policies? A Comparative Approach to Education Policy and Disability.* London: Falmer.

Hegarty, S. (1990) *Educating Children and Young People with Disabilities: Principles and the Review of Practice.* Paris: Unesco.

Jangira, N.K., Ahuja, A. (1992) *Effective Teacher Training: Cooperative Learning Based Approach.* New Delhi: National Publishing House.

Lipsky, D.K., Gartner, A. (1989) *Beyond Separate Education: Quality Education for All.* Baltimore: Paul H. Brookes.

Miles, M. (1989) 'The role of special education in information based rehabilitation.' *International Journal of Special Education*, **4**, 111–118.

Miles, M.B., Huberman, A.M. (1984) *Qualitative Data Analysis.* Beverley Hills: Sage.

Mittler, P. (1993) 'Childhood disability: a global challenge.' *In:* Mittler, P., Brouillette, R., Harris, D. (Eds.) *World Yearbook of Education 1993: Special Needs Education.* London: Kogan Page, pp. 3–15.

Pijl, S.J., Meijer, C.J.W. (1991) 'Does integration count for much? An analysis of the practices of integration in eight countries.' *European Journal of Special Needs Education*, **6**, 100–111.

Ross, D.H. (1988) *Educating Handicapped Young People in Eastern and Southern Africa.* Paris: Unesco.

Schon, D.A. (1983) *The Reflective Practitioner.* New York: Basic Books.

—— (1987) *Educating the Reflective Practitioner.* San Francisco: Jossey–Bass.

Skrtic, T.M. (1991) 'Students with special educational needs: artifacts of the traditional curriculum.' *In:* Ainscow, M. (Ed.) *Effective Schools for All.* London: Fulton, pp. 20–42.

Stoll, L. (1991) 'School effectiveness in action: supporting growth in schools and classrooms.' *In:* Ainscow, M. (Ed.) *Effective Schools for All.* London: Fulton, pp. 68–91.

Tomlinson, S. (1982) *The Sociology of Special Education.* London: Routledge.

Unesco (1988*a*) *Unesco Consultation on Special Education: Final Report.* Paris: Unesco.

—— (1988*b*) *Review of the Present Situation in Special Education.* Paris: Unesco.

—— (1993) *Education for All: Status and Trends.* Paris: Unesco.

Werner, D. (1987) *Disabled Village Children: a Guide for Community Health Workers, Rehabilitation Workers and Families.* Palo Alto, CA: Hesperian Foundation.

10
EDUCATION: THE EXPERIENCE OF THE KARNATAKA PARENTS' ASSOCIATION

Michael P.A. Mathias

The founders of the Karnataka Parents' Association for Mentally Retarded Citizens (KPAMRC) decided at its inception that it would follow the path of being a facilitator, a catalyst, to promote the growth of an expanding infrastructure to cater to the needs of persons with mental retardation. They decided that it would be a grass-roots movement, with its community of parents sowing the seeds of growth. KPAMRC has therefore never asked for, nor obtained, government funding. Perhaps the one singular characteristic of KPAMRC that distinguishes it from many other non-governmental organizations has been its positive intent not to become institutionalized. It runs no school to show as an edifice of its mission. It has no tangible assets in the form of land or buildings. It has no plush office with all the trimmings that go with it. Consequently, it has no bludgeoning overhead expenditure that could in time threaten its very existence.

KPAMRC has always maintained itself and ensured its growth through its members, its friends and the community. Consequently, it has always moved in the direction of involving the community, by establishing and spreading its roots in the community, and by drawing on and developing the resources of the community. There has been a continuous cycling of this process, with each cycle witnessing a resultant enlargement of its activities.

The common cause

From its inception, KPAMRC has worked together with other disability groups to formulate a joint approach towards ensuring the rights to education of people with disabilities. The methodology for educating children with various categories and levels of disability will vary, but the right to education is common. The terms of reference for the joint working also included the rights of these children to receive education based on the principle of 'normalization', that no child with disability should be distanced from a 'normal school environment', and that 'integrated education' in all its manifestations would be a goal to be achieved.

For some years this initiative received a very limited response. In October 1984, however, the government of India prepared a document entitled *Challenge of Education— a Policy Perspective*, aiming to meet the demands of the rapidly changing environment. It threw the document open to public debate. There were no provisions envisaged to meet the educational needs of children with disabilities. The document portrayed people with disabilities at the lowest spectrum of humanity, and it made references to the voluntary sector that were not in good taste. All this stirred the voluntary sector into action, and brought them together. Four principal organizations representing the physically impaired, the hearing impaired, the visually impaired, and KPAMRC came together under a banner called 'The Common Trust'. Through organizing a workshop for the four Southern States of India, with those attending including quite a few government personnel, and through a subsequent consultation exercise, a section on education for children with disability was included in the National Policy on Education (1986).

The educational system

Perhaps we should start by defining the term 'education'. Mahatma Gandhi said, 'By education, I mean an all-round drawing out of the best in child and man—body, mind and spirit.' We are thus led to believe that any form of education, if done well, be it formal or informal, whether it is done in a regular school, a special school or in an integrated system, will help in the integration of the child not only within her or himself, but also within the mainstream of the community and society at large.

We must consider the conditions prevailing in the educational system at large in India before attempting to find solutions to the problems being faced by the community of persons with disability:

- The number of children in a classroom could range from 50 to as much as 100. In many parts of rural India primary schools have just one teacher.
- Regular teachers are not given any information on the needs of special children. Even aspects concerning specific learning disability are new to them.
- We know today that 20–25 per cent of so-called 'normal' children studying in the educational mainstream have special needs. Our teachers are ill-equipped to deal with slow learners or those with emotional problems, with the result that children are thrown out of the educational system through no fault of their own.
- In addition, children come from vastly different backgrounds of culture, religion, language, and so on. They find it extremely difficult to adapt to a system that is not flexible enough to cater to their needs. Generally, everything is taught by rote, compounding the problem further. We do, however, see the beginning of change in this regard, particularly in urban areas.
- Primary education suffers from a want of adequate funding and political commitment. On the other hand, higher education is subsidized to the detriment of the vital area of primary education.
- Creating further confusion, each State in the country is fighting for education in its own regional language.

Integrated education

It is not fair to see special education versus integrated education as a polarized issue. Special education is an educational process of specially designed instruction to meet the unique needs of special children. The integrated education system should automatically take into account the principles of special education, depending on the individual needs of the child. The classical model of integrated education, where the child with a disability studies alongside her or his non-disabled peers, is an extremely difficult system to implement effectively. This is particularly the case in developing countries, where adequate support systems are not available. Therefore, we should consider more than just one model of integrated education.

KPAMRC has propounded the 'add-on principle'. This principle speaks of adding-on to an already existing facility, a facility for people with disabilities. This principle was first actively used in the attempt to promote more centres for special education. The case was made for a number of small special schools ('opportunity schools') to be integrated with schools for normal children scattered over Bangalore (the capital of Karnataka State). To have the special school in the same campus would ensure interaction between the children. Children with developmental disabilities, like all children, need to be accepted and to mix socially. Children without disabilities also benefit greatly, through learning to understand children who are less able than themselves.

Another reason for having small special schools throughout the city was the need to cater to the various communities, some of which showed very diverse ethnicity. Children with developmental disabilities cannot adjust to change easily and need an environment as unchanging and stable as possible, with the school environment being an extension of the home environment and vice versa. Therefore, it was imperative that special schools be started within each small vicinity, where it might generally be assumed that living habits, cultural habits, language and attitudes would be fairly consistent among the children.

The concept of opportunity schools has evolved over time, and is more easily understood as the term 'parallel education stream'. Thus, two schools are on the same campus, governed by the same management. In rural areas, a 'resource room' model, located in one school, or serving a cluster of schools, may achieve the same goals. Apart from the subjects dealt with in the parallel education stream, integration is sought through common transport, a common assembly, school day, sports day and other activities.

Those in charge of special schools often feel rather alarmed by these models of integrated education. Perhaps these schools could convert themselves into resource centres, particularly for early education, attending to the needs of young children with disability, to train parents and to bring children to a state of readiness to enter into integrated or parallel education.

Systematic planning is the essence of what could and should be done. The parallel stream should be adopted by clusters of good regular schools. Each school should be given the option of choosing to accomodate any one particular disability. They would then add this facility onto their existing infrastructure.

Support of various types will be needed. For example, children with hearing impairments require hearing aids and other equipment. Children with visual impairments require a host of aids in the form of talking books, books in braille, etc., and training in orientation and mobility. Those with locomotor impairments require prosthetic aids, and schools must be fully accessible to those with mobility problems. In developing countries, funds may not be available for the construction of ramps and escalators for access to upper storeys of a school building. An alternative could be found in rotating classrooms at ground level.

The add-on principle also applies to teacher training. The teachers and other staff in schools serving children with disabilities require training. Good educational colleges have been imparting training in education for many years in various disciplines. They now need to add on the facility of training teachers in special education as well. In addition, India has many medical institutions and engineering colleges throughout the country. These institutions could be considered as centres for the manufacture of aids and appliances, and for the training of relevant resource personnel. Again the add-on principle applies; resources are available, but need to be seen as resources that can be utilized for people with disabilities.

The underlying principle of the add-on process is to use the existing infrastructure wherever possible, rather than attempt to create resources from scratch. Developing countries cannot afford to do this, and neither is it advisable from the point of view of integration.

Teacher training

KPAMRC early on embarked on a teacher training programme for children with developmental disabilities. The fact that an association of parents decided to venture in this direction took most people by surprise, especially because it had entered a field that was considered the sole and private domain of 'experts' and the 'medical profession', and also because it would entail building an infrastructure from scratch. KPAMRC has trained an average of 17 teachers per year over a period of 14 years. Most of the teachers in the various schools offering special education in Karnataka State have been trained by KPAMRC. Links between past students and KPAMRC have been maintained over the years: we have always viewed them as a precious resource and keep in contact with them through a newsletter. The trainee teachers are spread over eight schools for practice teaching, with great commitment of the principals and staff of these schools. Theory classes are held in the afternoon in one such designated school. Except for incidental expenses and staff salaries, all services are given free by the community of schools and their staff.

KPAMRC has recently embarked on other programmes for training personnel, including one for teachers in the field of 'Learning Disabilities and Integrated Education'. The focus of this programme is to create expertise in the screening, diagnosis and remedial teaching of children with specific learning disabilities. Many of these children are presently in schools for special education of children with developmental disabilities, but should be studying in the regular educational stream and be integrated into regular classrooms with resource teacher support. There is also a programme of in-service training for teachers in regular schools in Bangalore. Two new training programmes commenced in 1990–91, the first to train teachers in 'Early Intervention for Children with Developmental Disabilities', and the second in 'Autism and Behaviour Modification'.

Conditions for implementation

The background realities prevailing in India and other developing countries have been enumerated, and a model for integrated education for children from all categories and degrees of disability presented. However, a great number of pre-conditions need to be met before implementation becomes a reality.

The thrust should cover all children with special needs, irrespective of category and degree. This includes those with developmental disability, those with sensory and locomotor impairments, those who have a specific learning disability, and those who are emotionally disturbed. A tall order perhaps, but unless we view the problem in totality nothing much can be achieved.

Assessments should be done from a functional point of view. Children with developmental disability should not be assessed on the basis of IQ, which is outmoded and has absolutely no relevance. It is only from functional assessments that Individual Educational Plans can be formulated (see Chapter 8).

Emphasis should be placed on the inclusion of special educational methods into the curricula for regular teachers, to cater to the 20–25 per cent of children with special needs in regular classrooms.

Teachers should be trained in larger numbers in the various disciplines of special education. The Unesco model of training the 'multi-category teacher' in one academic year, a teacher capable of teaching children drawn from all categories and degrees of disability, seems mainly to be a way forward where services are very underdeveloped. The experience of KPAMRC is that special education introduces concepts that are highly abstract in nature, and that trainees undertaking a training programme for teaching children with developmental disabilities take a full year to acquire even a basic working knowledge. Even this duration is insufficient.

We find in India that regular teachers who graduated many years ago have not kept abreast of modern teaching methods in their field. Teachers can never truly teach unless they are continuously learning themselves. As Rabindranath Tagore once said, 'A lamp can never light another lamp unless it continues to burn its own flame.' The same problem exists when it comes to teachers trained in special education. We see a vast difference between those trained a decade ago to those trained in the very recent past. The content of training programmes has improved greatly, based on current perceptions of what needs to be taught and put into practice. Teachers trained previously should be obliged to update their knowledge and to have refresher courses every three years or so, to renew their certificate of competency as teachers. This should particularly be the case when it pertains to special education.

Finally, it is imperative that all disability groups work together. They can learn from one another. They need to work in partnership with one another, in mutual trust and understanding. For long enough, the problems faced by people with disabilities have been viewed from a narrow perspective by individual disability groups, particularly in developing countries where resources both human and financial are extremely limited. The only sensible approach is to present a common front to government and other agencies. The past has shown us that, when individual groups approach government and other agencies, services become skewed in favour of one disability at the cost of another. This should be avoided especially where resources are limited, making it all the more imperative for these resources to be put to optimum use. In addition, it has been suggested that one in every ten persons in developing countries suffers from some form of impairment. Can we afford not to consider a joint approach to the situation?

'Together we can, holding in common the rights of persons with disability'—this should be our motto.

11
DISABILITY PROGRAMMES IN THE COMMUNITY

Gautam Chaudhury, Kalyani Menon-Sen and Pam Zinkin

Community-based rehabilitation (CBR) has been promoted over the past decade as the best way to meet the needs of disabled people in developing countries and to enable their social integration. It has been thought of as the best and most cost-effective way of helping the majority of disabled children and adults who at present receive little medical or social attention, and as a solution to a lack of suitably qualified and trained personnel and material resources.

What is CBR?
Protagonists insist that there is only one CBR but, in practice, there are many interpretations of the term and programmes vary considerably. Although the issues are important, discussion of the 'correct' definition is not fruitful and will not be entered into here. Instead, different programmes for disabled children will be described and some underlying assumptions discussed.

Community-based *vs* institution-based rehabilitation
Traditional societies have not created residential institutions (old people's homes, hostels for disabled people, long-stay psychiatric hospitals and so on) the way developed countries have. Those that do exist traditionally are religious institutions, such as Buddhist monasteries or Koranic schools.

However, in developing countries most services for disabled adults and children have been planned and delivered by Western-influenced professionals in hospitals, urban rehabilitation centres and special schools. Such institution-based rehabilitation has been able to reach only about 5 per cent of the children with impairments, mainly from the urban elite. Forty years after Independence in India, 95 per cent of blind children were not receiving appropriate education (Cutinha, personal communication 1990). Disabled children in rural areas are often not reached at all (Mia *et al.* 1981, Unesco 1988).

Children in both developed and developing countries who attend residential special schools have serious problems in re-integrating back into the mainstream of their communities, in spite of possible academic advantage. These difficulties in re-integration are especially important for children in developing countries, since institutions have several problems, including: (i) they are usually far from the family home, with inadequate and expensive transport precluding frequent family contact, especially for the poorest families; (ii) the positive benefits of peer group solidarity are lost once the child leaves residential school, as contact between distant communities is impracticable; (iii) the material standard of living to which the child becomes accustomed is often higher than that of the family or community; (iv) the methods of communication for deaf or blind children are not shared with or taught to the family or neighbours; (v) the children have not learned important living and social skills according to the traditional ways of their community.

There are ongoing discussions in developed and developing countries about the meaning and practice of integrated schooling (*e.g.* Miles 1985*a*, Hegarty 1993). In developing countries the organization of schools and current teaching methods remain inappropriate for children with impairments and work against their integration into mainstream schools or society. Separate classes, separate schools and in some cases even residential schools may be needed, but the trend is generally toward integration within the ideology of equalization of opportunities. Integration is *not* just physical presence, but implies that the child with the impairment can profit from the lessons and the school's social life. This in turn means modifying teaching and the learning environment so that the child with an impairment can also learn (see Chapter 9).

In countries with few resources the high proportion of a residential institution's budget which is used for non-educational aspects, such as building maintenance, paying cooks, laundry workers, gardeners, care staff, security guards, etc.—costs born by the home—must be questioned. In addition, experience from many countries suggests that sexual abuse is common in institutions, especially those for intellectually impaired and profoundly deaf children (Sobsey and Mansell 1990, Sobsey 1994).

Even where some institution-based help has been given, a typical outcome is described in the following case history (Williams and Williams 1993).

Alice lives in a rural area of the Solomon Islands about 100 km from the capital. She is the youngest of five children. Alice was detected by a medical team in 1987 when she was 4 years old. She had had poliomyelitis, both lower limbs were weak and wasted, and she could not walk. She crawled on the ground. After detection Alice was taken to a hospital in the capital for possible treatment and rehabilitation. After some months she was able to stand and could walk with a walker. She was then sent home with a walker donated to her by the Red Cross. The expectation was that she would walk unaided if she continued with exercises and physiotherapy at home.

Unfortunately, she was not given any physiotherapy and exercises although she used the walker to walk around the village. Able-bodied children from other families in the village were not taught how to behave toward a child like Alice. Every time they saw her using the walker they stared and laughed at her. They criticized and made fun of her. Boys joked with each other and said 'Hi! she's your wife, your wife!' Sometimes they quarrelled with her and said 'You polio! polio! polio! small leg!' and so on. Adults gossiped and said 'It's a curse from God because her parents didn't go to Church.'

All these unkind and negative attitudes toward disability caused great problems for Alice in walking around the village. Her parents were ashamed of her and would not allow her out of the house. The contractures developed further in her legs and she became unable to stand and once again reverted to crawling.

There was no follow-up from the medical team. Transport was difficult and expensive, and Alice's parents could not afford to take her back to hospital.

Clearly, a new approach, which takes the life of the disabled person in her/his own community into account is essential. Outreach services would not have solved Alice's difficulties, and hence a radical reorganization of services is required away from institutional care to a community-based approach in which professionals share their skills with disabled people, community workers and parents (Helander 1993).

Examples of CBR programmes
CBR programmes have begun in different ways but continue to evolve. The examples that follow have been chosen to illustrate lessons that people have learned as they went along. The learning process is demonstrated in greater detail later in this chapter in the children's stories and descriptions from the SANCHAR project, in which the first two co-authors of this chapter work. Many other CBR approaches and programmes in developing countries are described elsewhere (*e.g.* Thorburn and Marfo 1990, Save The Children Fund 1994).

1. World Health Organization (WHO)
WHO (Helander *et al.* 1989) described CBR as:

'. . a term used for situations where resources for rehabilitation are available in the community. There is a large-scale transfer of knowledge about disabilities and of skills in rehabilitation to the people with disabilities, their families, and members of the community. There is also community involvement in the planning, decision-making, and evaluation of the programme.'

Later a joint position paper from the International Labour Organization (ILO), Unesco and WHO (1994) defined the two essential elements of CBR:

'Community-based rehabilitation is a strategy within community development for the rehabilitation, equalization of opportunities and social integration of all people with disabilities.
'CBR is implemented through the combined efforts of disabled people themselves, their families and communities, and the appropriate health, education, vocational and social services.'

Much of the emphasis is on the community's responsibility to recognize the need for rehabilitation of their members who have impairments. Although it is accepted that 'community action for CBR is often initiated by a stimulus from outside the community, most likely from the ministry, committee or organization responsible for the programme', the paper states that 'it is the community which decides whether CBR will become part of its ongoing development activities.' While acknowledging that support from outside the community should be available, the joint position paper also states that 'there should be no support to the community unless it is willing to meet that need.'

   Pupulin (Chief Medical Officer, Rehabilitation at WHO) asserts that at community level CBR must mean that . .

'. . within their homes and communities, children and adults with disabilities have the opportunities to receive training for functional activities, including self care, mobility and communication; to have an education; and to work in the most productive way possible either within or outside the household.'

These opportunities occur in the community only if disabled people themselves, their families and other community members are active in the rehabilitation process (Pupulin 1992).

   The WHO programme is based on the manual *Training in the Community for People with Disabilities* (Helander *et al.* 1989) which consists of 30 training packages dealing with all aspects of impairment, and a set of four guides for use at community level by disabled people, teachers and a community rehabilitation committee. The manual is the fruit of experience and field testing, many experts having contributed to it. Its great merits are that (a) rehabilitation technology is demystified and made accessible, making the large scale transfer of professional knowledge and skills to disabled people, their families and CBR workers possible, and (b) conditions are classified simply as difficulties in function, *e.g.* a child with difficulty in hearing, an adult with difficulty in seeing, a person with strange behaviour, etc. Thus no medical or diagnostic knowledge is necessary before beginning rehabilitation. The manual has been criticized as being too rigid, prescriptive, and oversimplified (Miles 1985*a*, Jaffer and Jaffer 1990) but is defended on the grounds that technology should be standardized, although service delivery and management cannot be (Helander 1993). An excellent manual dealing with cerebral palsy, to accompany the original manual, has been produced (WHO 1993).

Typically, WHO programmes are integrated into primary health care (PHC). The community health worker (village health worker, family welfare educator or whatever name is used) is trained to carry out health tasks. In addition, CBR functions are taught using the manual as a technical tool. When criticized for taking a medical approach, WHO (Pupulin) explained that WHO's role should be mainly concerned with 'medical rehabilitation' directed toward alleviating the effects of the impairment, while collaborating with other agencies, such as education. Pupulin also states that, since the health sector may have personnel at the community level, it is often the most convenient service to promote rehabilitation, but this does not necessarily mean that it is the most important or only service.

Nevertheless, many CBR programmes have developed as 'one component of PHC' (Lundgren-Lindquist and Nordholm 1993), the work of CBR being integrated into the PHC workload. This has not always been successful for a variety of reasons, mainly that the infrastructure may be weak and many health workers are not oriented to rehabilitation, being more concerned with prevention and cure (Thorburn 1990).

2. Guyana Community Based Rehabilitation Programme
The Guyana project (O'Toole 1988*a,b*) began as a small local project, as an attempt to see if CBR was feasible in the Guyanese coastal community. Two groups of workers, volunteers and nursery teachers, were trained to work with young children and their parents. A home worker visited the child's home regularly, working with the child and parents, using an approach modified from Portage and the WHO manuals. The children's progress was examined using the Griffiths Mental Development Scales at six-monthly intervals. One of the main aspects of training was that, as many workers found learning from written materials difficult, local video material was developed. The emphasis was on practical training.

In Guyana the strong community spirit led to 100 volunteers applying for 25 places on a training course even though salary and travel costs were not paid. In the event, 30 were selected to take part in an 18 month experiment. After the 18 months, 28 of the original volunteers were left and of these 15 volunteered for a further period. In contrast, the use of the teachers was not effective. Although in theory they had time, as they only worked in the mornings, in practice they were not interested in the work. Later many teachers did become interested and volunteered, several becoming very active key workers and 'trainers' in the programme.

There were many successes, especially as far as the volunteers' work was concerned. It is important to appreciate that the volunteers were usually assigned to one or two families, in contrast with other projects where CBR workers commonly see many children. Most of the parents participated actively in the home programme although some found the role too demanding.

From the work of the volunteers, but not of the teachers, the community became involved and took responsibility for the CBR programme. O'Toole distinguishes the approach in the Guyana project from that of the WHO model, mainly with reference to the innovation package or manual. He suggests that the WHO method assumes that parents are waiting and eager for new ideas and if properly informed will change their behaviour. This approach does not acknowledge what the families are already doing, and may weaken local enthusiasm and creativity. In contrast, the goals in the Guyana project are focused 'on persons as the point of entry, rather than on goals and structures of the organisation. It is people who design, accept and implement changes' (O'Toole 1991).

The project began in a small way so that key aspects could be studied, and it receives substantial financial backing from an international organization. It is one of the few projects clearly to have addressed the question of costs. The cost per child was estimated at $48 per year in 1988, but O'Toole recognized that this did not include referral and estimated that the true cost of a CBR programme might be quite high. This may limit development, but at present barriers to expansion are organizational problems and lack of experience in running large programmes. The programme is currently being extended to a remote inland community, where a teacher, health worker and parent form a team. In these areas many local people thought that there were so few disabled children that the CBR programme should promote child development in general. This included reading and health education based on the Unicef 'Facts for Life' programme. Gradually the community realized that there were disabled children among them, and CBR has become the nucleus for development and for community activities. A change in government has meant that CBR is now being supported nationally although it will take time and careful planning before extending to all areas.

3. Uganda Community Development Assistant Programme

The Uganda National Programme began in three rural areas and reaches both adults and children (Department of Community Development 1992). The programme is based on the strength of the existing home care that the family give their disabled child. Although most parents of disabled children in Uganda care for their child themselves, they are not aware of what they can do to help the child. The programme gives additional training in disability to existing community development assistants (CDAs), whose general function in their area is to stimulate and support all aspects of that community's progress. Disabled adults, chosen by the disabled people's organization, train together with the CDAs but work mainly on community awareness and income generation. After an initial three weeks training, three months is spent back in their communities carrying out field work before returning with their own discovered needs for further training. The total course lasts six weeks. The Uganda programme has developed its own training material based on what the family is already doing and uses *Disabled Village Children* (Werner 1987; see p. 160) as a reference book. Following the training the CDAs work with children and adults with a range of impairments. The CDAs are able to teach parents simple techniques for helping their child with daily living activities, to make appropriate equipment from locally available resources, to liaise and work with disabled people, and to guide referrals. Initially, referrals have been mainly of children with club foot and cleft lip or palate, these being conditions that local medical services have the capacity to deal with, producing good results.

Since the CDAs' original training was concerned with promoting and assisting the whole community in all aspects related to the community's need for progress, they appear to have little difficulty with the concept of disabled children being integrated into school and all aspects of community life. However, many of the children have very severe impairments and need initial intensive help. In a few months CDAs have been able radically to transform the lives of many children.

Peter, a child with severe cerebral palsy, had for years been lying inside his mother's hut, unable to sit up or talk. The child was helped to sit in a corner seat, then in a chair with a table. He then managed to learn to walk between home-made parallel bars, and subsequently with crutches. All the equipment was made from locally available wood specifically for Peter, and there was no waiting list! He had quickly outgrown the first chair, but a second was made at once. After four months Peter was able to take himself to a latrine that had been made specially for him. He was learning to talk, and his family and their friends were learning to understand him. He was beginning to count and to recognize and name pictures drawn for him by the CDA. His mother had taught him to play a traditional harp and he accompanied other children while they sang.

A local health worker remarked that they had 'been waiting for him to die, but now he is a person.'

This programme envisages that some of the parents will take over the role of the CDAs to enable the latter to move on to help other children in their community.

Disabled people have taken on the task of raising community awareness. They have formed about ten cultural groups which have developed their own songs, poems and plays to entertain and educate local people. This activity is becoming so successful that it is now an income-generating as well as an awareness activity.

The programme is government-run but cooperates in all aspects with the National Union of Disabled People of Uganda (NUDIPO) and with non-governmental organizations (NGOs). It receives some financial support from an international NGO and will extend to more districts within the next year. NUDIPO does not have the resources to implement the programme, which it regards as a government responsibility (Msigye, personal communication 1993), but has consultative status, helps to determine policy, and has representatives both teaching on the course and having a fundamental role in evaluation.

4. Community Based Rehabilitation Alliance (Combra) (Uganda)
Most CBR programmes described are in rural areas. The Combra project is run entirely by

a local NGO in one of the poorest slums in Kampala, Uganda (Kangere, personal communication 1993). This is built on a swamp, subject to flooding, and homes are periodically washed away. The stagnant water, poor drainage and sanitation are responsible for a high incidence of malaria and diarrhoeal disease and there is a high prevalence of AIDS-related illness. There are many single parents and orphans, and other parents have to work in the city, leaving many young and disabled children in the care of their older siblings or grandparents.

The project is an association of disabled people, the elderly, their families, friends, the community and professionals. It was begun by committed Ugandans who were unpaid and who had no financial backing. Work is conducted in a tiny lock-up 'office' similar to the row of commercial stores alongside. There is only room for a chair, a small table and a bench. Posters and educational material line the walls.

Initially people from the community sought financial help from the project, but since the project received no foreign or government funding, they later asked only for advice and practical help. The team carried out home visits and held group discussions, and as their work became known they formed an association. The team found that the community were most concerned about two adult brothers who were aggressive and out of control. Through medical contacts the brothers were seen by a psychiatrist who visited once and prescribed treatment with psychotropic drugs. This has been maintained by the workers and has proved so effective that the brothers come of their own accord for treatment and are actually helping some of the old people by carrying water for them. This success was one of the factors which helped the team to be appreciated and gain acceptance in the community.

Another factor was the teams' recognition of the community's needs which were not directly related to disability. For example, many impoverished grandparents look after disabled and non-disabled grandchildren, since many of the parents were either killed in the war, or died from diseases, including AIDS. The team tried to improve the health status and the economic situation of grandparents. This was extremely difficult in a poor community where everyone is struggling to make a living. The first idea was a charcoal-vending cooperative project. None of the old people could keep accounts, so help was given by a community member. As the old people came to understand accounts and cash flow, they realized that they were not making a profit so they themselves worked out a maize buying and reselling scheme, which they predicted would be more profitable. A volunteer paediatrician helps with the old people's medical needs as well as seeing the children.

Care for disabled people in the community is 'home'-based, but the community members support and help each other. Day care is beginning once a week for intellectually impaired children in a small community centre, furnished only with mats. A teacher has agreed to spend a weekly session with the children.

A 9-year-old boy with athetoid cerebral palsy, who has learned English as well as his own local language, is trying to write with his foot, and would obviously benefit from educational help. His father died recently from an AIDS-related illness, and his mother and younger sister are HIV-positive. There is no money for special school fees and his needs cannot yet be accommodated in the overcrowded local school.

The government recognizes the value and experience of the programme. Its initiators help government staff in training programmes for the CDAs and in the participatory evaluation that government has carried out in its own scheme. It now has some financial backing for staff salaries from a US-based organization.

5. Project PROJIMO (Mexico)

Project PROJIMO (an acronym, also meaning 'neighbour' in Spanish) began in relation to a long-standing primary health care project in a rural community in a mountainous area of Mexico (Werner 1993). There were no doctors, and villagers chose health workers who took short training courses (Project PROJIMO, undated). When the training began, villagers often selected a disabled person because disabled people were more likely to be available. They were not usually involved in working in the fields and were often unmarried due to local prejudices. However, the villagers found that many disabled people made outstanding health workers with more empathy for those in trouble, attributable to their own experiences as disadvantaged persons.

Arising from the health programme's experience a programme was initiated, mainly by disabled villagers, concentrating on the needs of young physically disabled people. The project workers learned most of their skills through a hands-on, problem solving approach during short-term visits by rehabilitation professionals, many of whom were themselves disabled, and who willingly shared their skills. The team discovered the measures that were effective for each individual through a process of consultation, *as equals*, with that disabled person. They learned to make splints, callipers, wheelchairs, and so on. They built a 'model' home where wheelchair users were able to carry out all household activities. The difference between this ideal home and those often found in other centres is that it is based on the local village houses and the adaptations are all made from locally available material. Thus these adaptations can easily be copied in local houses.

The centre has developed particular skills in the rehabilitation of young people with spinal injury. Children with different impairments are brought for consultation or for short-term visits. They are attended by a team consisting mainly of disabled people.

The village-based rehabilitation centre *is* a centre, but it is fundamentally different from other centres in the following respects:
(1) The project is run by disabled people themselves, who, as a group, have rejected 'normalization' into a culture they regard as unjust. They see themselves as working toward a society which is more accepting of difference.
(2) Disabled people themselves take charge of their individual impairments.
   • They learn rehabilitation methods and skills from professionals, from traditional sources and through their own experience.
   • The underlying principles of treatment are that therapy is integrated into everyday life as far as possible and should be fun.
   • The conditions in the centre are similar to those found in local homes with locally appropriate adaptations.

An example of the approach is in the case of 'scissoring' in cerebral palsy. Whereas a specially manufactured 'corner' seat might be recommended by Western trained professionals and a simplified form of the same seat made using locally appropriate technology, in Project PROJIMO other ways would be looked for to achieve the same goal. These would be based on observing what children of the same age would be expected to do in the village culture. In other words, if the 'rehabilitation' aim is to keep the hips externally rotated and abducted, then, for example, such children could sit in a hole dug in the sand with their heels in holes, so that they could join other children outside, or could sit on a donkey in front of one or other parent. In the latter instance not only is the sitting position beneficial, but the child is also involved in a normal everyday activity (in the community) with her/his parent. This is not only cheaper and more readily available than a special seat, but also favours integration. This creative approach is one of the characteristics of the project.

In the PROJIMO project it was observed that disabled people and their families often found their own solutions to the difficulties of daily life without professional help. They were also able to show how disabled children can be integrated into families.

Helander (1993) considers that Project PROJIMO is complicated and 'medical'. However, the teaching material, which was produced in the form of a book (*Disabled Village Children*—Werner 1987), developed out of the practical experiences of the team members, the technical content being verified later by professionals. The project's declaration of principles states that 'simplified community based rehabilitation should be an essential part of primary health care everywhere.'

6. Samadhan (Delhi)

This project was initiated to help children with intellectual impairment, in the slums of Delhi (Balasundaram and Woods 1990). Basic assumptions underlying the project were that parents can be taught to train their own children and that a home-based learning intervention service can be delivered by minimally trained people. However, the attempt to introduce a modified Portage system into the children's homes ran into many difficulties, requiring radical revision of the material. There were problems, too, with the choice of volunteer worker. Initially the workers were from educated social groups, but the class and cultural divide was too great for their intervention with the families to be useful. In the second phase, young women who lived in the low income areas were recruited.

The difficulties met by CBR workers trying to introduce the modified Portage system into the homes of poor people in Delhi were often unrelated to 'rehabilitation' and included drunken husbands, mothers-in-law and over-curious neighbours. It was also found that many parents had to work, leaving the care of the child to an older sibling. Thus it seemed more appropriate to establish day centres for the children where care, stimulation and a meal were provided. The programme at the day centres also ran into difficulties. For example, an expatriate worker began toilet training but had not realized that there were no toilets at all in the slum.

The project leaders came to realize that the project and the community had to aim at complete social change rather than focus on disability. It was also realized that, within the slum communities themselves, the approach had to be different depending on the social, religious and cultural make-up of the particular community.

7. Los Hermanos de los Pepitos (Brothers and Sisters network—Nicaragua)*

Nicaraguan parents formed an organization, known as 'Los Pepitos', to help their children with cerebral palsy. Among the organization's many activities was a project involving brothers and sisters of disabled children, known as 'Los Hermanos de los Pepitos'. Its aim was to help the brothers and sisters to understand their sibling's impairment through workshops where they shared experiences and learnt about the impairment. They became involved with helping their disabled sibling at home, but also in raising awareness in school and in the community in general. This was done through a range of activities such as exchanges of sporting, leisure and cultural activities, *e.g.* birthday parties, camping trips, art groups, outings, athletic competitions and so on.

A pilot project which began in one of the districts of Managua, the capital, soon extended into other areas over four years. Other members of the family and of the community became involved, including school friends of the brothers and sisters, uncles, aunts, cousins and neighbours. Because of the wider involvement, the name of the project was changed to 'Youth Network'.

The aims of the network were to help in rehabilitation and integration of the disabled child, through promoting community awareness and supporting the struggle for the rights of disabled people. Members of the network took part in workshops and meetings run by other organizations working with children so that awareness of disabled children's needs and rights would spread to activities in these groups' domains. An example of this is their involvement in Child-to-Child programmes where groups of children work in health promotion and against violence and ill-treatment of disadvantaged children, such as 'street' children (see Chapter 15).

8. Action on Disability and Development (ADD–India)**

ADD–India is an independent NGO working in over 900 villages in southern India in cooperation with rural development organizations. These organizations include the Rural Development Trust, PREPARE (a local NGO working in social action and community health), and the Young India Project, which promotes action for the rights of poor people in rural areas (Coleridge 1993). ADD–India initiates the process by enabling such agencies to formulate policies which include development work with disabled people, to design a programme, to train their staff and to assist in networking, all within an agreed partnership.

ADD–India's work begins in a different way from most of the other programmes described and does not initiate services for disabled children. The basic philosophy is that disabled children should have the same things as all other children. ADD–India also believes that the needs of disabled people cannot be met by special services just for them since these create dependency. Instead disability issues should be built into every sector, be it banking, agriculture or government. Nothing should be separate for disabled people and existing structures should be used. The needs of disabled adults and disabled children should be met by each government ministry as appropriate and not by a special ministry.

---

*In part translated from a description by Juana Mercedes Delgado, January 1994, Managua.
**Derived from an interview with B. Venkatesh, Director of ADD–India, May 1994.

The role of professionals is to deal with the impairment, and disabled people themselves should decide whether suggested interventions will be useful for them.

Facilitators are trained to work in villages where the rural development organizations want to include disabled people in their work. The process begins with a detailed 'community analysis' of the political, economic and religious power structure of the community, the local pattern of disease, the local beliefs about such diseases, how the health centre functions, what is grown, the pattern of land distribution, how people spend their time and money, how money lenders operate, what credit facilities are available and what resources there are, both governmental and non-governmental, and so on. The information is gathered by talking to people in the community such as panchyat (rural council) leaders, teachers, shopkeepers and postal workers, and by observation, *e.g.* by sitting in the local liquor store to gauge its importance in the community. The findings are studied to see how social, economic and cultural factors affect the lives of disabled people in the community.

Information about disabled adults and children is collected as part of general information gathering, and thus the question of disabled people is raised as one of the topics of conversation in discussions. For example, when discussing the school or the balwadi (pre-school group), a question about the presence of disabled children is asked.

Community meetings are organized to debate issues which concern disabled people and to get community response and commitment to support the empowerment of disabled people. The field workers conduct these meetings involving disabled people as well as running poster campaigns through wall writing. Community members are invited to contribute money and materials to the organizations of disabled people (sangams) and to give disabled people the opportunity to train in agriculture, silkworm culture, and so on. The field workers also take classes on disability issues in village schools. As a result, non-disabled children take responsibility for bringing disabled children to school, assisting them in their studies and including them in play. A significant change is that disabled children are no longer called by the name of their impairment but are called by their own name.

Facilitators are trained to deal with many aspects of community development, and to understand the situation of disabled people in India and in the community in which they are working. One of the main training methods for facilitators is centred around stories of children with impairments: by asking 'Why did that happen?' and discussing the answer at each stage, the worker discovers the deeper causes of impairment and disability. Case studies of people with different impairments in different situations enable field workers to gain insights on the socio-political reality of disabled people in their families as well as perspectives on how disabled persons view themselves, their families and the outside world. The facilitators learn to use this 'but why' method with community groups.

It is only after this initial work of finding out about the community and being known in the community that the facilitators arrange meetings with groups of disabled people and parents. Before inviting disabled people to the first meeting, the field workers carry out detailed case studies of disabled people, establishing a one-to-one relationship with them. The case studies enable field workers to gain in-depth understanding of how disabled people live, what they cope with, how they feel about themselves, and how their family and the outside world views them. From these close relationships, the field workers grasp the root causes of disabled people's situations. Case work studies continue during the formation of the organizations. The next stage is usually to discuss individual problems as a group, but since sharing of experiences takes time, and initially their problems appear to have little in common, many people leave after the first meeting or so (many of these return later). Those that remain form a small organization or sangam.

The facilitators do not work *for* disabled people but help the group members to work together to analyse their problems, to find their own solutions, to be aware of their rights and to gain these rights through social action. ADD–India trains the groups in the field in management and administration, social analysis, communication and leadership skills. The aims of the groups are to enable disabled people to take action on their own behalf, and to use existing structures to secure benefits and services. ADD–India believes that struggles enable people to gain human dignity and create faith in themselves to bring about change in their own lives, however small that change might be.

The group members often perceive the attitudes of non-disabled people toward disabled people and of disabled people themselves to be a major problem. For example, Mira, who has cerebral palsy, was not accepted at the local school. Her mother was very, very poor but wanted her child to be literate. The sangam was just in the process of forming. Therefore the way this was dealt with at first was that the worker went to talk to the head teacher asking why Mira had not been accepted. The worker pointed out that there was no written rule by which the child could be excluded. The teacher thought that Mira would be a distraction to the other students and would need special attention. The worker said that they were not asking for special attention; the only thing that they asked for was that Mira should not be teased by the other children. The worker offered to help and used a Child-to-Child approach (see Chapter 15) to explain how hurtful teasing can be. As well as aiming to prevent teasing, the workers try to get the other children involved. One of the ways is for the non-disabled and disabled children to write plays and give puppet shows. Sometimes the children become activists in their community. Mira has settled into school and is now learning to read and write. Her mother is delighted, and is now one of the most active people in a strong sangam.

Another example of action by a sangam involves Ruma, who was begging outside the temple. The sangam members talked to her mother who explained that the family had to have the money that Ruma received in this way. She was reluctant but gave in to pressure and agreed to a trial of a different way of earning a living. The local women's group lent Ruma 200 rupees to start a very small shop. Ruma's mother became involved by being responsible for buying all the things needed for the shop. It is now making a small profit and Ruma's mother no longer sends her daughter begging.

The sangams deal with many different problems, and disabled people who left earlier often rejoin. The members begin to contribute a small agreed fee of, say, two rupees a month. This leads to working out how to keep accounts, how to open a bank account, what sort of leader is needed and many other organizational issues. The group find out what services are available locally and will help their members to use the services. For example, the sangam may pay fares, and a sangam member may accompany parents and their child to hospital appointments. The sangam would then help the family decide what treatments to accept.

The sangams have empowered themselves. They understand their situation and know what meets their needs; they can decide what they want from professionals. They are beginning to raise funds locally and to save. They have undertaken work for their villages on water, electricity, land and so on, sometimes taking the leading role in these common issues (see Chapter 15). Mira's mother said, 'What we want is not money. We want worldly wisdom. We want literacy. We should know more about the world. We must know how to help our children where we are.'

A note on industrialized countries

The 1994 joint position paper by ILO, Unesco and WHO (1994) points out that 'CBR is appropriate for both industrialized and developing countries. The broad methods used to implement it are applicable in either setting. However, the detailed methods of implementing CBR, and the resources available for it, will certainly vary among countries.'

For some years, the move in developed countries has been away from institutional care toward care in the community. Unfortunately, during this period of change there has not only been economic pressure, affecting poorer people and poorer communities, but also it has occurred at a time when government policies and practice encourage individualism. Many communities that existed, such as the mining communities, have been destroyed, and government actively encouraged people to leave their homes in search of employment elsewhere.

However welcome the move away from the medical model and from institutions has been, community care has led to a range of social and welfare interventions which do not necessarily lead to disabled people having more control over their lives. Since social and welfare service providers have a wider view than most medical people, it may actually lead to situations in which there are professionals and experts ready to advise and intervene in *every* area. 'The community worker [in Britain] is there to provide expert assessments and advice on nearly everything, from the architecture of the home, the whole range of equipment that all people need for modern living, to advice and counselling for intimate personal and sexual problems' (Finkelstein 1993*a*). Experts then see the lives of disabled people as a series of problems to be solved—by professionals—without changing the basic approach.

On the other hand, as residential hospitals for people with mental illness have closed, the financial resources and personnel have not been adequate to support people living in the community. 'Care in the community' in Britain often means home care by a woman on her own.

Primary health care

CBR is proving to have many of the same problems in interpretation and implementation as PHC. In international terms PHC is *not* family doctor based medical services, nor is it first contact care. PHC ideas were discussed and resolutions adopted at a meeting organized by WHO and Unicef at Alma Ata in 1978 (WHO and Unicef 1978). The goal was to achieve health for all people by the year 2000. 'Health for all' was defined as 'an acceptable level of health evenly distributed throughout the world's population.' It was recognized that improvements in health came about through economic, social and political changes and were not merely a result of medical services. PHC was the approach and process by which the goal could be achieved. PHC involved an integrated health sector (primary, secondary and tertiary care) involved with other sectors and with the community as a whole in the process of development. This process was seen as the key to attaining the goal as part of development and in the spirit of social justice. The *essential principles* of PHC were defined as:

(1) equity between and within countries;
(2) community participation;
(3) multisectoral collaboration.

PHC included promotion, prevention, curative care and rehabilitation. Eight *essential components* were listed:

- education concerning prevailing health problems and the methods of preventing and controlling them;
- promotion of food supply and proper nutrition;
- an adequate supply of safe water and basic sanitation;
- maternal and child health care;
- immunization against the major infectious diseases;
- prevention and control of locally endemic diseases;
- appropriate treatment of common diseases and injuries;
- provision of essential drugs.

After initial successes with the PHC approach in some projects and countries (Heggen-hougen 1984), the emphasis on economic adjustment programmes—largely determined by international monetary agencies and Western governments (Costello *et al.* 1994)—has forced cuts in government health spending and deterioration of health services in most poor countries. Thus PHC has been shifted away from its comprehensive base to separate programmes of selective technical measures, ignoring the basic principles (Newell 1988, Wisner 1988). Much of this shift was led by donor agencies whose need for measurable outcomes reinforced selectivity rather than steady comprehensive multisectoral development. *This makes selective primary care unlikely to be an effective base for disability programmes.* There are three underlying reasons for this.

First, equity, essential in CBR, is now rarely mentioned (Walt and Rifkin 1990). Health improvements depend on reaching those without access to resources necessary for health (not just medical services). A commitment to a redistribution of resources in Sri Lanka, China, Cuba and Costa Rica showed how health status improved without enormous financial resources (Rohde 1983). Over the past decade resource distribution has generally become more inequitable, with a widening gap between resources available in rich and poor countries and between rich and poor people within those countries (Hutton 1993). Rural and less influential populations, which include disabled people, have had diminishing access to services.

Second, community participation is often token and might include only 'patient compliance', 'mobilization' of the community in an aspect of a vertical programme such as immunization, and involvement in the selection of a volunteer village or community health worker (CHW). Broad participation implies a process of the community's active involvement in assessing its own health needs and, through its own health committee, control of the work and financing of CHWs (Bichman *et al.* 1989).

Recognizing the social determinants of disease, the CHW has been seen in some programmes as someone who would work with her/his community to deal with the root causes of ill health, as much as providing services (Werner 1981, Chabot and Bremmers 1988, Walt 1988).

Although there is diversity, CHWs are often volunteers who have undergone brief training and are seen as peripheral or at a 'lower' level of medical services. As such they are expected to deal with almost all the villagers' medical problems. They may be required to maintain themselves and their families or, alternatively, to be maintained by the community which selected them. The CHW's role in community participation is often confined to mobilizing the community to accept top-down planned 'health education' or immunization programmes, whereas most villagers want help for their immediate health problems. Although many poor communities can ill afford to maintain a health worker, the curative aspect of their work might be worthwhile if CHWs had adequate medical supplies and the backing of accessible and affordable referral services. These have rarely been available, and on the whole communities do not see PHC as effective (Walt 1988).

In any case, because of changes in land tenure and usage, migrant labour, urbanization and its consequences, and wars and conflict leading to large refugee and displaced populations, cohesive 'traditional' villages and communities may be disappearing.

The third factor concerns multisectoral collaboration. Although this has occurred in some places, and integrated rural development programmes often include health services, many plans are drawn up within 'PHC' programmes which ignore other sectors. For example, there are programmes promoting oral rehydration as a simple technological method of preventing deaths from dehydration caused by diarrhoea; however, without a comprehensive approach including water and sanitation (and soap) the incidence of diarrhoea remains unchanged.

There is an ongoing debate between those who do not envisage PHC being effective in dealing with the health problems of communities unless it is comprehensive and is based on the fundamental principles (Heggenhougen 1984, Wisner 1988), and those who suggest that in the present state of the world's economy, selective technical measures (such as immunization and oral rehydration) can be effective in reducing mortality (Walsh and Warren 1979, Cornia *et al.* 1987, Mosley 1988).

Although it is recognized by those working closely with children in developing countries that the state of the world's children has been threatened by the economic situation, and in particular by structural adjustment, the selective approach advocated has been challenged by those who see comprehensive primary health care as essential and possible even in the present climate (Segall and Vienonen 1987).

Given that CBR requires a wide range of services (not just in health), as well as changes in the environment and especially in attitudes of the community, of professionals and of authorities, it is obvious that basing it in selective PHC is unlikely to succeed.

The socio-economic determinants of *impairment* are similar to the determinants of disease and directly involve the whole community. PHC is appropriate to tackling problems at this level. However, the *disability* aspects of CBR require a focus on the community of disabled people and their families as well as a change in attitudes and a reorganization of the wider community, so that disabled people, one of the social groups of which it is composed, are taken into account.

What has become clearer over the decade is that CBR involves a social process that has to be reconsidered in the context of each country's and community's development; there is no quick cheap fix or universal solution. It cannot simply be added on as a centrally planned ninth component of PHC, alongside immunization or an essential drugs programme.

CBR is not second best

A community approach is not just a cheap alternative for developing countries. Whatever the present shortcomings due to political and economic considerations, major changes toward community care in Britain have come about in the past two decades or so largely through the disabled people's movement and parents' organizations. Disabled people themselves have explained how the present way in which society is organized 'disables' people with impairments—a social model, or construct, of disability (Oliver 1990).

Resources

Although some communities have shown a great capacity to mobilize resources from within the community, the premise that communities are always able to take responsibility for their disabled people ignores the real situation of many communities. It also fails to analyse preventable and social causes of impairment and to recognize that responsibility lies not only with the community but also with national and international policies and structures.

Doctors and other professionals often try to erase economic conditions and power relationships from their deliberations. It is assumed that there are scientific truths which are above these issues, or have nothing to do with them. Nonetheless, economic factors cannot be ignored when discussing community programmes for children. This is particularly so when parents, especially mothers, are expected to take on added responsibilities for care, education and therapy. In addition, communities are required to draw on their own resources and be self-reliant in almost every field—water supplies, health programmes, so-called income generation and so on. This is happening at a time when the economic and social forces are putting stress on communities and causing them to break up.

It is difficult to see how communities as poor as those of the Kampala and Delhi slums could be more 'responsible' or economically self-sustaining in respect of CBR as well as all the other programmes they are now expected to maintain, unless a more equitable distribution of resources were part of the agenda.

Where people's main concern is the right to eat, economic considerations apparently take priority. However, there is no evidence that economic advancement alone, without social change, leads to improvement in the life of disabled people or of other marginalized social groups.

Disabled people are often better integrated into communities in developing countries than they are in the more individualistic societies of the West, although their social status is usually low. Even in poor countries, removal of barriers can occur where the will and imagination exist. Examples of changes in the physical environment in poor countries are: ramps made out of sand and mud in Mozambique, special latrines for young children with cerebral palsy in Uganda, and a village community in Mexico working together to make a cement walkway so that wheelchair users (in Project PROJIMO) can reach the centre of the village.

The more difficult change is in the attitudes of the community, so that a child like Alice with poliomyelitis is not laughed at. 'Child-to-Child' programmes (Hawes 1988; see also Chapter 15) as part of their mission have worked to improve the understanding of non-disabled children so that they help a genuine integration of disabled children into local schools. The Child-to-Child programme takes the roles of older children into account in activity sheets that deal with ways of playing with, stimulating and caring for their younger siblings, In Nicaragua, Los Hermanos de los Pepitos have taken an initiative and shown that they can protect and care for the disabled children they know. Through talking to school friends and other children they increase understanding and change attitudes.

People do have enormous resilience and can be strengthened, but strengthening community resources for disabled people alone is unlikely to help their integration in the long term. In the Uganda slum project (Kangere 1993) workers found it unacceptable to concentrate only on disabled people and concluded that for CBR to work they had to think in terms of complete social change. This may seem idealistic, but it is no more idealistic and unrealistic than expecting the poorest communities and families to 'mobilize' non-existent resources.

The following case history from SANCHAR (1992), near Calcutta (see p. 175), shows how unrealistic this can be.

Sadhana's story is one we have often quoted as one of our successes.

Sadhana was born with 'brain damage' and as a result had severe spasticity. Sadhana's family —her parents, and three other children all younger than Sadhana—are very poor. Both parents work as daily paid labourers, at whatever work they can get. They live in the corner of the veranda of Sadhana's uncle's house after their own was swept away by the rains.

Sadhana, 10 years old when we first saw her, would spent the entire day sitting on a piece of sacking in this veranda. She could just manage to sit up by herself, but could not keep her balance. She was bathed and fed by her mother in the morning, and then left on her own. She would soil herself where she lay, and one or other of her parents would clean her when they found time. Sadhana's father told us that he had taken her to an orphanage run by a missionary group when she was a baby (the family are Christians) but soon brought her back again when he felt she was not being cared for properly.

Initially we developed a programme to help Sadhana sit up by herself. The process of designing and constructing a suitable chair attracted the interest of her father, who had initially pressurised us to arrange for sponsorship for his child, or some other financial help. Soon, the father became so involved that he took over from us and constructed an excellent seat by packing earth onto the side of the raised veranda, so that Sadhana could sit with her back supported and her legs dangling and separated. A bamboo table was made to fit across the front of this seat, so that Sadhana could feed herself off a plate. Within a year Sadhana was pulling herself around the courtyard on her stomach and elbows to where she would relieve herself, and was helping her mother by picking and cleaning the rice and the wheat for the family's meals, while sitting at her table. She had learnt to put on her pants herself, and could stand for some time with support. We planned to make a toilet for her—a pit over which she could squat while supporting herself holding onto a bamboo railing. We felt excited at Sadhana's rapid progress, and had great hopes for her future. We had grown to be close friends of the family, and felt that Sadhana's parents, seeing all she was learning to do for herself, were slowly beginning to think of her as something other than a burden. The child herself was bright and confident.

We were shocked when on one of our weekly visits, we found that on the previous day, her parents had given her away to Mother Teresa, after signing an agreement to relinquish all their rights to the child. We could not understand how Sadhana's father, who had brought his daughter back from an orphanage because, as he told us, he could look after her better than anyone else, could give her up once again. But as we spoke to Sadhana's mother about her difficult decision we began to understand the terrible strains of the situation. Sadhana's father, who had been working for some months in a steady job as a cook, had been dismissed by his employers and was now unemployed. The family were on the verge of starvation. Sadhana's father was becoming more and more frustrated. He would abuse and even beat Sadhana's mother in his rage, and she in her turn would sometimes slap Sadhana even when she realized the child was helpless. Neither of the parents had any time to help Sadhana learn anything new—all her learning and progress was made during our weekly lessons. The veranda in which they lived was breaking down—the roof and much of the floor had been damaged in the rains. There was very little work, and the family was reduced to eating only once a day. The parents sat up all night when it rained holding pieces of sacking over the children. We had to admit that, in this situation, it was inevitable that they could not care for Sadhana. As her father put it, 'at least in the Home, she will eat her fill every day.'

Women as carers

Professionals often plan programmes assuming that all disabled children live in two-parent or extended families. Thus most CBR programmes, such as the WHO, Guyana and Uganda national programmes and those based on Portage, rely on the mother or a 'trainer' who will be at home, and will be able to carry out various aspects of the training or stimulation programme. While most mothers attempt to carry out these roles, the social and economic aspects of people's lives are neglected.

Over the past decade women, the main carers, have suffered disproportionately as a result of economic 'adjustment' programmes. Devaluation and removal of subsidies have increased the prices of basic foods, and cuts in public spending have led to increased school fees and medical expenses. Most of the coping strategies that women have found have diminished the time and energy available for child care (Chinery-Hesse et al. 1989). For example, women have found it necessary to work for longer hours outside the home— in their fields producing more, in the market place, or less commonly in formal paid employment (Kanji and Jazdowska 1993).

In most countries in the world there is an increase in the proportion of female headed households. Estimates indicate that women are the sole bread-winners in about a quarter of the world's households. In another quarter of households women are working and contribute over 50 per ent of the family income. In Latin America and the Caribbean the proportion is as high as 30 per cent (Himes *et al.* 1992). In many countries migrant labour means that many households are headed by a woman for most of the year.

Social and cultural issues

Even if a mother is at home all day, she may not want to be her child's teacher or therapist to the extent that many programme planners hope. In home-based programmes, the mother generally operates in isolation with her child most of the time. Frequently, professional support is inadequate in quantity and sometimes in quality (see Chapter 5).

In poor countries few professionals are available and hence the usual strategy is to train helpers (community workers), as in the programmes described above, so that more disabled children can be reached. In many programmes the helper is a voluntary worker (as in Guyana where it works well), but practical problems often arise. Volunteers often live in the same stressed communities and have their own problems.

In all home-based programmes the identification of the key community worker determines the success or otherwise of the projects. The workers' own social position, their economic circumstances and cultural factors are all important. In many societies home visits by anyone other than family or friends are not acceptable. In other areas home visits are not welcome because they might draw attention to the presence of the child, where families do not welcome this for many reasons. It may be an impediment to marriage for unmarried sisters in some societies, or might be interpreted by neighbours as the family's failure to care properly for the child.

Frequently, older children, grandparents or other family members care for the child but few programmes take the needs of these carers into account and plan accordingly.

Economic issues

Government spending on health care fell in most Latin American and African countries during the 1980s (*Lancet* 1990, Marshall 1990, Fiedler 1991). Although women's education is one of the most important factors in child survival and limiting family size (Ratcliffe 1983), expenditure on education also fell. The International Monetary Fund's structural adjustment programmes insist on government spending cuts and retrenchment of public sector staff. This has meant that teachers' salaries have fallen in real terms to below the poverty level. Some teachers have left, teach in private schools or try to enhance their income in a variety of ways. Even where there are no direct fees, the cost to parents has increased dramatically in many developing countries. Faced with having to choose which of their children they can afford to send to school, families may well decide to send non-disabled boys to school and not their daughters or their disabled children.

The attitude of the World Bank to disabled people is shown by their use of the concept of 'disability-adjusted life years' in the *World Development Report* for 1993: 'In addition to premature mortality, a substantial portion of the burden of disease consists of disability, ranging from polio-related paralysis to blindness to the suffering brought about by severe psychosis. To measure the burden of disease, this Report uses the disability-adjusted life year (DALY), a measure that combines healthy life years lost because of premature mortality with those lost as a result of disability' (World Bank 1993).

The use of this measure suggests that the Bank considers that disabled people might as well be dead. It is hardly surprising that their economic programmes do not consider the value of disabled people. Any consideration is in terms of 'safety nets' for poor people, an ineffective charity way of reaching the 'poorest of the poor', particularly in those countries where the majority of the population is poor.

Implications of the social model of disability for children with impairments

The social model of disability views people with impairments as a group disabled by the current organization of society, which takes no account of people with impairments and thus excludes them from the mainstream of social life. The implications of applying this social model to the support of children with impairments is complex, both in developed and developing countries. Areas for discussion are as follows.

1. Adult disabled people as role models

The presence of competent and respected disabled adults as positive role models for children who are growing up with an impairment will help their self-esteem. In the PROJIMO project in Mexico run by disabled people themselves, disabled children and their families see disabled adults in active controlling roles, perhaps for the first time in their lives. The adults are in charge of the programme, some provide nursing and medical care, others are engaged in skilled work such as welding, making wheelchairs and mending bicycles for non-disabled villagers, others are engaged in earning their own living and raising their family. The way in which this affects the self-esteem of the disabled children has been observed. Many of the children make firm friends with adult disabled people.

The Disabled Children's Action Group in South Africa is a parent organization that recognizes the positive role of disabled adults. It was begun by parents and relatives (almost all women) of disabled children to promote and protect the rights of disabled children, especially those in difficult circumstances as a result of racial oppression, environmental location and/or severity of their impairment. This group is affiliated to Disabled People South Africa and appreciates the importance of adult disabled people as allies, employing a disabled woman as its national advocacy manager (Majiet-Chalken, personal communication 1994).

Another aspect of the importance of role models was exemplified by a hearing impaired man from France who explained, in a television documentary, that when he was a child being taken to the USA by his parents he saw a group of deaf adults at the airport communicating through signing. He later explained how excited he was because, up to that time, he had never seen deaf adults and therefore thought that deaf children did not grow up.

Children with impairments may only have seen adults with impairments in inferior and powerless positions, such as beggars. Consequently they are likely to have poor self-esteem, which non-disabled parents have difficulty counteracting.

Many non-disabled children, too, may only have seen disabled adults in inferior positions, being dependent, pitied or even reviled. A relevant example is of a little girl

171

who, when she saw an adult wheelchair user waiting to cross a road, approached him and gave him money (Finkelstein 1993*b*). Attitude awareness and media campaigns *may* help to change attitudes, but are not as important as personal experience. Had the girl's first contact with the disabled person been when he was working, her reaction would have been quite different.

2. The changing impairment and the developing child

In children the extent of disability changes as the child grows and develops and is not 'stabilized' as in most adults. It is difficult to determine the limits of the 'medical rehabilitation process' in a young child with cerebral palsy or learning difficulties, for example. The implication is that 'medical rehabilitation', developmental therapy and specific educational interventions continue until there is minimal change. This makes it difficult to judge how the gains in diminishing the impairment and its complications, through professional and skilled intervention, are to be balanced against the child's other childhood needs and the child's right to be accepted as someone who is different.

Also, a judgement has to be made as to when impairment-oriented professional interventions become an unreasonable attempt to make a child 'normal' and are part of the child's social oppression. It is relatively easy to make the judgement retrospectively, but difficult in advance. Parents, making such a choice, may be determining their child's whole social identity. For example, parents of a child with severe hearing impairment may have to decide whether their child will have signing as a first language, thus having a different social identity from theirs. Professionals can contribute to the judgement, but should not make the judgement alone. Disabled adults, who are able to analyse their childhood experiences, might be in a better position to advise parents. Older children themselves should be involved, but need much more information than is presently available to them.

As a second example, the emphasis that professionals and parents may put on a child's inability to walk at an expected age may lead them to provide helpful physiotherapy, but may also enforce a demanding regime on the child and parents. Parents and adult disabled people are not necessarily in agreement about the limits (Beardshaw 1989, Oliver 1989). This is especially so for children whose walking is delayed, for example because of athetoid cerebral palsy, and who consequently are engaged in long hours of therapy when they might be learning, playing or making friends. It may also detract from all the child's other qualities and abilities and affect the child's view of her or himself.

3. Parents' role in relation to the social model

All children need their parents' and families' care and support to grow and develop. Among their basic needs for water, food, shelter, protection and basic health care is the need for love and being valued as individuals. It is to be expected that parents look for ways of curing or mitigating the effects of any illness or impairment their child might have. And when the medical profession itself is unclear and so evidently fallible, there is no obvious reason for them to stop searching for cures, although where the impairment is permanent a relentless search will not be in the best interests of the child and the family.

Parents are part of society and will usually have the same attitudes to their child's

172

impairment as those around them; if disabled people around them are seen as objects of pity with few opportunities then it is a personal tragedy. It is hardly surprising that they do everything conceivable to remove their child from this 'inferior' group. This can lead to parents spending huge sums of money, even selling their home, to find a cure. They may also participate in extraordinary ventures for their disabled child which they would not do with their non-disabled children.

Even if parents conclude that cure of the impairment is not possible, the limits of their caring and protecting role in relation to their disabled child are not as readily defined as for non-disabled children. Parents are very rarely credited with getting the balance right and may be accused of rejecting their child if in the view of the professional they 'under-protect' their child, and of 'over-protection' if they offer more care than the professional thinks they should (Mittler *et al.* 1986). This is especially important where there are cultural differences in what is expected of a child at different ages. Children often have very little autonomy and even when adult are expected to obey their parents in all decisions.

While all children develop awareness of their identity as they grow up, children who are 'different' from their parents and siblings have a more complex process to undergo, influenced by other family members' roles, beliefs and attitudes.

Some aspects of this complexity in practice emerge from the following case history, adapted from SANCHAR (1993) (see below).

When we first met her Swapna was 10 years old. The oldest of four children, Swapna has severe spastic cerebral palsy. The family is comparatively well off—they live in a two-room mud hut on their own land, have some agricultural land and a fishpond. Apart from this, the father occasionally operates an illicit country-liquor still. Although, when we first met him, Swapna's father estimated his monthly income at about 600 rupees ($15), we found that he was able to employ labourers both to farm his land and run the distillery. He was the kind of person who sat at his ease and ordered others around, at home as well as at work. As for Swapna's mother, she was always busy around the house—in all the time we have known her, we have never once seen her resting or relaxing.

Swapna's mother told us that for a week after she was born Swapna ran a very high fever. When she was 1 year old her mother was concerned that she was not able to sit up by herself. She was taken to a doctor who told the parents that she would be able to walk at the age of 12. A series of visits to other doctors and hospitals followed, with no improvement in the child's condition. Finally the family gave up hope. When we met her, Swapna spent most of her time lying on a mat on the veranda of their house. She was able to drag herself, or roll around on this veranda, and sit for some time if she had something to lean against, but with great difficulty. She could feed herself with her left hand while lying on her side. She had bowel and bladder control, her hearing was normal and she could speak well enough to be understood although her speech was slurred.

Swapna, we soon realized, was an exceptionally intelligent child. She understood and deeply resented the fact that she was unlike other children and that many people reacted to her with pity or distaste. She felt that her parents thought of her as a burden, and would 'punish' them for this attitude in various subtle ways, like complaining to us about them, and spending as much of her time as possible with her maternal grandparents who lived nearby. Her grandparents, especially her grandfather, doted on Swapna and did everything they could to spoil her. Swapna had something of a royalty syndrome and insisted on having everything done for her. She refused to make an effort to help herself and was demanding and bad tempered most of the time.

Many of Swapna's feelings of dissatisfaction and depression came from her sense of being deprived of many things—being 'normal', being rich, living in a city, having an exciting time like the girls of her age in the video films she watched at the village video parlour. Swapna told us that her parents thought her a useless burden, that they would be happy if she died. We put the situation to her as a challenge—we told her that she would have to convince her parents that she was capable of doing a lot. We would help her, but the main job would be hers.

Initially Swapna's father was very aloof and distant with us. His attitude seemed to be that nothing could be done with the child, but that we were welcome to try. On most of our visits we would find Swapna at her grandparents', and it was the grandfather who initially became our friend and partner. Swapna was a fast learner and was soon bathing herself, and dressing and undressing on her own. It was decided that she could learn to sweep the house. Her grandfather made a special small broom for her and she started learning to use it while walking on her knees. Swapna was, however, adamant on one point—she would sweep her grandparents' house, but not her own!

Since Swapna found it very difficult to sit up without support, we decided to make a chair for her with a backrest and a kind of table in front. Although Swapna's father was an interested observer during our discussions about the design of the chair, it was her grandfather who had most of the ideas. However, Swapna's father got together the materials required to construct the chair—something that gave us hope that his attitude was changing.

Swapna's father was now taking more interest in us and our activities. He was very curious and would bombard us with questions. Did we all have college degrees? How much did we earn? Did we have contracts with the government? Could we arrange some 'grant' for the child or an allowance for the family? He and his wife had initially wanted to put Swapna in a Home where she would be looked after, but when he saw how much Swapna had learnt and changed, he began to feel interested in her as a person. Swapna's mother began to ask her to help with simple chores like cleaning the rice or sorting vegetables, and praising her for being able to bath and dry herself, dress and undress, and get on and off the veranda steps on her own. Swapna began to feel proud of her achievements and told us she wanted to learn to read and write. She struggled to learn how to hold a pen and was soon writing her name and doing simple sums.

Then, when we visited the house, Swapna's father would come and watch the exercises we helped Swapna to do to release the spasticity in her limbs and to help her to use them. We had been talking for months about making a table for Swapna, at which she would be able to sit and eat. Swapna's father would keep promising to get the required materials, but kept 'forgetting'. Finally, more than a year later, we found that a table had appeared—Swapna's father had hired a carpenter and spent a considerable amount of money to get it built. Now, when we told Swapna that her parents loved her and cared about her, she responded with smiles and not her former scepticism.

Things were changing—Swapna's father nagged us into getting a wheelchair for her in which he himself would wheel her to her grandparents. Her mother was brighter and more open with us, and was teaching Swapna to mop the floor. We had discussions with her parents and grandparents about what Swapna could do to earn her own living when she was older—the idea of a small poultry farm was mooted. Swapna herself was a different person—cheerful, confident and eager to learn and do more and more.

One day, about a year ago now, Swapna's father told us that her grandfather had met a man who promised to cure Swapna and make her walk after a massage with holy oil. To our dismay we found that Swapna was quite convinced that she was now going to be like other children—she told us that she would do nothing more than bringing water and sweeping the house after she was 'well'. Once again we spent many hours with Swapna's parents and grandparents going over the situation. Swapna's mother told us that she was back to her old self—sulking and refusing to do anything for herself. We all sat together and talked to Swapna, and helped her to understand that if she did not do things for herself she would never be able to learn, and that she had to take the responsibility for herself. It was painful for us all, most of all for Swapna, to think that one day she would be left alone, with no parents to look after her, and how she managed then depended on her making an effort now.

Swapna agreed, although reluctantly, to learn new skills and struggle to become self-sufficient.

In the last year, Swapna has made great strides. She is now eager to start working and contributing to the family income. We are exploring the possibility of helping her to start a small backyard poultry unit. We are also trying to create opportunities for her to move around more and meet more people. We feel that meeting and talking to her can help people recognize the potential of other children with disabilities who need help and support from the community.

In developing countries the issues of the social model in relation to children have not been fully studied and debated. We have made an initial attempt to signal some of the issues, albeit from the point of view of non-disabled professionals.

The question of any disadvantaged group empowering itself in the prevailing socio-economic conditions may seem completely idealistic, where conditions in the communities are like those of Sadhana's family. However, the sangams supported by ADD–India provide a successful example.

Empowerment in SANCHAR in India

SANCHAR is an organization which works with some of the poorest families living around Calcutta: the staff include the first two co-authors of this chapter. The workers are tackling some of the fundamental issues concerning empowerment and attitudes in a very poor community. A detailed description is here presented of the ways of working in the organization, and also of the relationship between aims and working practices, showing how lessons have been learned along the way.

The team tries to enable poor people with impairments to gain control over their lives. SANCHAR believes that, given support, disabled people and their families are capable of understanding and analysing their situations, and working out the best way to tackle their own problems. The SANCHAR team act as facilitators in this process of analysis and problem solving and believe that *the way we work is as important as what we do'.* SANCHAR tries to work through processes which are enabling and empowering, and which help persons with impairments and their families to recognize, strengthen and build on the positive aspects of the situation.

The work is predominantly with children. No formal surveys are conducted in the villages where the work is carried out. The team comes to know of disabled children through contacts, formal and informal, with members of the women's groups, teachers at local schools and pre-school groups, other children, neighbours and health and community workers in the area. Sometimes, parents of the child contact them directly.

SANCHAR works through their relationship with the child and the parents and family of the child. The first step is usually to help the parents accept that their child is perhaps never going to be completely 'normal'—that there is no magic cure. It is only after reaching this understanding that the team and the parents together move to an appraisal of the child's major problems and potential for becoming a member of the family unit on equal terms with everyone else. This analysis forms the basis for working out a plan for each child based on the parents' expectation and the child's ability and condition. The next step is to design activities and programmes which are implemented in the child's home in partnership with the parents.

Interventions may vary from a long-term learning process for the child, to referral for surgery where this is appropriate, or help in procuring and getting used to orthotic and prosthetic aids and appliances. Children with specific medical problems like epilepsy or tuberculosis are referred to specialists or other institutes. Individual learning programmes are implemented through weekly visits to the child's home, with the parents and families continuing and following up the 'lessons' on other days of the week. The emphasis is generally on helping the child to become independent in activities of daily living, and to become a confident, self-reliant person. Wherever possible the children are encouraged to attend normal schools, help with household chores, work in family enterprises or become wage-earners.

Practical learning about poverty
Most of the families and children are very poor, and have family incomes of less than 1000 rupees (~$25) per month. This poverty affects every aspect of their lives.

SANCHAR's experience has been that most parents feel a strong sense of guilt, as if in some way responsible for their child's impairment. This feeling is usually stronger in the mother, who is inclined to attribute the impairment to a fall or illness during pregnancy, complications during delivery or a lack of care during early childhood. This feeling is often reinforced by relatives and even health workers in the community and may be a powerful barrier to being able to make a realistic assessment of the child's problems, as well as affecting the child's self-image and the way in which the child and the parents relate to each other.

Like anyone else, poor families and parents are prepared to try anything to help their disabled children. However, for these very poor families, access to the specialists and institutions in the city is limited because the cost of travelling and 'treatment' is more than they can afford. The fact that many such 'specialists' continue to hold out hopes for a cure (for conditions such as cerebral palsy or intellectual impairment) while prescribing expensive and useless vitamin tonics, makes matters worse. The family often sells land and assets to buy these medicines which, of course, make no difference to the child's condition. Finally, when the money runs out the 'treatment' is stopped and the parents continue to think that it was only because of their poverty that the miracle eluded them. This is the state of mind in which the families are often found when work is begun with them.

The ways in which families deal with the situation of a child with an impairment are also affected by their poverty. Caring for the child is difficult since both parents have to go out to work, and responsibility for looking after the daily needs of the child is taken over by another child, usually an older sister, who then becomes the key person for work with the child. Even in families where the mother is at home all day, the burden of household chores leaves her with little time or energy to devote to the child. In such cases, helping the child to become independent in the activities of daily living has immediate short-term benefits for the mother, apart from the long-term gains of increasing the child's confidence and self-image.

However, for a very poor family the disabled child may come low on the list of priorities, as described in Sadhana's story. It has been painful but essential to understand that when the parents are not sure where the next meal for the family is coming from, and have no security of any kind even for basic needs, it becomes impossible for them to have any confidence in their capacity to change their situation.

The experiences of SANCHAR are not unusual and show that it is *essential* to understand the situation of families and communities in 'models' of CBR.

Rehabilitation as part of community development
SANCHAR's approach to disability and people with impairments has grown and deepened. A changed perception has come about through a collective learning process rooted in the work itself and in understanding development as a people-centred and people-controlled process of social, economic and political change. To achieve a change in the situations of disabled people, interventions need to be seen in this broader context.

We see society as composed of inter-related groups, and the nature of a particular society as determined by the nature of these relationships. Our present society is characterized by unequal relationships, with certain groups being deprived of resources, basic rights, and opportunities to acquire these rights and resources, which are concentrated in the hands of other powerful groups. The latter, even though they are numerically in the minority, dominate and control the structures and systems of society and use these to perpetuate their control. The landless, wage-workers, artisans, tribal people and women are all members of oppressed and deprived groups. Disabled people, when situated in this framework, can be located at the bottom of the heap in each group—doubly oppressed by virtue of belonging to a deprived group, as well as by their 'incapacity' in their own eyes as well as in the perception of others.

'Development' is understood as involving a change in the situation of deprived and oppressed groups in the direction of more equity in relation to other groups. SANCHAR's experience, and that of others, has shown that for changes of this nature to be lasting and deep, they must come about through the conscious and collective action of those who are to benefit from the change. In other words, development for a particular group has as its imperative the active involvement of members of that group, as actors in the process of change rather than as its objects. The SANCHAR collective believes that people have the capacity to play this active role—to comprehend and analyse the reality of their situation and to plan and implement strategies to change that situation.

Thus work with disabled people should focus on helping them to gain control over themselves, their lives and their situations. SANCHAR aims to help them to analyse their situation collectively, although in villages disabled adults and children are geographically scattered so it is difficult for them to meet in one place on a regular basis.

What are the dimensions of empowerment for a person with an impairment? The work of SANCHAR has focused on a step-by-step progression, from understanding and controlling the body and day-to-day life, to control at the level of the family and the community. It seems obvious that such processes are more likely to be controlled at the level of the community rather than in the cocooned environment of institutions. Therefore CBR is seen not as an alternative to other valid strategies but as the only strategy with potential for bringing about lasting changes in the lives of disabled people.

The role of professionals

Most CBR projects, where medical rehabilitation of the impairment is prominent, are ultimately run by professionals. Since the entire superstructure of disability work has evolved from an institutional base, it is inevitable that professionals and institutions exemplify the same world view, and that they be designed to meet each others' needs. Merely transposing a professional rehabilitation worker, or one trained by them, from an institutional setting to a village will not automatically create a faith in the capacity of disabled people to take control of their lives, or even the conviction that it is necessary and desirable for them to do so. A people-centred holistic perspective needs more than the addition of certain 'participatory' elements onto a diametrically opposing world view. If professionals have had no personal experience of the process of collective empowerment, even in another context, they are unlikely to understand this dimension of work with families and disabled children (see also Chapter 9).

While 'empowerment' in all contexts is an ideal, the only real empowerment is by the individual or the social group. The reality for any individual with an impairment is that several forms of control are being exercised simultaneously. SANCHAR workers took the role of facilitators but found it was difficult not to assume a controlling role. In day-to-day work it was impractical to wait for each decision to be taken independently so that it was a step forward in the process. Instead, the SANCHAR workers found themselves becoming the decision makers and starting to exercise control over the person with the impairment, the family, and by extension the community.

Changing to group work

A more detailed analysis of how difficult it is to avoid the controlling role of the professional came from experience of group work. The earlier strategy of visiting each family separately and building up partnerships on an individual basis led to some practical problems. As each worker had to interact with four or five children during the weekly visit to the village, the time available for each family became short. In addition, energy and enthusiasm were reduced with subsequent sessions, so that the interaction with the last family to be visited became qualitatively poorer. The child worked and learned alone, and did not have the opportunity to feel enthused and stimulated by other children tackling similar situations.

The child and the family developed a deep relationship with the person who was 'their' worker, which facilitated their learning. However, this relationship often had an element of dependence, so that if, for any reason, that particular worker was substituted by another person, the child found it difficult to learn.

The first attempts to develop a collective approach were a response to this situation. SANCHAR had been working with a home-based approach in the first 20 villages in the field area. Recently, when activities were initiated in ten new villages, meetings were organized in a central place where all the parents came with their children. In day-long sessions the children were assessed and strategies discussed with their parents. It was finally agreed that, on one fixed day of the week, the child with the parents, or primary caregiver, would come to the centre for the learning session. The session would be attended by as many field workers as practical, with at least two always there. This has been the working method for some time now, and it is found that the children of these villages are stimulated by being in a group. Also those parents who come to the session spend the time talking with each other and are gradually building a relationship. As in the Samadhan project (see p. 160), many parents of children with severe impairments who need constant attention also appreciate the respite. With the children working in groups at approximately the same stage of learning, more time and attention can be given to each group.

However, this group approach has its own limitations. The SANCHAR team found that the relationship with families in villages where the group approach was adopted was qualitatively poorer than in the earlier home-based programme villages. Although an initial visit was made to each home, subsequent interactions have been with one member of the family, often a different person each time, and in particular very few fathers come. The disabled child may be brought to the group by an older sibling, who goes off to play until it is time to take the child home. The team member is not part of the families' daily life and struggles, as happened with families visited in their homes.

When working with groups, team members have found themselves getting more technical. Perhaps because the relationship with the family is felt to be more superficial, there was a tendency to focus exclusively on the needs of the child to determine the learning agenda. This reduced the extent to which individual programmes were tailored for each child. Instead there was a tendency to 'market' approaches which were found effective with other children. For instance, a functional literacy package for all the children with hearing impairments in the group may be recommended, or a particular set of exercises for all the children with cerebral palsy.

Another important insight was that, when the members were in a group, interactions tended to be more with each other than with the parents. In home-visiting, care would be taken to avoid using terms which the parents and family would not understand and which increased the 'expert' aura. In speaking to each other the team was not always so careful.

A combination of the two approaches is now planned. A strong relationship with the family will be built up through working with the child at home during the early stages. It is only after the initial period of mutual adjustments, when a solid basis for partnership with the parents has been established, that the move to working in groups will occur. Even afterwards, individual contact will be maintained by visiting the parents at home at frequent intervals.

Empowerment
Ways of strengthening the collective process so that it leads to a greater degree of control by the persons concerned are being sought. Experience with parents so far has been that the process by which confidence is gained to plan and implement strategies independently is a slow and painful one. Although there are notable exceptions, the majority of parents have not gained the confidence to implement a learning programme entirely on their own, even when the skills being taught are simple ones like feeding, bathing or dressing. All parents teach these skills to their other children, but in the case of the child with an impair-

ment, the fact that the child is older and learns so much more slowly seems to make the process alien and artificial, so that parents think of it as a special job.

However, when parents have gained confidence in their skills they have become excellent teachers. For instance, in the case of a child learning a family trade in which a high degree of skill is required, some parents can plan and implement an entire learning programme, breaking up the necessary skills into smaller units, teaching each of them step-by-step and monitoring the child's progress. It is interesting that the professional's lack of skills in this area seems to be a factor in increasing the parents' involvement and confidence.

Specific steps have to be taken to make stronger the link between the child's learning processes and the family's process of gaining control over their lives and situations, as well as to ensure that this enhanced control leads to a collective process of analysis and action.

SANCHAR's experience of working as a collective has taught the team something of the practical difficulties of working in this way. Concepts such as collective leadership and collective decision making appear to presuppose a group of similarly conscious and empowered individuals. In practice, there are wide variations in the degree to which each person is prepared to assume the responsibility for her/his own life. Efforts to 'fill in the gaps' lead almost inevitably to concentration of power and control in the hands of a few decision makers.

SANCHAR recognizes that a change in the unequal relationship between professionals and disabled people is fundamental. This will inevitably lead to changes in the basic fabric of society. How valid are efforts to rehabilitate individuals into a social structure which is basically unjust, unless they are also questioning society?

Conclusion

There is no blueprint for disability programmes for children in developing countries. We are at the stage of trying to examine and evaluate what works, but adequate tools for the evaluation of community-based disability programmes have yet to be developed. We are faced by the challenge of looking beyond old frameworks through a process of collectively sharing and learning from each others' experience.

REFERENCES

Balasundaram, P., Woods, P.A. (1990) 'A home-based system of service delivery; some difficulties and lessons learned.' *Paper presented at the CAMHADD/Unicef Workshop, Male, Maldives, 1990.*
Beardshaw, V. (1989) 'Conductive Education: a rejoinder.' *Disability, Handicap and Society,* 4. 3, 297–299.
Bichman, W., Rifkin, S.B., Shrestha, M. (1989) 'Towards the measurement of community participation.' *World Health Forum,* **10**, 467–472.
Chabot, H.T.J., Bremmers, J. (1988) 'Government health services versus community: conflict or harmony.' *Social Science and Medicine,* **26**, 957–962.
Chinery-Hesse, M., Agarwal, B., Ariffin, J. (1989) *Engendering Adjustment for the 1990's. Report of a Commonwealth Expert Group on Women and Structural Adjustment.* London: Commonwealth Secretariat.
Coleridge, P. (1993) *Disability, Liberation and Development.* Oxford: Oxfam Publications.
Cornia, G., Jolly, R., Stewart, F. (1987) *Adjustment with a Human Face.* Oxford: Clarendon Press.
Costello, A., Walker, F., Woodward, D. (1994) *Human Face or Human Facade? Adjustment and the Health of Mothers and Children.* London: Centre for International Child Health.

Department of Community Development (1992) *Guidelines for Community Based Rehabilitation Services.* Kampala: Republic of Uganda Department of Community Development, Vocational Rehabilitation Section.

Fiedler, J. (1991) 'Child survival and the role of the Ministry of Health in Ecuador: progress, constraints and reorganization.' *Health Policy and Planning*, **6**, 32–45.

Finkelstein, V. (1993a) 'The commonality of disability.' *In:* Swain, J., Finkelstein, V., French, S., Oliver, M. (Eds) *Disabling Barriers—Enabling Environments.* Milton Keynes/London: Sage Publications with The Open University, pp. 6–16.

—— (1993b) 'Review of disability, liberation and development.' *Disability News*, (November).

Hawes, H. (1988) *Child-to-Child. Another Path to Learning.* Hamburg: Unesco Institute for Education.

Hegarty, S. (1993) *Educating Children and Young People with Disabilities. Principles and the Review of Practice.* Paris: Unesco.

Heggenhougen, H.K. (1984) 'Will primary health care efforts be allowed to succeed?' *Social Science and Medicine*, **19**, 217–224.

Helander, E. (1993) *Prejudice and Dignity: an Introduction to Community-based Rehabilitation.* New York: United Nations Development Program.

—— Nelson, G., Mendis, P. (1983) *Training Disabled People in the Community.* Geneva: WHO.

—— Mendis, P., Nelson, G., Goerdt, A. (1989) *Training in the Community for People with Disabilities.* Geneva: WHO.

Himes, J.R., Landers, C., Leslie, J. (1992) *Women, Work and Child Care. Innocenti Global Seminar Report.* Florence: Unicef/ICDC; New York: Unicef.

Hutton, W. (1993) *The British Economy and Third World Debt. Conference Report.* O'Connell, H. (Ed.) London: One World Action, pp. 24–25.

ILO, Unesco and WHO (1994) *CBR. Community-based Rehabilitation For and With People with Disabilities. Joint Position Paper.* Geneva: WHO, ILO; Paris: Unesco.

Jaffer, R., Jaffer, R. (1990) 'The WHO–CBR approach: programme or ideology: some lessons from the CBR experience in Punjab, Pakistan.' *In:* Thorburn, M.J., Marfo, K. (Eds.) *Practical Approaches to Childhood Disability in Developing Countries: Insights from Experience and Research.* St Johns, Newfoundland: Memorial University, Project SEREDEC; Spanish Town, Jamaica: 3D Projects, pp. 278–292.

Kanji, N., Jazdowska, N. (1993) 'Structural adjustment and women in Zimbabwe.' *Review of African Political Economy*, **56**, 11–26.

Lancet (1990) 'Structural adjustment and health in Africa.' *Lancet*, 335, 885–886. *(Editorial.)*

Lundgren-Lindquist, B., Nordholm, L. (1993) 'Community based rehabilitation—a survey of disabled in a village in Botswana.' *Disability and Rehabilitation*, **15**, 83–89.

Marshall, J. (1990) 'Structural adjustment and social policy in Mozambique.' *Review of African Political Economy*, **47**, 28–43.

Mia, A., Islam, H., Ali, S. (1981) 'Situation of handicapped children in Bangladesh.' *Assignment Children*, **53/54**, 199–214.

Miles, M. (1985a) *Children with Disabilities in Ordinary Schools.* Peshawar: Mental Health Centre.

—— (1985b) *Where There Is No Rehab Plan.* Peshawar: Mental Health Centre.

Mittler, P., Mittler, H., McConachie, H. (1986) *Working Together. Guidelines for Partnership between Professionals and Parents of Children and Young People with Disabilities. Guides for Speical Education No.2.* Paris: Unesco.

Mosley, W.H. (1988) 'Is there a middle way? Categorical programs for PHC.' *Social Science and Medicine*, **26**, 907–908.

Newell, K.W. (1988) 'Selective primary health care: the counter revolution.' *Social Science and Medicine*, **26**, 903–905.

Oliver, M. (1989) 'Conductive Education: if it wasn't so sad it would be funny.' *Disability, Handicap and Society*, **4**, 197–200.

—— (1990) *The Politics of Disablement.* London: Macmillan.

O'Toole, B.J. (1988a) 'Development and evaluation of a community based rehabilitation programme for pre-school disabled children in Guyana.' PhD thesis, University of London.

—— (1988b) 'A community-based rehabilitation programme for pre-school disabled children in Guyana.' *International Journal of Rehabilitation Research*, **11**, 323–334.

—— (1991) *Guide to Community-based Rehabilitation Services. Guides for Special Education No.8.* Paris: Unesco.

Project PROJIMO (undated) *Project PROJIMO: a Villager-run Rehabilitation Program for Disabled Children in Western Mexico.* Palo Alto, CA: Hesperian Foundation.

Pupulin, E. (1992) 'CBR: where we are now.' *Paper presented to the Rehabilitation International Seminar, Limuru, Kenya, September 1992.*

Ratcliffe, J. (1983) 'Social justice and the demographic transition: lessons from India's Kerala State.' *In:* Morley, D., Rohde, J., Williams, G. (Eds.) *Practising Health for All.* Oxford: Oxford University Press, pp. 64–82.

Rohde, J. (1983) 'Health for all in China: principles and relevance for other countries.' *In:* Morley, D., Rohde, J., Williams, G. (Eds.) *Practising Health for All.* Oxford: Oxford University Press, pp. 5–16.

SANCHAR (1992) *Annual Report 1991–1992.* West Bengal, India: SANCHAR.

—— (1993) *Annual Report 1992–1993.* West Bengal, India: SANCHAR.

Save The Children Fund (1994) *Children, Disability and Development: Achievement and Challenge. Conference Report.* London: Save the Children Fund.

Segall, M., Vienonen, M. (1987) 'Haikko Declaration on actions for primary health care.' *Health Policy and Planning,* **2**, 258–265.

Sobsey, D. (1994) *Violence and Abuse in the Lives of People with Disabilities—the End of Silent Acceptance?* Baltimore: Paul H. Brookes.

—— Mansell, S. (1990) 'The prevention of sexual abuse of persons with developmental disabilities.' *Developmental Disabilities Bulletin,* **18**, 51–65.

Thorburn, M.J. (1990) 'Practical aspects of programme development. (2) Training, resource mobilization, public education, and programme assessment.' *In:* Thorburn, M.J., Marfo, K. (Eds.) *Practical Approaches to Childhood Disability in Developing Countries: Insights from Experience and Research.* St Johns, Newfoundland: Memorial University, Project SEREDEC; Spanish Town, Jamaica: 3D Projects, pp. 55–72.

—— Marfo, K. (1990) *Practical Approaches to Childhood Disability in Developing Countries: Insights from Experience and Research.* St Johns, Newfoundland: Memorial University, Project SEREDEC; Spanish Town, Jamaica: 3D Projects.

Unesco (1988) *Review of the Present Situation in Special Education.* Paris: Unesco.

Walsh, J.A., Warren, K.S. (1979) 'Selective primary health care: an interim strategy for disease control in developing countries.' *New England Journal of Medicine,* **301**, 967–974.

Walt, G. (1988) 'CHWs: are national programmes in crisis?' *Health Policy and Planning,* **3**, 1–21.

—— Rifkin, S. (1990) 'The political context of primary health care.' *In:* Streetland, P., Charbot, J. (Eds.) *Implementing Primary Health Care: Experiences Since Alma Ata.* Amsterdam: Royal Tropical Institute, pp. 13–20.

Werner, D. (1981) 'Village Health Worker: liberator or lackey?' *World Health Forum,* **2**, 46–54.

—— (1987) *Disabled Village Children: a Guide for Community Health Workers, Rehabilitation Workers and Families.* Palo Alto, CA: Hesperian Foundation.

—— (1993) 'Enabling primary health care through disabled people.' *In:* Rohde, J., Chatteerjee, M., Morley, D. (Eds.) *Reaching Health for All.* Delhi: Oxford University Press, pp. 87–102.

WHO (1993) *Promoting the Development of Young Children with Cerebral Palsy—a Guide for Mid-level Rehabilitation Workers.* Geneva: WHO.

WHO and Unicef (1978) *Alma Ata: Primary Health Care. Health for All Series, 1.* Geneva: WHO.

Williams, L., Williams, G. (1993) 'A situation analysis and action plan for community based rehabilitation for disabled people in the Solomon Islands.' *Action plan submitted for the Diploma for Teachers and Planners of Community Based Rehabilitation.* London: ICH.

Wisner, B. (1988) 'GOBI versus PHC? Some dangers of selective primary health care.' *Social Science and Medicine,* **26**, 963–969.

World Bank (1993) *World Development Report 1993. Investing in Health. World Development Indicators.* Oxford: Oxford University Press for the World Bank.

12
GROWING UP DISABLED

Joseph Kisanji

Society and disability

Studies in anthropology, history and community health have shown that the presence of people with impairments is part of the normal pattern of society (Okeahialam 1974, Groce 1989–90, Ingstad 1990), yet society has tended throughout history to exclude people with impairments from its mainstream (Pritchard 1963, Scholl 1986, Walker 1986). This chapter is concerned with the experience of growing up disabled in sub-Saharan Africa, but the issues raised have a wider relevance.

Transmission of culture

The ways in which people with impairments are viewed in various societies depend on complex factors, and they change over time in parallel with societal changes such as industrialization, the spread of formal education, and changes in the age distribution of the population. In order to gain a deeper understanding of disability issues in African culture, we must first clarify Western perceptions and stereotyping.

Racially biased suggestion of intellectual inferiority or superiority has long been exposed as scientifically fraudulent (Gould 1981). However, the culture of a people does have a significant effect on their thought processes. In a review of the literature, Evans (1970) investigated the belief that:

'. . different thought systems are the results of customs and traditions produced by and perpetuating the existing social and political system. In an analysis of African philosophy, Brelsford showed that the African sees himself as part of a total system which includes other individuals as well as spirits and things, and he accepts the universe rather than challenging it.'

Both parts of this can be challenged. The first part deals with the influence of culture on people's thinking. However, the reverse is equally true, as ideas can and do shape culture (Skrtic 1991).

The second contention requires a closer look. The traditional African community had the political and religious systems vested in one leader, be it chief, king or queen. All the community members as individuals or clans were part and parcel of the religious matrix (Datta 1984). However, this should not be interpreted as inability to control the physical, social, religious and political factors within the environment. Examples of environmental controls and changes include the organization of communal farming, and technological innovations such as yarn making and cloth weaving equipment and the production of hoes with wider blades and longer handles. The communities responded to their changing social, economic and political needs, even if this meant fighting for them. The informal education system that existed in traditional societies transmitted to the young generation the knowledge, values, beliefs and skills developed over the years. The skills so gained could be improved upon and therefore take the community a step forward (Kenyatta 1965).

The role of education in the maintenance of culture has been extensively described (Fafunwa 1967, Nyerere 1967, Fafunwa and Aisiku 1982, Holmes and Hurst 1983). However, traditional, informal, primarily oral education does more than maintain culture. Nyerere in his book, *Man and Development* (1974), clearly defined the role of education as a tool for the liberation of both the individual and groups of people mentally, socially, physically and politically as well as from the inhospitable environment. Freire (1972) also stressed these roles of education through his participatory approach. Although Nyerere and Freire refer mainly to the Western-type formal and informal systems of education, these roles were also conceived in the traditional education in Africa. Thus, Belsford's contention (Evans 1970) that the African accepts, but does not challenge, the environment is not true.

The thesis of this discussion is that even in the least developed communities in the world there exists a knowledge base and activity to ensure self-maintenance and development in all spheres of their life, including the disability area, within the limits of their resources.

Societal integration
Available literature on disability in developing countries takes the viewpoint of Western education and culture and emphasizes the presence of negative attitudes toward impairment and disabled people (Marfo *et al.* 1983, 1986). However, viewed from within communities with a high level of illiteracy and a subsistence economy, the general pattern of overt community reaction has been one of sympathy and acceptance, providing all the basic needs—food, shelter and clothing—at the extended family level, and allowing people with impairments to participate in the community institutions and activities within the limits of their abilities. Personal observation and communications in Africa show that people with hearing, visual and physical impairments are relatively well integrated in society. In comparison with the demands of sophisticated technological societies, in subsistence economies people with specific learning difficulties and mild or moderate intellectual impairment encounter fewer problems. It is to be argued, therefore, that for such communities integration and 'normalization' are not new concepts.

Western influence has caused disabled people to be gathered together, seen and presented as a group or groups, in playgroups, early stimulation centres, preschools, schools or rehabilitation centres and programmes. Although this practice has brought about several benefits, such as literacy, recreation and leisure time activities (as in Deaf clubs), and the development of disabled people's organizations as pressure groups, it has eroded their sound base of normalized living as valued people.

The following vignettes drawn from the village community of the author illustrate these points.

Ndaya was born deaf. After a short illness at the age of 4 years, he became lame as well. He could not go to school because of his communication difficulties. Many able-bodied children were not attending school anyway. As he grew up, other children imitated his gait and high-pitched and unintelligible speech as well as his gestures. Ndaya was strong and hard-working. Although children caricatured his speech and movement, he was well respected by adults and village leaders. He earned this respect by his assertiveness, diligence and independence. By village standards, he was a skilful, hard-working and competent builder and farmer. Living in a fishing community, he also became skilful in making and using river and lake fish traps.

Ishila had a clumsy gait. It was not known how this clumsiness developed. In addition she had intellectual impairment and drooled. She played with children much younger than herself. Both children and adults teased her. At such times she would merely chuckle back innocently. Her parents loved her, and by village standards she was fed and dressed well. Ishila moved freely in the village and was accepted in all gatherings, be they social, political or for communal work.

Kibwana was popular with all age groups. He played all kinds of games with other children. He could ask adults any question, including personal questions which young people of his age did not dare to ask. He could do anything that both his peers and older people asked him to do, especially things that were socially unacceptable, such as calling names and stealing food items from other people's farms. Kibwana was not taken seriously because he was considered to be 'stupid'. The plump, happy-go-lucky Kibwana spent most of the time laughing and slapping his behind, producing a loud sound which attracted much laughter. He acted like a jester. Kibwana was clothed well, although when annoyed he would strip off and throw away his clothes. He had many friends, both boys and girls.

These three examples illustrate that persons with impairments may not be marginalized in village society. However, attitudes toward disabled people in many African communities vary according to type, cause and severity of the impairments. The author's personal experience provides another dimension.

I contracted measles when I was about 2 years old, while living with my grandmother, and this resulted in corneal scars, hence opacities, in both eyes. The scar in the right eye covers only a small part of the pupil, while that in the left lies squarely on the pupil. As such I have relied on the visual function of the right eye since early childhood, making the left eye go 'lazy' (amblyopic).

I lived with my grandmother until I was 8, in the small village of Isonganya near Mwambani, which is a large village and the then seat of our chieftaincy, in Chunya District in Tanzania. She was very fond of me. She never wanted me to go out to play with other children, lest they took advantage of my poor eyesight and hurt me. After a long time she came to trust a neighbour's son to whom she gave instructions about what types of play we could engage in. Boisterous play, which I wanted to join in, was proscribed. I became so close to Daudi that I felt lonely when he had to go to school. My unhappiness made my grandmother allow me to follow Daudi to school, eight miles away. (I do not remember why I was not supposed to go to school then. It could have been that I was too young to attend school. Daudi was older than me. It could also have been due to my grandmother's over-protectiveness.) We ran most of the way, both ways, even when there was heavy dew on the tall savanna grass which overhung the footpath. Daudi usually held my hand according to instructions given him by my grandmother.

An important aspect of my life in my grandmother's house was the application of some very tiny seeds, from a wild sweet smelling plant locally known as ivumbasya, in my eyes. I had to close my eyes for long hours. It was believed that these seeds would remove the scars; unfortunately they did not.

I felt independent when I left my grandmother to live with a paternal uncle. He did not want me to go to school. Instead, he made me look after cattle. I could now play boisterous games. I gradually began to understand why my grandmother had protected me from joining other children.

185

Boys would make fun of my eyes, imitate my head tilt and the way I walked. It was very painful at first. I remember one day a boy forcing me to look at myself in the mirror he had brought from home for the purpose. Since then mirrors have made me feel uncomfortable. Due to such incidents, I remember that at times I withdrew from the group and cried; sometimes I sobbed openly. As time went by, I learned to accept my impairment. But what became important to me was the fact that I was an accepted member of the group and had friends. When I was gored by an angry cow, they visited me almost every day after taking the cattle home.

I began formal schooling when I was 9, after my father returned from training as a Rural Medical Aid. I had no problem following school work, although my eyesight had to be supported by spectacles from the age of 12. But I abandoned them twice when I felt my vision had improved. I was not informed about my infantile cataracts until long after I had finished school. School friends accepted my impairment more readily than the herdboys. This may have been due to my good academic performance. This, too, earned me some trouble, as a number of older boys who were not doing well in the Middle School grades ganged up against me for putting them to academic humiliation!

I had gained through play, schooling and household responsibilities (as a first born, looking after my young brothers and sisters when my parents were away) a high tolerance for frustration. However, my self-image was shattered three times when girlfriends told me they could not marry me because I was 'not seeing well', 'likely to go blind' and/or 'ugly'. It took me three years to risk entering any private relationship with a woman after the last episode. The satisfaction I derived from my work as a teacher, the two men and a woman with corneal scars like mine whom I had met, the five visually impaired students admitted to the secondary school where I was teaching and whom I volunteered to assist, and the training in special education, helped to restore my self-esteem.

This personal account shows that for my visual (and in fact mild) impairment, the problem lay with the protective attitude of my family rather than with the general public. Had it not been for joining the cattle herding group, dependency and helplessness would have been created. The herdboys and the girlfriends made me see reality and learn from it. I came to recognize and accept my impairment and its inherent limitations. I therefore concentrated on what I could do rather than on what was impossible, and this facilitated the development of self-confidence, competence and a sense of personal worth.

Public attitudes were, and are, more negative in relation to some types of impairment than has been illustrated in the experiences described above. Some impairments have been, and still are, so resented when they occurred that those affected were either rejected or viewed with fear. Leprosy, multiple impairments and albinism are cases in point. Leprosy is contagious and was recognized as such. It was difficult to cure the disease which, for lack of a scientific explanation, could only be attributed to a curse from God or the gods or to witchcraft. To get rid of this menace the society resorted to ostracizing the lepers as well as 'witches' and 'wizards' who could have caused it (Institute of Education 1984).

The effect of the presence of a person with an impairment on the family is well known and well documented. The demands that profound multiple impairments entail are enormous. This applies to all families and communities whatever their status. It is therefore not surprising that persons with such impairments were sometimes considered subhuman, or of an undefined human status (*e.g.* the *baana ba kilema* or 'faulty children' of East Kasai, Zaire, whose 'naming means that their body is characterised with [*sic*] a fault (kilema)'— Devlieger 1989), or were simply killed at birth (Chowo 1978, Walker 1986).

Albinism is a condition that is not readily accepted. In illiterate communities its cause is not understood. It is, therefore, feared. In some societies it is attributed to reincarnation (van Pelt 1982, Devlieger 1989), while in others it is taken as a bad omen. As a result people fear coming in contact with albinos. In some communities in Tanzania and Zambia, for example, expectant women avoid seeing albinos for fear of giving birth to an albino child (Possi 1988).

The above beliefs have implications if any Western-type service is to be started in such communities. The overall cultural base must be explored, capitalizing on what the given community knows and cherishes, and gradually dismantling the spiritual cloak of fear of the unknown.

Schools and disability

Society's attitudes toward disabled people determine the kind and level of services that are developed at any point in time. However, attitudes change over time as they are moulded by such factors as exchange of new ideas and success stories, formation of formal and informal, national and international interest and pressure groups, worldwide socio-political changes, improvements in health services, the general increase in the level of education, and the expansion of the concept of individual worth and human rights (Gearheart and Weishahn 1976).

Special education is one area of services that has been affected by such changes in attitudes. For instance, Onwuegbu (1988) argues that 'special education is the result of four unrelated, even sometimes antagonistic factors or what one may term human charac-teristics' of superstition, wickedness, sympathy and curiosity. It is worthwhile, therefore, to examine special education in Africa against this background of 'human characteristics' and global socio-cultural factors.

Education and vocational rehabilitation of persons with impairments was started by churches and other voluntary organizations (Unesco 1981, Abosi and Ozoji 1985, Ross 1988, Dery 1991). These organizations established schools for disabled children and young people without the involvement of the local community. Evangelism, along with the dishing out of free clothing and food, and digging of village wells or provision of piped water, so sparing the community the bother of having to travel long distances to fetch water, were enough to entice the community to accept the establishment of ordinary and special schools. In addition, the church had the support of the colonial government whose directives the village could not reject (Datta 1984).

Justification for early special schools

The first schools for children with impairments were segregated and residential, because not every village had an ordinary school and formal education for disabled young people was a new idea to be tried in demonstration centres. However, the most important factors were that this was the form of provision in the home countries of the colonial pioneers of special education, and there were very few missionaries who were qualified special education teachers (see also Chapter 11). The special school was to combine the work of teaching children and training local teachers. Furthermore, the teachers had knowledge and skills in only one type of impairment. Working in an ordinary school would have brought them in contact with children for whom they were not prepared.

Unesco (1986), in a worldwide survey in 14 countries, showed that teachers who are not trained in special education feel uneasy about accepting disabled children in their classes (see Chapter 9). In a recent study by the present author (Kisanji 1992), the views of ordinary classroom teachers on integration in Tanzania were sought. It was found that almost half recommended special school placement mainly because they were not specially trained. The irony of this, however, is that the same teachers are being successfully involved in a community-based rehabilitation (CBR) project.

Parents and school placement
Parental expectations are that the school will bring about noticeable improvements in their child within a short period. When this does not happen, they may withdraw the child from the school or transfer the child to another similar or different school (Kisanji 1985, 1991). Sometimes, when the child is treated inappropriately, parental action is completely justified, as when a deaf child is considered 'mentally handicapped', or a slow-learning child is retained in the same class for as long as ten years (Mwangi 1983).

Community-based services
The child who is born with or who acquires an impairment early in life may be lucky to find her or himself in a family of accepting parents and in an area where rehabilitation programmes exist. In such a case the family may receive guidance and counselling from the community health worker, family welfare educator, social worker, community rehabilitation worker, rehabilitation assistant, educational assessment and resource teacher or itinerant teacher, depending on the service and terminology used in the locality or country. However, the presence of health centres and clinics does not always guarantee an advisory and/or therapeutic service. Bennett (1981) has lamented that these facilities are concerned merely with the weighing of babies. This picture is not entirely true in view of the existence of close collaboration between teachers and nurses at the community level in some countries such as Botswana, Kenya, Tanzania and Zimbabwe (Unesco 1981, 1989; Kisanji 1991), where community nurses and teachers work hand-in-hand in the assessment of children with impairments and in subsequent interventions. In Tanzania, for example, nurses were able, with some training, to set up an assessment centre at an ordinary primary school, as a result of which special classes for intellectually impaired children have been established (Unesco 1989).

Medical, educational and vocational rehabilitation services are now available in almost every country, although coverage is far from complete. The implementation of CBR takes various forms in different countries (O'Toole 1990, Kisanji 1995) (see Chapter 11). Although there are differing child-rearing practices, and medico-spiritual beliefs leading to hiding or overprotection of disabled children in Africa (Walker 1986, Devlieger 1989, Ingstad 1990), many children and young people are reached by some form of service in their community. However, they are often not included in educational and medical statistics.

Attempts have been made in several countries to evaluate the effectiveness of projects and programmes, such as CBR in Kenya and Zimbabwe (AMREF 1987, O'Toole 1991), daycare centres in Botswana (Otaala *et al.* 1989) and an itinerant teaching service for children with visual impairment in Kenya and Malawi (McCall and Best 1990, 1993). These project and programme evaluations identify their viability and areas of strength and weakness. However, it is also important to look at specific intervention measures which have affected the individual disabled person.

Experiences of disabled young people

The account that follows is the result of personal observation and interviews with young people who have impairments, and with their parents, as well as with teachers and community rehabilitation workers, in Botswana, Kenya, Malawi and Tanzania from 1987 to 1992. The experiences are presented to reflect successful and unsuccessful interventions. The focus is on adolescents and young adults, which has the added benefit of allowing sufficient time for reflection on what services may have achieved for individuals.

1. Mambo is 18 years old. He started to speak only at the age of 4 years. He could not follow even simple instructions at home. His parents and elder brother and sister thought he was deaf. The village dispensary had advised the parents to take him to the district hospital where he was also diagnosed to be deaf, but nonetheless he was referred to the national hospital for further check-up. As a school for the deaf was nearer than the hospital, his parents decided to seek admission to the school which accepted children as early as 5 years of age. After several tests, Mambo was declared to be hearing and, therefore, was not accepted by the school. A visit to the national hospital was now unavoidable. The ear, nose and throat (ENT) specialist confirmed the diagnosis made by the school and referred Mambo to the Psychiatric Unit where intellectual impairment was suspected. He was referred to the only special school for 'the mentally handicapped' in the country. His parents were reluctant to part with their child because the school was residential. As Mambo's condition was not as severe as that of most children in the school, he was transferred after two years to a special class which had just opened in a town far from his home village, where he lived with relatives. He was placed with children in Level 2.

He remained in that class for ten years. His parents were very disappointed as they expected Mambo to develop like other children, though not as fast. In addition it was expensive for them to visit Mambo several times a term. Last year a special class for children with learning difficulties was opened in a nearby town. His parents decided to transfer Mambo to this unit. To their surprise, Mambo is making a lot of progress. He can now read and write fluently and neatly. He has also been made one of the school prefects.

2. Kalinga and Haswa, 16, are visually impaired twins and both in their final year at an ordinary junior secondary school. They were admitted into Grade 1 at the age of 6 years. However, when their father, as the village headman, was first contacted to identify visually impaired children to be enrolled in a new special school to be opened in a neighbouring village, he had dismissed the foreign (White) teachers with the excuse that there were no such children in his village. Kalinga and Haswa were then about 2 years old. Acting on a tip they had been given by local colleagues, the teachers continued visiting the headman until one day, when he was with them, the two children crawled out from their confinement in a neighbouring room. It then became easy to negotiate with him for their education. The two White teachers took turns to visit the family with a local teacher they had identified to train in order to work with them in the new special school. They helped the headman

to try to understand the causes and effects of blindness as well as how to train the children at home. When the school opened, he was taken to see for himself what and how blind children were being taught. When his two children turned 6 he agreed to send them to the special residential school for the blind.

3. Musasa, 15, was born deaf. His mother suspected something was amiss because he lay quietly for long hours when left alone unless he was wet or hungry. His father would boast of this behaviour, as he recalled being told by his parents that he had been a very quiet and peaceful child. However, Musasa's mother confided only in her own mother, lest she created problems with her husband if she mentioned her suspicion. She noted that Musasa was not able to talk at $1^1/_2$, nor at 2, nor at $2^1/_2$ years. His only means of communication were pointing at objects, pulling his mother and elder sister, and crying. Finally at some point his mother decided that she had to consult one of her husband's elder sisters who, it was agreed, should make Musasa's unusual development 'officially' known to him. This had to be done with caution and circumlocution, using many proverbs, metaphors and riddles. It took several weeks for the man's sister to come to the point of Musasa's problem. However, once she had told him he said that he understood his wife's predicament and assured her that Musasa's condition would not affect their marriage. They took Musasa to the local medicine man and the dispensary, but never beyond this. As the nearest school for the deaf was about 120 kilometres away they did not bother to take Musasa there. However, Musasa made friends as he grew up and followed them to the local school, against the wishes of his parents who wanted him to help in the house, with the cattle and in the banana grove. Teachers in the school did not know what to do with Musasa, and he consequently dropped out of 'the school adventure'. Today he communicates by means of gestures and a kind of sign language understood by his family and by other deaf people in the community, and he is actively involved in the agricultural activities of his parents.

4. Ganga, aged 20 years and physically impaired (with wasting of the lower limbs), went to ordinary primary and secondary schools. He started school at the age of 6. He crawled on the rough village road 3 km to and from the nearest primary school. At the age of 12 he performed highly in the primary school leaving examinations and was selected to join a residential secondary school away from home in another region of the country the following year. He had to contend with the hustle and bustle of travelling to and from school each term covering a distance of over 400 km, by the often crowded buses and train with the help of a relative or school friends. Ganga had to be carried onto vehicles and into buildings with stepped entrances. School friends were always ready to assist Ganga, including with washing and ironing. He has always had friends of both sexes. He is now in his second year at university. Early this year he was presented with a wheelchair bought with contributions from second year students.

5. Jahazi, now 19 years old, went blind in one eye ten years ago. When he went to hospital his eyeball was removed. Since then vision in his other eye has steadily deteriorated. His academic progress regressed with the gradual loss of vision. The ordinary school he attended did not make any special support arrangements for his learning. He performed very poorly in the leaving examinations at the end of primary school. Jahazi has now been in hospital for two months; the eye specialists have not as yet decided what to do with him. His attempts to find out the nature of his visual problem have been fruitless. Jahazi is interested in going to a special school or vocational training centre for visually impaired persons where he may learn braille reading and writing as well as a trade, but hospital staff have not been able to advise him.

6. Papa, aged 12 years, who has hearing impairment, was enrolled in the local CBR project when

he was 4. The community rehabilitation worker used to work with Papa's grandmother on his communication skills, social skills and the 'three Rs' (reading, writing and arithmetic). She made arrangements at the city's general hospital for Papa to see the ENT surgeon. She accompanied them on the first two visits, during which the grandmother was shown how to clean his ears and to administer medication and asked to bring Papa back to the hospital once a month for check-up. However, he was taken to hospital only once after this. The grandmother claimed she had no money to pay for transport, which was less than five pence in local currency at the time, and that she had no-one to look after her stall where she sold vegetables from her garden. In the meantime the community rehabilitation worker arranged for Papa to be placed at a local preschool. A visit to the school showed that Papa played alone. Pus was oozing from his ears and produced a bad odour. The teachers had appealed several times to the grandmother to take Papa to hospital but with no success. The CBR project, which was paying Papa's school fees, had to resume attending to his health. Papa is now in Grade 6 in the community primary school.

7. Zara could not walk until the age of 5 years. Even at age 15 she is still drooling and not completely toilet trained. Her parents have taken her to a number of witch-doctors and herbalists as well as to Christian crusade prayer meetings in search of a cure. Several appointments at the hospital showed that very little medical help could be given. Schools for children with learning difficulties to which she was referred could not admit her because she was not toilet trained. Finally at the age of 10 she was recruited into the local CBR project. The rehabilitation worker visits Zara twice a week but works with her alone. Her mother goes to the market in the morning leaving her by herself at home; her father disappeared to an unknown place when she was 6 years old. Activities during the visits are centred around greetings, singing, arithmetic and writing, but Zara has not learned to cook and cannot keep herself clean.

8. Maua, aged 16 years, was admitted into a CBR project four years ago. She was discovered by a community rehabilitation worker during one of her visits to another child in the neighbourhood. Maua is the elder of two children, her brother being 10 years old. She has never learned to stand on her own and appears to have a hip dislocation. Her legs are thin and cannot stretch. She moves by crawling. Maua underwent an operation last year to release the leg contractures, but still cannot use her legs. She now uses knee and hand pads made from old car tyres to help her move comfortably and safely on rough ground. She is too old to be accepted at the local primary school which her brother attends. Instead she sells charcoal outside their house to supplement her mother's income. Her mother, a single parent, is an office messenger in a large town and after office hours sells fried fish in the slum area where they live. The community rehabilitation worker used to visit Maua once a week to help her with physical exercises, but had to stop when Maua started selling charcoal as the visits would have interrupted Maua's working hours and she could not afford to miss a single customer.

9. Iganga is now 20 years old. He went to a special school for children with learning difficulties for ten years. Five years ago, he made friends with some children older than himself in the neighbourhood and refused to continue going to school. Since then he has been roaming the streets with his friends. Last year Iganga was arrested for attempting to steal a bag at a bus station. His friends ran away and left him behind. In court, he could not be well understood, and even when his parents explained their son's condition to the police, they were not listened to. Iganga himself claims that he did not know what was going on at the bus station. He only saw his friends running away. Apart from his parents, no-one, not even the local association for persons with 'mental handicap', was prepared to help Iganga out of this mess. He was convicted, together with the friends who were caught through him.

10. Mapesa, 20, attended ordinary primary and secondary schools with attached residential resource rooms for the blind. Although Mapesa has some residual vision, he was taught to read and write braille. Teachers discouraged him from using his sight, but he learned to read inkprint with the help of classmates. He can write a few words, and is very proud that he can write his name and recognize his signature. Mapesa speaks highly in favour of integration, but is unhappy that the schools did not give him enough typing skills. He had to consolidate these in teacher training college.

Mapesa has prepared two weddings which did not materialize. He met the first girlfriend at a pub where she worked. Within three months, he proposed marriage to her. He informed his relatives, but when wedding arrangements had begun, his close friends told him that his fiancée was flirting with three different men. The second attempt came a year later, with a girl he met at a friend's house. She was a secretary in one of the government departments in a nearby town. She backed out of the marriage arrangements because she did not want to live in the village where he was teaching.

11. Mitimingi, 20, and Mikoche, 18, are both deaf. They attended the same special primary school for children with hearing impairment. After the ten years of primary education, they both secured places at the vocational training centre run by the same agency which runs the school. They got married last year and now have a baby boy. The agency helped them to rent a house in town not far from the school. Every day during the rainy season, after work at the training centre, the new couple used to go to their farm. They had a good yield of maize and beans last season and they planned to increase the acreage under crop this season. Mikoche spends most of the time with their baby now, something which Mitimingi is unhappy about. For three days he emphatically asked his wife not to eat because she had not been working on the farm with him. A person eats after working hard! Mikoche had to seek advice from the headteacher of the special school on what to do, as her husband does not understand the important role she is now playing in the family. The headteacher and one of the senior male teachers have gone to the family twice to talk to Mitimingi about family roles and responsibilities. The headteacher plans to increase the amount of time spent on family education and homecraft in the curriculum.

Reflections on the experiences

The experiences of the young people described here raise some salient issues of growing up disabled in a developing country. The discussion below focuses on the family structure, religion, child-rearing practices, parental expectations, school effectiveness, community-based services, collaboration between parents and professionals, social relationships, employment opportunities and quality of life in general. All these issues must be seen within the context of continual, and sometimes rapid, cultural change. Culture, then, forms the important backcloth so often ignored by Western rehabilitation experts (Miles 1989).

The family structure

The developing countries of Africa and Asia differ from the Western world in the dominant family structure, and this in turn affects the source of support for a disabled person that may be readily available or easily solicited. In Europe and North America the unit is mainly limited to the nuclear family. In Africa and Asia the aunts and uncles are as important as, sometimes more important than, the biological parents. Aunts, uncles and grandparents have specific roles to play, especially at puberty and in initiation and marriage ceremonies (van Pelt 1982). The extended family system in developing countries places the respons-ibility for the care, education, welfare and employment of children and young people on competent members of the large matrix of relations (Sechrest *et al.* 1973, Datta 1984, Bickford and Wickham 1986, Salia-Bao 1989).

Although culture is constantly changing (Carrithers 1992), the extended family system may be difficult to dismantle altogether in view of its origins and its intricate links with indigenous religious beliefs and politico-economic factors. Salia-Bao (1989) provides a useful description of the origins and the contribution of the extended family system to communal life. He writes:

'It is the intermingling of the father's 'spirit' with the mother's blood (in the sense of kinship) which is believed to form the child. This explains Africans' belief in communal life and the extended family system. Its most important expression is the system of lineage. By extension, this spiritual entity explains inherited characteristics and creates a type of group personality, which gives a certain formalism to the larger society and lays the foundation of the community personality.

'Lineage ties form the basis of communal life, which is the main source of economic and polit-ical life. For example, members of a lineage own land together through the eldest parent and chief. They help one another to build houses, make farms and in many other ways. Lineage heads have the duty of maintaining peace and unity within the co-operating group. The lineage tie is important in understanding the settlement pattern of the people, their concepts of land, and their ways of using land resources and developing people for various services.'

With lingering poverty in the developing countries exacerbated by unjust world trade, policy imposition in the form of structural adjustment and general global economic re-cession (Seidman and Anang 1992), it is difficult to believe that in the foreseeable future the extended family system will be completely eroded, despite such signs in urban centres.

Parents of disabled children in developing countries experience the same emotional states as their counterparts in developed nations. However, despite the gross underdevelop-ment of Western-type support systems, they have the benefit of sharing the responsibilities involved in caring for the child within the extended family structure. This is evident in the case of Mambo and Papa, both of whom lived with relatives in cities during at least part of their school career.

The movement of people from rural to urban areas has also meant separation from the close-knit support system that would otherwise be available to parents of disabled young people in the rural communities. In a typical extended family set-up Zara and Maua could not have been left on their own and seen by the community rehabilitation worker in the absence of another adult family member.

Disabled young people and their parents in urban centres, especially those in the poor city slums, have a double disadvantage. They receive nothing in the form of support. They have no support from relatives, most of whom live in the rural areas. Those relatives who may be in the same towns are poorer than those in rural areas because they have no farms, but instead have poorly paid, often menial jobs. They cannot find time and money to help a needy relative. At the same time most developing countries do not have an elaborate system of social and community workers or respite care, or of social security payments, as found in developed countries.

Religion

Traditional African religion is a ubiquitous life factor which cannot be unravelled or separated from any aspect of human activity. Drawing heavily from J.S. Mbiti's *African Religions and Philosophy*, Salia-Bao (1989) writes:

'Mbiti believes that 'African religion' has no definition because it is limitless. Because traditional religions permeate all areas of life, there is no formal distinction between the sacred and the secular, the religious and the non-religious, the spiritual and the material. Wherever Africans are, there is our religion: we carry it to the fields to sow seeds or harvest a new crop; to the beer party or to attend a funeral ceremony; those engaged in education take religion to the examination room at school or university; politicians take it to parliament. Although many African languages do not have a word for religion as such, it nevertheless accompanies the individual from long before birth to long after death. In modern times these traditional religions have not remained intact, but they are by no means extinct. They often come to the surface in times of crisis, or people revert to them in secret. . . Traditional religion is not primarily for the individual, but for the community to which he or she belongs.'

This vivid description implicitly and rightly suggests that religion is taught and learned, by tradition, in folk tales, songs, proverbs, riddles, dances, rituals and ceremonies, virtually in every activity. Religion, as it was introduced by missionaries as supporters of the colonial administration, had a pacifying effect, leading to the acceptance of the status quo and sometimes complacency. However, as Salia-Bao points out, "African traditional religion is deep-seated in African culture, and it forms the basis of the extended family system, chieftaincy practices, the land tenure system and all socio-political practices. . . Cameron and Dodd warn that, despite a century of imperialist cultural aggression in various guises, 'the persistence today of indigenous cultural processes should not be underestimated'."

The birth of a child is a religious event because it is the product of the 'mixing of the father's spirit with the blood of the mother'. Hence ceremonies surround the birth. However, the birth of a child with an impairment (or becoming impaired later in life) is viewed with suspicion, as this may be due to the wrongs committed by the parents or grandparents against God, the gods or the ancestral spirits. Efforts to trace the wrong-doer often lead to blame falling on one spouse, usually the woman. This is the kind of situation that Musasa's mother found herself in. Her husband had boasted of being a quiet child and was not deaf. Why had Musasa developed this problem?

Traditional education was mainly oral and people learned by doing (Nyerere 1967). This form of learning also applied to religion. Proverbs, riddles and songs carried religious and other messages. Musasa's aunt used these successfully to win her brother's understanding of Musasa's condition and his wife's predicament.

Perhaps the most significant effect of religion on disability is the motivation it provided to seek a cure, redress with God, the gods or ancestral spirits, to 'neutralize' the 'bad eye' of non-well-wishers and to counteract the effects of witchcraft and sorcery. This was the case with Zara. Her parents consulted witchdoctors and herbalists and when this failed they went to the Christian crusade prayer meetings which, unfortunately again, did not yield the expected outcomes. The motivating religious beliefs are so deep-rooted that most parents and relatives, at some point or other, openly or secretly, consult and seek the services of witchdoctors, herbalists, fortune-tellers, fetish priests and others thought to be of possible help in removing the impairment and/or ameliorating its effects (Okeahialam 1974, Walker 1986, Kisanji 1993). The spread of conventional medicine, community health and literacy has had merely a superficial effect on this belief system.

Child-rearing practices
Walker (1986) cautions against assuming homogeneity of African customs and attitudes toward disease and, by extension, disability. The caution is pertinent also to other developing countries, even those strongly characterized by the extended family structure.

The growing child becomes acquainted with the customs and values cherished by the community, including those related to disability. Disabled children assimilate the language used and actions of all around them. Generally, those who survive, whatever their condition and severity, tend to be given extra care and protection by family members. The hiding away of the children reported in literature is often explained away by parental shame and guilt (Sauter 1978, Walker 1986, Onwuegbu 1988). Overprotection is perhaps the largest single factor which results in hiding and refusal to send disabled children to school and other services (Lowenfield 1972).

Kalinga and Haswa may have been affected by parental overprotection. The confinement within the house may also be a reflection of the fact that responsibility for their children is seen to lie with the family. Strangers were not welcomed. This possibility can be deduced from the fact that community members knew about the existence of Kalinga and Haswa. They had tipped off the White teachers before the latter visited the headman.

Overprotectiveness is also vividly described in the case of my own experience while in the care of my grandmother. I was not allowed to play away from home, and only passive and less boisterous play was prescribed. This was an unfortunate situation in view of the importance of play, also acknowledged in indigenous education, for the growing child (Fontana 1988, Salia-Bao 1989). Thus children and young people who have impairments, whose parents and relatives or guardians provide little or no exposure to play and other forms of environmental stimulation, are likely to be physically, socially, emotionally and intellectually stunted. Luckily Kalinga, Haswa and I were not adversely affected, at least intellectually.

Naming of children according to their impairment ('Mpofu'—blind; 'Mapula'—deaf) may inflict a sense of helplessness. Apart from the labelling effects on the expectations of parents and service providers, such names may have negative influence on the development of self-concept and self-esteem of the growing child (see Chapter 2).

Western society has generally become more permissive in its child-rearing practices despite the expected community and family variation. It emphasizes and 'fosters a growing degree of independence and of choice' (Wolfson 1976). The extended family in Africa is founded on authoritarian hierarchy, from the chief or clan head to the youngest members. Busia (see Salia-Bao 1989) believes that 'African society is founded on duties rather than rights', duties that are both ritualistic and humanistic. These duties are fostered through socialization in the home, at play and during dances, rituals and ceremonies. Serpell *et al.* (1993) support this view, saying that, 'Whereas Western theories of socialization have

195

tended to place a great deal of emphasis on the promotion of autonomy, African parents tend, by contrast, to be more preoccupied with the cultivation of social responsibility and nurturance.'

They also cite authors who describe the 'complete' or 'educated' individual in the African sense as one who has 'good manners or tact, sociability, self-awareness in relation to oneself, one's brother, one's family and the community, self-control and mastery of one's emotions [and] tenacity of character.' Thus, respect for age, responsibility and social status, prescribed roles of boys and girls, and participation in family and communal activities were enforced within set standards by all elders and through peer pressure.

These duties applied to all members of the community, including disabled people. However, the expected level of competence would differ according to the individual's physical and intellectual ability. This expectation may be summed up by the following proverbs, translated into Kiswahili, used among the Wapare and Wakerewe of Tanzania respectively: *Hata kama ni jinga, litengenzee upinde,* which literally means 'Give him a bow and arrow even if he is a fool'; and *Asiyekiuno naye huvua,* meaning, 'A person without a waistline [considered to be ugly in the given community] takes off clothes to take a bath like others' (Omari *et al.* 1978). These proverbs are used to tell people that every person, whatever her/his limitations, is capable of contributing something to community life.

Interviews with parents and teachers about young people who have impairments often begin or end with what the individual can or cannot do according to age and sex. Musasa's parents want him to look after cattle and help in the banana grove because they know he can do this; they are not sure he can succeed in school which, in any case, is located 120km away. The importance of a girl learning to cook is reflected in the story of Zara. Even at the age of 15 she was not able to cook a meal. In most African homes, girls are able to cook, wash clothes, clean the house and generally look after their younger brothers and sisters as early as 7 to 8 years.

Parental expectations
Parental expectations may be reflected in child-rearing practices, gender stereotyping and the kind and level of competences demanded of young people. In many instances parental expectations are very clear—as in the cases of Mambo, Musasa, Ganga and Zara—namely, to have a good formal education, to acquire skills relevant to life in the community, and to be able to contribute to family upkeep through learning by doing. When these expectations are not met, parents give vent to their dissatisfaction in a number of ways such as withdrawing children from, or changing, schools or programmes; refusing to register them into school or service; not participating in home visits in CBR programmes or in meetings with professionals; and joining pressure groups with interests similar to their own. Some of these reactions can be observed in the experiences of Mambo (changing schools), Musasa (refusal to send to school) and Zara (non-participation). Many parents who are members of associations of parents of disabled persons are motivated by the expectations they hold for their children, although associations are a very recent development in many countries.

School effectiveness

As in the case of Mambo's parents, one area of concern is the school. Special schools and units in many countries are few and far between. Parents who do not want to part with their disabled children for any considerable period of time, and especially those who are not convinced of the benefits to them of formal education, would resist sending them to school. Interviews conducted by the special education team in rural villages in Tanzania in 1980 during a Unesco/World Bank Education Sector Study (Kisanji *et al.* 1981) showed that parents were not prepared to send their children to special schools located in other regions of the country.

There are a number of problems which impinge on the effectiveness of special education. The motivation of teachers in special education in many African countries leaves much to be desired. Demands for extra allowances and better conditions of service continue to rage on in a number of countries including Botswana and Tanzania (Kisanji 1991, Mkaali *et al.* 1992). The effectiveness of special education is also affected by inadequate financial and human resources. Teachers in special education are not only in short supply but their quality is also, in many countries, of particular concern. For instance, writing from his experience in Kenya, Mwangi (1983) observed:

'. . in many classes opportunities for pupils to learn and master new skills are not adequately provided. . . some teachers have lower and negative expectations as to what their child [*sic*] can do. Therefore lessons are not well prepared, their presentations are generally poor and children are not appropriately reinforced. The result of all this is that children have remained in a class for many years having learnt little in the area of academics [*sic*] and social competence.'

A situation such as this points to the need for better training of teachers (see Chapter 9).

In addition, many special schools and units in developing countries have classroom arrangements in which pupils continue to be seated in rows, with non-interactive teaching methods and culturally inappropriate curricula (see Chapter 9). Malbran and MacDonagh (1993) have highlighted similar criticisms of curricula in special education in Ibero-American countries, namely: a lack of ecological validity resulting from the adoption of models, methods and materials produced in developed countries; non-functional learning, *i.e.* learning not directly applicable to common daily task demands in the natural and social environment; training in unsuitable skills, not based on an analysis of cultural context and projected future needs; and a lack of balance between academic, recreational, socio-cultural and vocational skills training. 'These inadequacies', they claim, 'affect motivation and expectations about the validity of special education.' Mwangi (1989) gives an example of inappropriate curriculum when he describes a classroom situation in Kenya in which adolescents with learning difficulties are made to count bottle tops as part of number work or to work on light bulbs for a Philips factory. Instead they could be learning to sell charcoal or to roast maize which is a popular snack in both rural and urban areas.

Against this background, it may not be possible to explain Mambo's progress in his last school by a single factor. The encouragement and support of his parents when they were able to see him more often and regularly, the school ethos and innovative teaching methods, curricular relevance and age-appropriateness, and Mambo's increased disposition to learn may all account for his success.

Collaboration between parents and professionals

The success of modern rehabilitation services implies a partnership of all stakeholders, namely, disabled people, their parents, the immediate and wider community and the professionals. Unfortunately, the most important stakeholders, the disabled people themselves, have for far too long been 'objects' rather than part of the rehabilitation process. For instance, people with low vision have been restricted to learning to read and write braille (Corn 1986), those with hearing impairments have had to be taught with varying levels of success to speak (Unesco 1984), and those with 'mental handicap' brushed aside as incapable of making decisions (Mittler 1993). However, thanks to pressure from associations of disabled people and advances in psychology, technology and medicine, the global trend is changing positively. Programmes for people with low vision are gradually being introduced in many developing countries so that people like Mapesa will not in future be unnecessarily subjected to learning braille.

The economic status and type of the family may often determine whether a family member will play a leading role in the training and education of their child in partnership with a trained home visitor. Absence of extended family support in an urban setting and social pressures on single mothers often frustrate the efforts of those professionals who would like to work in partnership with families. Maua, Papa and Zara suffered from insufficient input from family members. However, partnership should mean that the times of visit and/or consultation should take into account the convenience of the caregivers. Zara would probably have gained more if the training had been carried out in the presence of her mother who could have suggested the most appropriate skills for her daughter.

Partnership also raises the issue of mutual trust as a basis for collaboration. Mambo's parents wanted to see quick outcomes from schools; Zara's parents did not believe in what the hospitals told them and instead sought a cure from traditional healers and prayer meetings; and Papa's grandmother did not think it was worthwhile taking him to hospital repeatedly for cleaning his ears. Professionals should learn to negotiate with parents and families and to provide information in ways they can assimilate. Mittler (1993), after presenting the summary of the results of a Unesco survey of partnership between parents and professionals, concluded:

'We need to reappraise the whole basis of our relationships with parents; to see them as equals and as partners, to listen to them and consult them from the outset, not only about their child but about the nature of our programmes and what we have to offer. This applies equally to all countries but particularly to societies where few or no resources are available to disabled children.'

Social relationships

The experiences of Iganga, Mapesa, and Mitimingi and Mikoche are perhaps not unique to disabled people, but they point to the degree of relevance of current education and rehabilitation programmes as preparation for social integration and meaningful life in the community. An unsuccessful education career caused, among other factors, by a curriculum that is unresponsive to the specific needs of disabled young people can lead to their being unscrupulously exploited and abused by both their peer group and older people. For a social system that is not alert to the specific needs and rights of disabled people and to the prevalence of physical, sexual, economic and psychological harassment, exploitation and abuse, disabled people, such as Iganga, continue to 'suffer without bitterness'. Think also of the many disabled children, women and men who are planted in the streets to beg in order to fatten the pockets of their so-called 'kings' every evening in return for an assured daily meal! The story of organized street begging in Lagos (Okoli 1993) can be repeated for many developing countries.

Indigenous education was rich and relevant in that it covered all aspects of community living. Story telling, riddles, proverbs and songs by the evening fire, in dances and during ceremonies touched on morality and the consequences of wrongdoing, bad and good company, bravery, the unwritten law, social and political unity, sex roles, duties and responsibilities, courtship, the bride-price and marriage, homecare and child-rearing, polygamy and the dangers of promiscuity, care of the sick and the aged and death (van Pelt 1982, Datta 1984, Salia-Bao 1989). This informal system of education persists today in both rural and urban areas. Except for those with profound impairments, all young people underwent the initiation ceremonies including endurance tests, sex education, circumcision or clitoridectomy and adult role training. (For a description of social participation in some West African countries for people with intellectual impairment, see Serpell *et al.* 1993.)

Mitimingi paid the bride-price before wedding Mikoche, and Mapesa would have to pay it, at least in part, before the wedding. Disability is no licence to remission of the bride-price.

Conclusion

Growing up disabled in a developing country may appear to the Westerner as desolate and gloomy. Indeed the critical indicators of human development such as infant and under-5 mortality rates, immunization coverage, life expectancy at birth, net enrolment ratios, literacy, urbanization and the gross national product per capita (Grant 1992, United Nations Development Programme 1992) present a gruesome picture. The chances of survival for the children with impairments who require specialist medical care are low, and when they survive there are no assurances that they will receive proper medical care and education (see Chapter 1).

However, in the midst of the struggles for economic survival and well-being, the general practice in developing countries is to raise disabled young people as accepted members of the community. They grow up within a social world which includes the meaningful messages of the lullaby on the mother's back, fetching of water from the family or communal village well, moonlight play of hide-and-seek, initiation into adulthood, looking after farm animals and crops, possibly choosing a partner and making a home. Disabled people share in these social experiences with varying degrees of accomplishment. This quality of life could be improved by raising the living standards of the population in general. The question still remains: how can disabled people have equal opportunities in developing countries in the face of rapid cultural change, worldwide recession, armed conflicts, continued imbalance of trade, structural adjustment and the ongoing rapid technological advances of the modern world?

REFERENCES

Abosi, O.C., Ozoji, E.D. (1985) *Educating the Blind—a Descriptive Approach.* Ibadan, Nigeria: Spectrum Books.

AMREF (1987) *The Nairobi Family Support Service. A Participatory Evaluation Report.* Nairobi: African Medical and Research Foundation.

Bennett, F.J. (1981) 'The role of health services in the early detection of impairments, disabilities and handicaps.' *Paper presented at the Unesco Seminar on Planning for Special Education, Nairobi, 20–30 July.*

Bickford, T., Wickham, E. R. (1986) 'Attitudes towards the mentally retarded—results from six countries.' *In:* Marfo, K., Walker, S., Charles, B. (Eds.) *Childhood Disability in Developing Countries—Issues in Habilitation and Special Education.* New York: Praeger, pp. 251–262.

Carrithers, M. (1992) *Why Humans Have Cultures: Explaining Anthropology and Social Diversity.* Oxford: Oxford University Press.

Chowo, H.T. (1978) *Survey of Disabled Children in 29 Villages with Community Schools.* Dar es Salaam: Ministry of Education. *(Research report.)*

Corn, A.L. (1986) 'Low vision and visual efficiency.' *In:* Scholl, G.T. (Ed.) *Foundations of Education for Blind and Visually Handicapped Children and Youth: Theory and Practice.* New York: American Foundation for the Blind, pp. 99–119.

Datta, A. (1984) *Education and Society: A Sociology of African Education.* London: Macmillan.

Dery, S.E. (1991) 'The education of visually handicapped children: an African perspective.' *Kenya Institute of Special Education Bulletin,* (April), 16–19.

Devlieger, P. (1989) 'The cultural significance of physical disability in Africa.' *Paper presented at the Annual Meeting of the Society for Applied Anthropology, Santa Fe, New Mexico, USA, 5–9 April.*

Evans, J.L. (1970) *Children in Africa: a Review of Psychological Research.* New York: Columbia University, Teachers College Press.

Fafunwa, A.B. (1967) *New Perspectives in African Education.* Lagos: Macmillan.

—— Aisiku, J.U. (Eds.) (1982) *Education in Africa: a Comparative Survey.* London: George Allen & Unwin.

Fontana, D. (1988) *Psychology for Teachers, 2nd Edn.* Leicester: British Psychological Society/Macmillan.

Freire, P. (1972) *Pedagogy of the Oppressed.* New York: Continuum.

Gearheart, B.R., Weishahn, M.W. (1976) *The Handicapped Child in the Regular Classroom.* St. Louis: C.V. Mosby.

Gould S.J. (1981) *The Mismeasure of Man.* London: Penguin.

Grant, J.P. (1991–1993) *The State of the World's Children, 1991; 1992; 1993.* New York: Unicef.

Groce, N. (1989–90) 'Traditional folk belief systems and disabilities: an important factor in policy planning.' *One in Ten,* **8–9,** 2–7.

Holmes, J., Hurst, P. (Eds.) (1983) *International Handbook of Education Systems. Vol. II. Africa and the Middle East.* Oxford: Oxford University Press.

Ingstad, B. (1990) 'Disability and culture.' *In:* Bruun, F.J., Ingstad, B. (Eds.) *Disability in a Cross-cultural Perspective. Working Paper No. 4/1990.* Oslo: Department of Social Anthropology, University of Norway.

Institute of Education (1984) *Development of Special Education in Tanzania.* Dar es Salaam: Institute of Education.

Kenyatta, J. (1965) *Facing Mount Kenya.* London: Vintage Books.

Kisanji, J. (1985) *Report to the Ministry of Education, Science and Technology on Visits to Special Education Programmes in Kenya.* Nairobi: Unesco.

—— (1991) *A Review of Special Education in Botswana and Recommendations for a National Policy.* Gaborone, Botswana: Ministry of Education. *(Consultancy report.)*

—— (Ed.) (1992) *Basic Facts About Special Education in Tanzania.* Dar es Salaam: Ministry of Education and Culture.

—— (1993) 'Special education in Africa.' *In:* Mittler, P., Brouillette, R., Harris, D. (Eds.) *World Yearbook of Education: Special Needs Education.* London: Kogan Page, pp. 158–172.

—— (1995) 'Understanding CBR models.' *CBR News,* No. 19, p. 4.

—— Nchimbi, J.E., Maggs, A. (1981) 'Special education for the handicapped.' *In:* United Republic of Tanzania *Development of Education: Opportunities for External Funding. Report No. 39.* Paris: Unesco, pp. 223–253.

Lowenfield, B. (1972) *Our Blind Children: Growing and Learning with Them. 2nd Edn.* Springfield: C.C. Thomas.

Malbran, M.delC., MacDonagh, M.I. (1993) 'Special education in Ibero-American countries: current situation and tendencies.' *In:* Mittler, P., Brouillette, R., Harris, D. (Eds.) *World Yearbook on Education: Special Needs Education.* London: Kogan Page, pp. 141–157.

Marfo, K., Walker, S., Bernard, C. (1983) *Childhood Disability in Developing Countries: Towards Improved Services.* Edmonton, Alberta: Centre for International Education and Development, University of Alberta.

—— —— —— (1986) *Childhood Disability in Developing Countries: Issues in Habilitation and Special Education.* New York: Praeger.

McCall, S., Best, T. (1990) *Itinerant Teaching Services in Kenya/Malawi.* London: Royal Commonwealth Society for the Blind. *(Research report.)*

—— —— (1993) 'Planning mainstream education services for children with visual impairments in developing countries.' *In:* Mittler, P. Brouillette, R., Harris, D. (Eds.) *World Yearbook of Education: Special Needs Education.* London: Kogan Page, pp. 65–75.

Miles, M. (1989) 'The role of special education in information based rehabilitation.' *International Journal of Special Education,* **4**, 111–118.

Mittler, P. (1993) 'Childhood disability: a global challenge.' *In:* Mittler, P., Brouillette, R., Harris, D. (Eds.) *World Yearbook of Education 1993: Special Needs Education.* London: Kogan Page, pp. 3–15.

Mkaali, C., Kulwa, B., Kisanji, J., Eklindh, K. (1992) *Policy Guidelines for the Development of Special Education in Tanzania.* Stockholm: Swedish International Development Authority for the Ministry of Education, Dar es Salaam, Tanzania.

Mwangi, P.D. (1983) 'The curriculum not the hindrance but the teachers!' *Special Education Bulletin for Eastern and Southern Africa,* **1** (3), 5.

Nyerere, J.K. (1967) *Education for Self Reliance.* Dar es Salaam: Printpak.

—— (1974) *Man and Development.* Dar es Salaam: Oxford University Press.

Okeahialam, T. (1974) 'The handicapped child in the African environment.' *In: The Child in the African Environment: Growth, Development and Survival. Proceedings of the 1974 Annual Scientific Conference of the East African Medical Research Council.* Kampala: EAMRC, pp. 371–377.

Okoli, C.I.B. (1993) 'The menace of organised street-begging in Lagos, Nigeria.' *Disability Awareness in Action Newsletter,* **10** (September), 3–4.

Omari, C.K., Kezilahabi, E., Kamera, W.D. (1978) *Misemo na Methali toka Tanzania.* Arusha, Tanzania: Eastern Africa Publications.

Onwuegbu, O.I. (1988) 'Development of special education in Nigeria.' *In:* Abosi, O.C. (Ed.) *Development of Special Education in Nigeria. Papers in Honour of Peter Mba and Samuel C. Osunkiyesi.* Ibadan, Nigeria: Fountains Books, pp. 5–12.

Otaala, B., Njenga, A., Monau, R. (1989) *An Evaluation of the Day Care Programme in Botswana. A Consultancy Report for the Government of Botswana and the United Nations Children's Fund (Unicef).*

O'Toole, B. (1990) 'Community based rehabilitation: the Guyana Evaluation Project.' *In:* Thorburn, M.J., Marfo, K. (Eds.) *Practical Approaches to Childhood Disability in Developing Countries: Insights from Experience and Research.* St Johns, Newfoundland: Memorial University, Project SEREDEC; Spanish Town, Jamaica: 3D Projects, pp. 293–346.

—— (1991) *Guide to Community-based Rehabilitation Services. Guides for Special Education No. 8.* Paris: Unesco.

Possi, M.K. (1988) 'Some aspects for the education of albino children in Tanzania.' *Tanzanian Teacher,* **1**, 15–20.

Pritchard, D. (1963) *Education and the Handicapped.* London: Routledge.

Ross, D.H. (1988) *Educating Handicapped Young People in Eastern and Southern Africa in 1981–83.* Paris: Unesco.

Salia-Bao, K. (1989) *Curriculum Development and Africa Culture.* London: Edward Arnold.

Sauter, J.J. (1978) *Causes of Blindness Detected in 19 Schools for the Blind in Tanzania. Final Report.* Dar es Salaam: University of Dar es Salaam.

Scholl, G.T. (Ed.) (1986) *Foundations of Education for Blind and Visually Handicapped Children and Youth: Theory and Practice.* New York: American Foundation for the Blind.

Sechrest, L., Fey, T., Zaidi, H., Flores, L. (1973) 'Attitudes towards mental disorder among college students in the United States, Pakistan and the Philippines.' *Journal of Cross-Cultural Psychology,* **4**, 342–359.

Seidman, A., Anang, F. (Eds.) (1992) *Twenty-first-century Africa: Towards a New Vision of Self-Sustainable Development.* Trenton, NJ: Africa World Press.

Serpell, R., Mariga, L.. Harvey, K. (1993) 'Mental retardation in African countries: conceptualization, services, and research.' *International Review of Research in Mental Retardation,* **19**, 1–39.

Skrtic, T.M. (1991) 'The special education paradox: equity as a way to excellence.' *Harvard Educational Review,* **61**, 148–206.

United Nations Development Programme (1992) *Human Development Report 1992*. New York/Oxford: Oxford University Press.

Unesco (1981) *Sub-regional Seminar on Planning for Special Education, Nairobi, Kenya, 20–30 July*. Paris: Unesco.

—— (1984) *Consultation on Alternative Approaches for the Education of the Deaf. Final Report*. Paris: Unesco.

—— (1986) *Helping Handicapped Children in Ordinary Schools: Strategies for Teacher Training*. Paris: Unesco.

—— (1989) *Sub-Regional Project for Special Education in Eastern and Southern Africa: Project Findings and Recommendations*. Paris: Unesco.

van Pelt, P. (1982) *Bantu Customs in Mainland Tanzania, 4th Edn*. Tabora, Tanzania: Tanganyika Mission Press.

Walker, S. (1986) 'Attitudes towards the disabled as reflected in the social mores in Africa.' *In:* Marfo, K., Walker, S., Charles, B. (Eds.) *Childhood Disability in Developing Countries: Issues in Habilitation and Special Education*. New York: Praeger, pp. 239–250.

Wolfson, J. (1976) *Personality and Learning 2. A Reader Prepared by the Personality and Learning Course Team at the Open University*. London: Hodder & Stoughton with Open University Press.

13
VIOLENCE AND DISABLED CHILDREN

Naomi Richman

The needs of disabled children are basically the same as those of other children, but in situations of violence and conflict it becomes more difficult to ensure that these needs are met, and that adequate protection is provided for more vulnerable children.

There is very little written about disabled children in conflict situations, but we would expect conflict to increase the numbers of physically impaired children, and to make life more difficult for those with existing conditions. Their problems are exacerbated because most conflicts occur in developing countries, where children are already at a higher risk of impairment due to poverty and limited health care, and where resources for disability services usually do not have priority.

The disabling *psychological* effects of conflict have received more interest than the physical effects, and we can only speculate about the interaction between psychological and physical factors in these situations.

Effects of violence and conflict

The increasing impact of modern conflict on the civilian population has been noted by many authors (*e.g.* Zwi and Ugalde 1989). It is common for up to 80 per cent of casualties to be civilian, with the majority being women and children. This holds true whatever the type of organized violence: 'conventional' combat, repressive regimes, civil war, wars of liberation and insurgency, or so-called 'low intensity' warfare. Terrorizing the population has become an important weapon in many conflicts, and chemical warfare, defoliants and bombs reach civilians either deliberately or coincidentally. In particular the various types of modern land-mine, often laid without any regard for civilians, are an increasing long-term menace (Human Rights Watch Arms Project 1993).

Even after direct conflict is over, poverty, destruction of the economy and of the infrastructure, and other constraints such as sanctions, continue to affect the health of large sections of the population (Lee and Haines 1991). It is the poorest who are most affected by war and its aftermath (Zwi and Ugalde 1991), as is also the case in disasters such as earthquakes (Cuny 1983).

Prolonged situations of violence often lead to a gradual 'militarization' of society, with freely circulating arms and a social acceptance of violence. Coupled with social and economic disruption, this is a potent brew in which criminal violence flourishes, often linked with drug dealing. Family tension, alcoholism and domestic violence also grow when there is poverty and social instability.

In the post-war period, returning soldiers face a difficult readjustment to family life, especially if they are disabled and unemployed. Young people frequently form a high proportion of the armed forces: they encounter special problems in readjustment because they have had few chances to learn about the social skills for civilian survival. Their situation is especially precarious when they have no family.

In all these situations children with impairments are more vulnerable as they need extra care and time, and so are an added strain on the family. However, even in the most desperate situations parents do find ways of giving this care.

Conflict and disability

Conflict affects the occurrence of impairment in a number of ways. First, we have seen that children's well-being is affected by poverty and social disruption. Second, basic health services are disrupted directly, and resources for preventive and curative health care are reduced, because they are directed toward oppression or conflict (Zwi and Ugalde 1991). The activities of existing maternal and child health programmes, such as immunization, are disrupted or even disappear completely (Dodge 1990, Cliff and Noormahomcd 1993). Malnutrition increases, and specific nutritional deficiencies (*e.g.* iodine, vitamins) are not addressed.

Children thus become more susceptible to a variety of infections such as measles, poliomyelitis and diarrhoeal diseases, and are less able to resist their effects. An increased incidence of conditions such as motor impairment, hearing and visual problems following measles, and cerebral damage due to malaria, ensues. Intellectual impairment is increased because of lack of stimulation and deprivation, and because of direct insults to the brain, including nutritional deficiencies, infections and injury.

Disabled children are also less likely to escape during an attack, especially if they have a motor or learning difficulty or for other reasons are unable to look after themselves. A girl affected by poliomyelitis in Mozambique described to me how she had to be carried away by others whenever her village was attacked. Although she praised the concern of her relatives and neighbours, she became increasingly anxious about her situation and was eventually placed in an educational boarding school far from her family.

Special efforts may be made to protect such children, but sometimes this is impossible because only the toughest survive the hardships of flight. Parents have to make agonizing decisions as they flee, about how many children, and which children, they can manage to protect. Children, too, are consumed with guilt about siblings they had to abandon during flight.

The number of disabled people found in refugee camps will depend on the age of the camp, and the standard of living available. It is unusual to meet disabled people in newly arrived populations, presumably because they did not survive, but as time goes on, and provided that nutrition and care are reasonable, the numbers will probably rise.

Incidence and prevalence

Although the *incidence* of impairment increases in war, affected children are less likely to survive due to inadequate health care, so that the overall *prevalence* probably falls.

It is difficult to investigate the prevalence of impairment during times of war. Most conflicts occur in developing countries and we would expect to see similar patterns to those found in peace time plus war injuries (see Chapter 2). The type of conflict obviously affects the nature of injuries incurred. These vary from the effects of aerial attacks, chemical weapons and conventional warfare, through to those of 'low intensity' warfare, which might include deliberate mutilation of children.

The most common problems found in a survey of children in two provinces of Cambodia in 1986 affected hearing and speech, motor performance and learning capacity. The most frequent cause of motor impairment was poliomyelitis, followed by land-mine injuries and other accidents, and cerebral palsy. The overall rate of disability in children aged 0–15 years was estimated to be 2.57 per cent (Ministry of Health, State of Cambodia 1992) (see Chapter 1).

War wounds, including those resulting from land-mines, produce large numbers of physical injuries including amputations, as well as conditions like blindness, deafness due to perforated ear-drums, head injuries and facial disfigurement. Mines continue to cause injury long after the end of conflict. They can remain active for more than 70 years and pose a long-term threat both to individuals and to economic recovery in countries such as Cambodia, Afghanistan, Angola and Mozambique. Because mines remain lethal for long periods and because by their nature they are indiscriminate in their targets, it is now argued that under the UN convention on weapons their use should be banned (Human Rights Watch Arms Project 1994).

A study in Cambodia by King (personal communication, 1992) suggested that children were less likely than adults to be involved in land-mine accidents. However, this is surprising since children are more likely to run around over a wide area, tending animals or going into the bush to collect firewood. When a child steps on a mine and is wounded, the injuries are likely to be fatal or at least more severe, because of the child's size. The long time taken for civilians to reach medical care and the lack of adequate acute services add to the death toll.

Psychological consequences of conflict

Investigation of the psychological consequences related to conflict is more complex than for physical impairment, because it requires careful and culturally relevant interview techniques. Studies of adults suggest that following conflict, rates of psychological problems are higher than those of physical ones (Summerfield and Toser 1991).

There is little adequate information about the psychological consequences in children. Recent studies have looked especially for evidence of post-traumatic stress disorder (PTSD) related to specific 'traumatic' events such as witnessing the murder of a relative (American Psychiatric Association 1987). Symptoms of the disorder include intrusive images of the 'traumatic' events in the form of dreams or sudden vivid memories (flashbacks), avoidance of reminders of the events, and somatic symptoms.

This emphasis on symptoms of PTSD as the *sole* indicator of the disabling effects of conflict has been questioned for a number of reasons (Richman 1993*a*). Although surveys have described severe psychological effects following exposure to conflict, these studies have based their findings on brief questionnaires about symptoms. However, mere symptom counts based on questionnaire data cannot indicate the degree of *functional* impairment, and it is difficult to know the effect this has on their everyday lives.

205

In addition. focusing on PTSD ignores both the importance of chronic stress such as lack of food and recurrent threat on children's psychological state, and also the results of loss and bereavement as major influences on their adjustment.

A group of 60 children in Mozambique who were displaced inside the country because of fighting were interviewed about their views of the conflict and their emotional state (Richman *et al.* 1989). They described anxiety and fear, often precipitated by possible threat such as groups of men in the distance or sudden loud noises; difficulties in sleeping and nightmares; sadness related to loss and violence; and somatic symptoms such as fatigue, headache and stomach ache, limb pains, or unpleasant bodily sensations. Approximately a quarter were markedly affected by their symptoms. The majority were living in very bad conditions, suffering from separation from family, continuous threat and deprivation. None of these children were physically impaired, although many suffered from malnutrition and chronic ill-health due to bilharzial or other infections.

When estimating the extent of psychological impairment it is important to know how long symptoms persist, but this may be difficult to do in war situations, and most studies have relied on cross-sectional data. In another study of 60 Mozambican children, one year after the initial contact (Draisma and Richman 1992), threat of attack had diminished and the general situation was calmer. In those re-contacted there was a considerable reduction in somatic symptoms and anxiety, overall mood had improved, and they were generally more optimistic. One of the group was now dependent on crutches following an attack of poliomyelitis. However, it was only possible to contact about half of the original children, as many had returned to their home villages.

The severity of emotional distress experienced by children in situations of war and disaster depends on a variety of factors. These include the degree of threat; the intensity of exposure to violence, especially towards family or self; the extent of bereavement and loss; and whether protective adults are available. Young children are particularly distressed if they become separated from all familiar adults (Raphael 1986).

Most children appear to recover their equilibrium over a period of months if they are in a reasonable environment with a caring family, and are not subject to threat of attack. Unfortunately many children continue to live in harsh and threatening circumstances and this prolongs their distress.

Unaccompanied children

Death of relatives or separation from family are probably the most serious consequences of conflict for children. Children with no family (orphaned, separated or abandoned) are especially vulnerable. Their intellectual and emotional development is likely to be affected if they have no adult(s) consistently to provide emotional and physical care, when they will also be at risk of emotional and sexual abuse. Abuse can occur in any kind of social situation, but children in institutions or in foster families where there is inadequate super-vision are particularly at risk. Disabled children are more often picked out as victims because they may be less able to defend themselves.

Prevention of separation should be a priority, and any steps that separate a child from the family, even if this is supposed to be temporary, require careful consideration (Ressler

1992). There is often pressure from outside the country to evacuate children to safety or for medical reasons. Sometimes this benefits the children, but often the results are unfortunate and the relationship between the child and the family is seriously affected. The child and family may remain apart for long periods, perhaps for ever; or the conditions of care for the evacuated may turn out to be poor and the children suffer misery and feel abandoned. Children evacuated for medical treatment, either within their own country or abroad, may then be unable to rejoin the family, because transport home is impossible, the war zone changes, or because the whereabouts of the family is unknown. It is common for such children to languish in hospital for months, or even years, like a boy in Mozambique who had already been in hospital for over a year following an amputation after a land-mine injury (Human Rights Watch Arms Project 1994).

It can be a difficult ethical issue to decide whether evacuation for medical treatment will be in the best interests of a child with impairment. If it is decided to send children away for treatment they should be accompanied by a relative or at least an adult whom they know. The details of the child and family should be thoroughly documented so that there will be a good chance of reuniting them should communication be broken for a time. This may seem obvious but can easily be forgotten in acute situations in hospital emergency departments, for example. When children are evacuated there must be adequate supervision at the point of arrival and afterwards because there is a risk that they will be exploited: for example, used as prostitutes or as servants.

Ideally, unaccompanied children should be placed in foster families or small group homes while attempts are made to locate relatives. Such a programme of family tracing was initiated in Mozambique during the recent war, combined with a policy of not building extra orphanages for these children. There were only one or two small orphanages per province, and many children were spontaneously fostered. However, adoption or fostering of children with impairments is difficult, especially in times of social unrest and if there is no assistance for the extra costs incurred. There is a risk that some children will be taken in by families with the aim of exploiting them: for example, for begging purposes, or to obtain extra food.

Orphanages tend to have a concentration of disabled children because the children are more likely to be left there by parents wanting to give them a better chance of survival. Once accepted they are unlikely to leave because the family will not reclaim them.

Usually orphanages provide a poor environment for children especially when they are young or have special needs. Staff have had no training in understanding the needs of children with impairments and are poorly paid. The lack of individualized attention to the children and of permanent affectionate ties impairs their emotional and intellectual development (Aberg 1991). When the time comes eventually to leave the institution they have no family or community in which to integrate.

Due to the disadvantages of orphanages and the difficulties of arranging adequate alternative care, it is of the utmost importance to prevent separation, and where it has happened, to try to find the family. The possibilities and difficulties of tracing relatives should be carefully explained to the child, and the mechanisms set in motion as soon as possible (Williamson and Moser 1987). It must be borne in mind, of course, that some families are unwilling to receive their children.

Psychological effects of disability

Various factors influence the psychological state of disabled children—the type of impairment; how and when the impairment was acquired; the attitude of the community; family resources; and the resilience and resourcefulness of the child.

Type of impairment

Western studies indicate that any kind of chronic illness increases emotional difficulties. The causes are multifactorial and include the effects of hospitalizations and unpleasant treatments, upset about limitations on normal activities, anxieties about future well-being and life chances, and parental responses. These last may vary from extreme over-protectiveness to ignoring or denying the child's needs.

It appears that organic brain conditions increase vulnerability in children already at risk because of difficult social situations. Children with epilepsy and organic brain disorder, for example following head injury or infection, or with severe learning difficulties, have the highest rates of psychological impairment (Rutter *et al.* 1970). Problems with hearing, speech and communication are also associated with high rates of psychological difficulties.

In developing countries it is common for parents to hide away children with severe physical impairment or severe learning difficulties, who then have no opportunity to develop their capacities. However, we have little information about how they are affected emotionally by this situation. When the family does not accept an impairment, as when parents continually look for a healer with an effective cure for epilepsy or slow learning, this places further strain on a child (see Chapter 14).

How and when the impairment was acquired

The shock of receiving an injury may be long-lasting. One boy aged 5 years was present when his house was attacked and his father was killed before his eyes. He himself suffered a deliberately inflicted gunshot wound to his right arm which had to be amputated. On leaving hospital he went to live with his uncle in a safer place. Initially he was terrified of men, especially those in uniform, did not play and would not use his left arm: he had been right-handed. Over a period of more than a year he lost his fear of unknown men, began to attend school, made friends and studied, and was cheerfully using his left hand. However, he still had difficulties falling asleep, and his impairment was a constant reminder of the attack and the loss of his father.

Community attitude

Chapters 11 and 12 have discussed the powerful effects of community attitudes to disabled children on their adjustment. In some situations the war wounded hold a special place in society, as for example Palestinian youth honoured in the fight for national independence, and youths in various political struggles who have been detained and tortured. Permanent injury inflicted because of brave resistance will earn a child great esteem, as happened to a boy in Mozambique who had the fingers of one hand and both ears cut off because he refused to disclose his father's whereabouts. However, such honouring can gradually fade, and the pride of disabled children in their sacrifice also fades if the long-term prospects of work and marriage are minimal, or the results of sacrifice do not bear political fruit.

The side on which a person fought often determines their future, depending on which group ends up with power and the degree of national reconciliation. Even those who became disabled in defending their country may find that they are marginalized once peace comes, and resources to help them are scarce (Zinkin 1993). Others, who were involved in committing atrocities, might be ostracized and forced into a marginal existence or even criminal activities.

When nearly everyone is living through hard times, and when the war wounded are a common sight, community support for an individual child may lessen, from both adults and other children. Even when the impairment has obviously been acquired in war, if the ultimate causal explanation of their injury is seen as sin, fate or witchcraft, there may be lack of will to help.

The family

Whatever the particular causal explanations understood by a family, their capacity to accommodate a child with an impairment will depend a great deal on their resources, both personal and material. Those in the process of resettlement, or dealing with instability and poverty, will have less capacity to help. During conflict more fathers are away fighting or working, or perhaps dead, and more households are headed by women who have to earn a livelihood as well as bring up children. Economic difficulties, exacerbated by war, make it harder for families to look after their disabled children: the provision of resources and means of livelihood for such families helps to create a more positive attitude and lessens the risk of the child being abandoned (see Chapter 11).

The child

We have described how an impairment adds to a child's vulnerability in dangerous situations. However, children vary in their responses and their capacities to cope with danger and their impairment. They often show great courage in facing hardship, and it is no service to pity them rather than promote their independence. One boy who had a damaged leg following a bullet wound had worked out very carefully how he would escape should an attack materialize. A girl who used crutches to get around looked after three younger brothers and sisters and went to school, as well as doing odd jobs for money.

Factors that are related to children's resilience in the face of adversity include having a range of coping strategies which they can use flexibly. When action is required they will be able to make a realistic plan and execute this. Where action is impossible they can resort to useful mental mechanisms to help them cope with their situation, such as daydreaming, fantasy, distraction, blocking out unpleasant thoughts, or mentally rehearsing possible responses to the situation.

Coping capacity is to some extent learnt through adult example and personal experience, and children can be helped to improve their skills through discussion of their anxieties and of coping strategies.

Promoting coping skills
Disabled children affected by conflict need similar support to that required by other children, especially the possibility of confiding in an understanding adult.

Information and participation
Adults are often reluctant to speak with children about their situation or their impairment. This is excused by saying that the child is too young to understand. The child is left with anxieties unexpressed, or lacking essential information, for example about the feelings associated with a phantom limb, or the degree of improvement expected after poliomyelitis.

In busy clinics, especially in conflict situations, no-one has responsibility for explaining the condition and possible future help to the child or the family. Indeed, health workers may not be able to speak the child's language, or be familiar with the culture, so that opportunities for essential explanations and follow-up are lost. This communication is particularly important for conditions like epilepsy, where often ideas about causation militate against adequate treatment.

Trained health advocates, who need not be health workers, could convey these important explanations, and provide information to relatives about how they can help a child with an impairment.

Wherever possible, children should be involved in making decisions themselves, for example, about fitting a prosthesis, or about where they are going to live.

Working with the family
In situations of war or in refugee camps it is not easy to initiate programmes of support for disabled children, but it is important to do as much as possible, otherwise valuable time is lost, during which the child should be learning and developing. Discussions with local communities may bring up useful ideas about what would be feasible.

Most families are very pleased to have the possibility of help providing it is relevant to their needs: for example, a day centre so that mothers can work; physiotherapy advice; and practical aids, exercises or occupation for a child. At the very least, discussions could aim at encouraging adults to communicate with children about their situation, and ensure their integration and participation in the wider community, particularly if schooling is available.

A variety of initiatives have been described for supporting women affected by conflict, especially those with children. These include involving mothers in group discussions or activities such as setting up and running preschool centres (Fozzard and Tembo 1993). In this way the morale of the mothers is raised and they are more able to respond to the needs of their children.

Promoting integration
Whenever possible, disabled children should be involved in normal activities with other children. Even during situations of conflict it is possible to train teachers, and community workers and leaders, so that they will be sensitive to the needs of disabled children, and

ensure they are not marginalized, and that their capacities and special strengths are promoted.

Programmes in which children help each other, as when older children help those who are younger, or in Child-to-Child programmes focused on understanding other people's feelings and needs, could be used to promote integration of disabled children (Child-to-Child 1993—see Chapter 15).

Responding to the child's emotional distress

In some cultures it is not customary for people to talk about how they feel; they appreciate concern expressed through practical help that provides prospects for the future. However, some children have emotional problems related to their impairment, their family and the sufferings of war and separation. They need the opportunity to express their feelings and anxieties to an understanding adult who is open to whatever they want to say (Richman 1993*b*).

Sometimes group discussions are helpful, when participants can see that they have common concerns, and can talk about practical matters related to coping with discrimination or violence, or ways of contributing to the family or community when physical work in the fields is not possible.

Children with persistent distress related to experience of war need special attention, as well as care for their material needs. Even in situations of continuing conflict it has been possible to develop programmes of response to children's psychological needs. Common elements are the provision of as normal a routine of life as possible, especially schooling; recreational and creative activities like sports, games, art and drama; opportunities to talk and express their feelings; and working with parents (Gustafsson 1986; Ministry of Education, Mozambique 1990).

These kinds of programmes are relevant to the needs of all children whether they have impairments or not. Their value can be extended if linked with the training of teachers, health workers or volunteers in simple counselling skills to support children and families (Metraux 1988, Nikapota and Samarasinghe 1989, Richman *et al.* 1991, Jareg 1992, Metraux and Aviles 1992). Training should include raising awareness about disability and disabled children (Richman 1993*b*).

Conclusion

The situation of disabled children in times of conflict needs to be explored further. We need to know more about how they, their families and communities cope with disability in different settings. We also need to explore what kinds of help have been developed locally for disabled children caught up in conflict, and what initiatives it might be useful to try out in the future.

Although conflict situations make it difficult to provide for disabled children, there are a variety of actions that can promote their well-being. These include:
• reducing the number of unaccompanied children by avoiding separation from family, careful documentation of those who are separated so that relatives can be located, and establishing a programme for tracing families and reunification;

- sensitizing parents, the community, teachers and others about the needs of all children for supportive adults who are prepared to listen to their concerns;
- integrating children with impairments into ordinary life as far as possible;
- developing schools, leisure and creative activities from which all children can benefit;
- international advocacy to ban the use of land-mines completely—an urgent priority.

REFERENCES

Aberg B.G. (1991) *The Process of Change at a Children's Home.* Stockholm: Radda Barnen.

American Psychiatric Association (1987) *Diagnostic Statistical Manual III, Revised (DSM-III-R).* Washington: APA.

Child-to-Child (1993) *Helping Children in Refugee Camps.* London: Child-to-Child.

Cliff, J., Noormahomed, A.R. (1993) 'The impact of war on children's health in Mozambique.' *Social Science and Medicine,* **36**, 843–848.

Cuny, F. (1983) *Disasters and Development.* Oxford: Oxford University Press.

Dodge, C.P. (1990) 'Health implications of war in Uganda and Sudan.' *Social Science and Medicine,* **31**, 691–698.

Draisma, F., Richman, N. (1992) *School Based Programme for Children in Difficult Circumstances. Final Report 1988–1992.* Maputo, Mozambique: Ministry of Education.

Fozzard, S., Tembo, L. (1993) 'Promoting a caring environment for the children. A community based model for intervention.' *In:* McCallin, M. (Ed.) *The Psychosocial Well-being of Refugee Children. Research, Practice and Policy Issues.* Geneva: ICCB, pp. 130–147.

Gustafsson, L.H. (1986) 'The STOP sign—a model for intervention to assist children in war' *In: Action for Children: NGO Forum on Children in Emergencies.* New York: Radda Barnen, pp. 20–26.

Human Rights Watch Arms Project (1993) *Landmines: a Deadly Legacy.* New York/London: Human Rights Watch.

—— (1994) *Landmines in Mozambique.* New York/London: Human Rights Watch.

Jareg, E. (1992) 'Basic therapeutic actions: helping children, young people and communities to cope through empowerment and participation.' *In:* McCallin, M. (Ed.) *The Psychosocial Well-being of Refugee Children. Research, Practice and Policy Issues.* Geneva: ICCB, pp. 206–214.

Lee, I., Haines, A. (1991) 'Health costs of the Gulf war.' *British Medical Journal,* **303**, 303–306.

Metraux, J-C. (1988). *Los Niños. Victimas de la Guerra. Manual de Atención Psico-social para Promotores.* Managua: Centro de Publicaciones INIES.

—— Aviles, A. (1992) 'Training techniques for non-professionals: a Nicaraguan preventive and primary care mental health programme.' *In:* McCallin, M. (Ed.) *The Psychosocial Well-being of Refugee Children. Research, Practice and Policy Issues.* Geneva: ICCB, pp. 226–243.

Ministry of Education, Mozambique (1990) *Helping Children in Difficult Circumstances. A Teacher's Manual.* London: Save the Children Fund.

Ministry of Health, State of Cambodia (1992) *Transitional Health Plan. Part 1. Health Situation Analysis.* Phnom Penh: Ministry of Health.

Nikapota, A., Samarasinghe, D. (1989) *Training Manual for Helping Children in Situations of Armed Conflict.* Colombo, Sri Lanka: Unicef.

Raphael, B. (1986) *When Disaster Strikes.* London: Unwin Hyman.

Ressler, E. (1992) *Evacuation of Children in Emergencies.* Geneva: UNHCR/Unicef.

Richman, N. (1993a) 'Children in situations of political violence.' *Journal of Child Psychology and Psychiatry,* **34**, 1286–1302. *(Annotation.)*

—— (1993b) *Communicating with Children. Helping Children in Distress. Development Manual 2.* London: Save the Children Fund.

—— Ratilal, A., Aly, A. (1989) *The Psychological Effects of War on Mozambican Children.* Maputo: Ministry of Education.

—— Mucache, E., Ratilal, A. (1991) 'A school based community mental health programme.' *Paper presented at the 3rd International Conference Concerned with the Care for Victims of Organized Violence. November 1991, Santiago, Chile.*

Rutter, M., Tizard, J., Whitmore, K. (1970) *Education, Health and Behaviour.* London: Longman.

Summerfield, D., Toser, L. (1991) '"Low intensity" war and mental trauma in Nicaragua: a study in a rural community.' *Medicine and War*, **7**, 84–99.

Williamson, J., Moser, A. (1987) *Unaccompanied Children in Emergencies. A Field Guide for Their Care and Protection.* Geneva: International Social Service.

Zinkin, P. (1993) 'War, disability and rehabilitation in Namibia.' *In:* Preston, R. (Ed.) *The Effects of War in Namibia.* Windhoek, Namibia: Namibian Institute for Economic and Social Research, pp. 7.1–7.29.

Zwi, A., Ugalde, A. (1989) 'Towards an epidemiology of political violence in the Third World.' *Social Science and Medicine*, **28**, 633–642.

—— —— (1991) 'Political violence in the Third World: a public health issue.' *Health Policy and Planning*, **6**, 203–217.

14
RIGHTS NOT CHARITY

Leonard Williams

Across the world the common experience of disabled people like myself is that we are seen as having little to offer our communities. Non-disabled people determine what our needs are and how they should be met. Anger about this devaluing of disabled people's lives, and frustration at the control that non-disabled 'experts' and 'service providers' have over the quality of our lives, led to the foundation of an international disability rights organization in 1981—Disabled People International (DPI). More than a decade later, DPI goes from strength to strength. Those who are involved are the kind of people who would have been written off as incapable and uneducable, confined in institutions, neglected and left to die. Yet these are the people who, having taken control over their own lives, are now working at grass roots, national and international levels to bring about changes which will enable other disabled people to determine the quality of their lives.

DPI is now made up of National Assemblies representing over 90 countries, including the Solomon Islands. This means that within each country, organizations of disabled people are affiliated to one national body, which represents its country's disabled people within DPI. In turn DPI represents disabled people's interests at an international level in many contexts, including various United Nations organizations.

In addition to its international work, DPI has played a major role in encouraging disabled people's organizations at grass roots level. In each country disabled people face the problem that organizations *for* disabled people are run by non-disabled people. (This is particularly so in the Solomon Islands.) These organizations take it upon themselves to determine what is best for us. In many countries these are the organizations which are recognized and funded by the government rather than organizations of disabled people. (In the Solomon Islands, the Disabled Persons Rehabilitation Association is recognized by the government but receives no direct annual grants.)

Disabling society
Disabled people are fighting for a society which celebrates difference—a society which does not react to physical, sensory or intellectual impairments, or emotional distress, with fear and prejudice. We want a society that recognizes the difficulties we face but also values us for what we are as human beings.

Our hopes for the future are based on the justice of our wish for control over our lives, the strength of our demands for equal participation, and the passion of our belief in the value of our contribution to the communities in which we live.

Across the world, disabled people are struggling for access to education, jobs and housing, for the right to express their sexuality and to have children, to participate in political and social life, and in the development of our communities. However, the world is a disabling place, and millions of us experience the effects of it every day of our lives. At best we are pitied and patronized, at worst we are feared and vilified. We have been denied education, employment, a family life, human dignity—all in the name of what is 'wrong' with us.

An impairment affects the way our bodies and our minds work, but it is society's reaction to impairment which determines whether we may have a good quality of life. Disabled people are increasingly challenging the attitude which says that if you cannot walk then your life is not worth living. To do this we make a distinction between the way our bodies function, such as not being able to walk, and the way that society reacts to us.

This helps us to see that it is not the injury to the brain at birth which denies children with cerebral palsy access to the same schools as their non-disabled brothers and sisters. It is not the inability to see which denies a blind person access to higher education. It is not epilepsy which prevents someone from working. It is not a learning difficulty which denies the expression of sexuality. It is not the inability to get out of bed without help which incarcerates or imprisons someone within an institution.

Instead it is the way society reacts to physical, sensory and intellectual impairment which limits our possibilities. Most schools do not cater for children or adults who use wheelchairs, most employers refuse to offer a job to anyone who has a speech impairment. Many social service authorities choose to spend money on institutional care rather than provide physical assistance in someone's home.

These restrictions on our lives and our rights are based on many things. They arise from a complex mish-mash of good intentions, incomplete understanding, and unwillingness to identify with our lives. People are afraid of incapacity and dependency, afraid of difference. They find it difficult to put themselves in our place and cannot or do not want to identify with what it is to be like us.

A recent questionnaire survey of first year nursing students in the Solomon Islands looked at knowledge and attitudes toward various impairments, including blindness, paralysis, mental retardation, deafness and leprosy (Hill 1992). Students were most informed about and had most rehabilitation ideas for people with blindness. They had the least knowledge or ideas about rehabilitation for people with leprosy.

The students generally had fairly positive attitudes toward helping disabled people. The most common suggestions were to teach skills, give physical assistance and provide special equipment. They mostly identified paid professionals, family members and community members as the people who should do these things. However, some students recommended that special institutions be built for disabled people. For those with leprosy, the most frequent suggestions were to give medical help and to segregate 'leprosy victims' from society, showing that traditional attitudes are still very much alive in a young and educated group in the country.

Unequal opportunities
Disabled people experience a much higher level of unemployment than non-disabled people, and the majority who do find work are only offered low-paid, low-skilled jobs. Not

only do employers discriminate against disabled applicants, but non-disabled employees often create an unwelcoming, sometimes hostile environment for disabled co-workers. For example, the Disabled Persons Rehabilitation Association office shares accommodation with an organization whose staff have shown little or no recognition of the particular needs of wheelchair users who work in the office, nor of those with other impairments who regularly call in to the office for services.

A failure to make buildings accessible, or to provide readers for blind people and sign language interpreters for deaf people, creates a life of unemployment and poverty. It also means that society is poorer, for it loses the contribution that we have to make.

Denying our disability

Many people assume that the best thing for us is to be cured of our 'suffering', and that if this is not possible then there is little that can be done to enhance the quality of our lives, and our lives are hardly worth living. The media—newspapers, radio, advertising—promote the idea that we are to be pitied for our condition. This can severely undermine our self-esteem. We underestimate ourselves, feel neglected and shy. If we are mere victims of a physical or mental condition and desperate for cure, how can we also be competent parents, valued employees, loving partners, equal citizens? We often feel we have to deny any difficulties that we have, to deny our impairment itself, in order to assert that our lives have value.

As a young adult, I pretended that I was not disabled. The education system contributed to this denial, and society in general forced me into a position where in order to be 'able' I had to strive not to be disabled. Now I realize that I was denying I am a man. Having an impairment is an integral part of me and I found it so valuable to be able to 'come out' from isolation into the community.

When a mother says that she loves her child in spite of that child's impairment, she is saying that she does not love that part of her child. When our achievements are applauded as overcoming all odds, the disabled part of us is being denied and diminished. Valuing us as people should not mean ignoring the things about our bodies which make us different. In asserting our rights we also want to take pride in ourselves. We cannot do this unless our pride incorporates the way we are different.

Experiencing disabilities

To experience physical, sensory or learning impairments, or mental health problems, is to experience the vulnerability and imperfection of the human body. This indeed is what makes people afraid of us, for it is an experience which they do not want for themselves.

Our history is hidden from us. There have been many disabled people engaged in political struggles, many disabled artists, writers, musicians. But history has been written by those who believe that disability is a personal tragedy, that if disabled people achieve anything it is in spite of their disability.

Now, however, we are exploring and expressing the experience of disability on our terms, rather than on the terms of the non-disabled world. We are part of a social and political movement which is changing our present and making sense of our history.

Segregation and dependency trap

Some non-government charities run by non-disabled people, which raise money for disabled people, are based on segregation and dependency. Instead of enabling us to participate on an equal basis in our communities, charities sadly separate us out into categories based on medical definitions of 'what is wrong' with us. Money is raised in our name through the creation of feelings of pity or fear, and it is spent on things which non-disabled people consider to be 'best' for us. We have no control over what is done to us but are expected to make the gift of our gratitude to those who receive both financial and emotional rewards out of apparently doing good.

We can find it difficult to resist the relationship which charities force us into, because some individuals involved in charitable activities say that they are doing what they can from the best of motives. The charity trap is very much an issue about control. Who has the right to say what we need? Who has the right to say how we should be presented to the public? Who has the right to say how money raised in our name should be spent? Non-disabled people take all these decisions with little reference to those of us whose very existence has given them their jobs, their salaries and their feelings of self-righteousness.

Power to control self

The disability movements demand 'rights not charity', which sums up the alternative vision which we are posing to a world where, as tragic victims of our bodies' suffering, we wait passively and gratefully for good people to do their good deeds.

Our vision is of a society where disabled people are not segregated but instead have the right to a home of their own. It is of a society where we have as much right to use public transport as non-disabled people, where we do not have to rely on the benevolence of others for equipment which may be needed to carry out ordinary daily activities. It is of a society which recognizes our rights and our value as equal citizens rather than merely treating us as the recipients of other people's goodwill.

To live independently we need to have control over our daily activities and to be able to choose our lifestyle. One of the early struggles by disabled people for control over their lives took place in Berkeley, California. In the late 1960s a group of disabled people who had been confined to a hospital setting because they needed help with daily physical tasks, started to assert their rights to live in their own homes. As a result they set up the first Centre for Independent Living (CIL). This is an organization of disabled people for disabled people, concerned with access to suitable housing and personal assistance.

The CIL now provides practical and emotional support, as well as taking on wider issues of access to transport, education, employment and all the other things which make equal participation in the community possible. Although when it started the CIL mainly helped people who were blind, deaf or had physical impairments, the organization now covers the full range of impairments, including learning difficulties, head injuries and psychiatric conditions.

Today the principle of independent living for all provides an inspiration for many groups of disabled people in other parts of the world. The movement may have found its earliest expression in the USA, one of the richest nations of the world, but its roots are also to be found in the aspirations of disabled people in developing countries including the Solomon Islands.

The Disabled Persons Rehabilitation Association (DPRA) helps people who need personal assistance to control how that assistance should be provided. This means recruiting and managing disabled employees, negotiating funding, dealing with tax and so on. These skills disabled people acquire and pass on to others. It is all about taking control of our own lives.

Alongside the DPRA, organizations of disabled people provide practical support which, together with campaigning activities, helps to further the cause of community-based independent living and make it a practical reality.

The Disabled People's CBR Project, for example, provides interest-free loans for disabled people who are keen to utilize their skills in innovative self-help programmes in the community. This project aims to increase the self-confidence of disabled people whose experience of segregation and dependence within an institution or family setting often leaves them ill-equipped to make the transition to an independent adult life.

Disabled people are demonstrating that we are the 'experts on disability', that we know best what our needs are and how they should be met.

REFERENCE

Hill, L. (1992) *Rehabilitation Policy*. Honiara, Solomon Islands: Ministry of Health and Medical Services.

15
CONCLUSIONS

Helen McConachie and Pam Zinkin

How shall we conclude such a diverse book? It has ranged across continents, types of impairment, and professional outlook; from personal statement to closely referenced review; from innovative responses to particular circumstances in developing countries, to synthesis of experience and research from developed countries. What we aim to do in this final chapter is to examine further the factors which limit both how children with impairments live and efforts to support them and their carers.

Social and political context

Disabled people argue that strong anti-discrimination legislation is needed in order to establish equity in employment, education, housing, transport, and so on. In developed countries, much forward-looking legislation has been passed but has then had its purposes undermined by a lack of required funding by government (*e.g.* Disabled Persons Act 1986 in Britain). Many developing countries do not have legislation which enshrines the right to education of *all* children. Even when the right to education for all disabled children is recognized (*e.g.* in Britain since 1971; in USA since 1975) an individual child's right to an *appropriate* education is not in practice guaranteed. For example, some education authorities will allocate hours of classroom assistance on the basis of the average of available resources rather than of children's individual developmental needs. Recent Education Acts (1988, 1993) in Britain have instituted devolved budgeting with the consequence that children who are 'expensive' in terms of the resources they require are less welcome as pupils in mainstream schools, and special schools are keen to increase their school rolls. Therefore the debate over integration versus segregation comes to be biased by the amount of resources and by political decisions on the manner of their distribution.

At an international level, Article 23 of the UN Convention on the Rights of the Child (1989) concerns disabled children. No mention is made of children having the *same* rights; instead the text emphasizes 'the right of the disabled child to special care'. However, the qualifying clause 'subject to available resources' effectively absolves governments of responsibility. A statement of rights should be just that, setting an agenda and priority objectives.

Readers might quibble about the influence of *economics*. It might be suggested that economic growth is a prerequisite both for improving attitudes and for increasing special provision. Generally it is true that facilities for disabled people are enhanced with more resources, *e.g.* new buildings have ramps and induction loops, schools better meet children's specific needs. However, this is not a complete picture: there are countries which are successful economically where attitudes and practice toward disabled people are

219

frequently rejecting and controlling. The Industrial Revolution created conditions which prejudiced the quality of life of people with impairments who would have a valued place in a more varied agricultural community (Ryan and Thomas 1980, Oliver 1993). Where social conditions reward conformity, the diverse qualities and contribution of all members of society are deprecated rather than celebrated.

For disabled people in developing countries the overwhelming issue is poverty (see Chapters 2 and 11). When basic needs are not met, when there is limited access to food, water, shelter, health care, etc., then the community is concerned with survival.

'Ramps and lifts for wheelchair accessibility are of low priority for persons who don't have a wheelchair—nor enough to eat. Such basic needs are becoming more and more difficult to meet for all poor and marginalized people—including disabled people, most of whom are also poor and marginalized.' (Werner 1993)

Disabled people are increasingly active in political movements which combine their aims with those of other deprived communities or devalued people. For example, in one of the areas where ADD–India worked with the Young India Project (see Chapter 11), 40 landless disabled people joined in the struggle for land along with an agricultural labourers union. The disabled people added strength to the movement through their numbers and organization. If the issue had been over a small piece of land, not enough for everyone, then probably disabled people would have been marginalized. However, a large area was demanded and the disabled people shared in its distribution. If there had been different unions, such as the Union of Women, the Union of Disabled People, the Union of Agricultural Labourers, they would have been fighting among themselves. Strength came from there being only one union of poor people.

Political empowerment also leads to questioning of professional services (see Chapter 14).

'What kind of 'rehabilitation efforts' would be most appropriate? Clearly, ones that enable us. That help us to empower ourselves, so that we can join with other disadvantaged and socially concerned groups, locally and globally, to work toward changing the power structures that deny us our basic rights to meet our needs and potentials.' (Werner 1993)

Culture is another factor in the framework for disability. Attitudes about gender roles, attitudes about the causes of impairment (see Chapter 12), attitudes about 'cure' and about receiving services, all affect disabled children's views of themselves, their families' morale, and the strategies to be adopted by those planning services. For example, where there is a strong culture of pride in extended family self-sufficiency, offering advice on how to bring up a child with an impairment becomes a major exercise in family diplomacy (Lynch and Hanson 1992). These are issues for service providers in any multicultural society, not just for those in developing countries. Culture is not static; there is an interaction between economic status, the resources available in a community and cultural attitudes. What is important is adequate knowledge and preparation, respectful listening and flexibility. Then it is possible to harmonize intervention ideas with the positive frameworks of belief of that community, such as the spiritual support offered by traditional healers.

Gender issues may be even more crucial in developing than in developed countries. Being a girl may influence access to schooling and rehabilitation services more than factors such as severity of impairment or class. In all countries, disabled women are doubly disadvantaged. Professionals should be involved in working for fundamental change in gender relations in general, and in attitudes toward disabled women and girls in particular.

Funding

Many initiatives in rehabilitation in developing countries are financed by external governmental or non-governmental organizations (NGOs). These sources of funding can bring with them their own problems through imposition of conditions for receipt of the aid. It is quite appropriate to want to know that resources will be used wisely, but the conditions are frequently nothing short of imperialistic. Western government aid is tied to the receiving country having 'sensible economic policies'. Some NGOs assert their own religious and ideological views in deciding where to allocate funds. For example, the President of World Vision International has been quoted as saying, 'We analyse every project, every programme we undertake, to make sure that within that programme evangelism is a significant component. We cannot feed individuals and let them go to hell' (Hancock 1989). Aid organizations tend to impose their own consultants on the developing country programme even where there are experienced local professionals. These consultants are likely to receive higher salaries than the local rates and to be ignorant of the local cultural conditions which determine appropriate intervention strategies. Many foreign-based NGOs tend not to cooperate with the national government and may operate in a way that undermines national sovereignty, which would not be tolerated for an instant were the roles to be reversed. The NGOs frequently provide generous but short-term funding so that the project cannot continue when funds are withdrawn. Helander (1993) estimates that annually over 300 million dollars are spent in developing countries on about 4000 projects for disabled people. Therefore most projects are small-scale, leading to duplication of administrative costs. Where the funding agencies concentrate on single disability groups, their efforts tend not to be coordinated with others thus using available resources inefficiently. It is also clear that almost all of the donor money is controlled by able-bodied foreigners (Hanlon 1991).

A few NGOs have learned from past mistakes, but may then implement progressive conditions in a rigid way, leading in turn to other difficulties. For example, it may be insisted that a rehabilitation project be led by disabled people in order to receive funding; however, a disabled people's organization in a particular country may not have developed the capacity to take on provision of services. Overall, the merits of organic growth of a project which has been carefully instituted with community support through local sources of finance are more important than risking its rapid expansion and later demise through the hazards of external funding.

Programme goals

In any intervention project it is necessary to be clear about goals. In programmes for children with impairments, it is important to avoid misunderstandings between project workers and parents (see Chapter 9). For example, a programme for young children who have motor disorders may have the goal of helping them to function better in activities of daily living, but may be judged a failure by parents if they had expected the children all to learn to walk. It is therefore better to start in a small way, to listen to the aspirations of children and their families, to come to an agreement on feasible goals, and ideally to consult with disabled adults as advisers and role models.

Many projects in developing countries have attempted to import methods from developed countries, without looking carefully at the needs of the community in which they are based, and the particular goals for living of the children and families (see Chapter 12). A special teaching method may seem well packaged, or a therapy approach may have strong advocates, but the application of these in a different economic and cultural context may impose narrow and inappropriate goals. However, there is also an issue of a child's right not to have particular methods imposed. Many adult disabled people look back on the time they spent in therapy, the pain and effort they endured, and express resentment, feeling that they knew all along just what could and could not be achieved. In addition the 'therapy' rules may get in the way of play, fun and important relationships. Busby (personal communication, 1992) has spoken of the immense pleasure of being tossed around as a child by his father, a pleasure possibly heightened by the knowledge that it was 'forbidden' as it would raise his muscle tone. Diamond (1981) has written of her frustration at being constantly reminded to sit 'properly' when playing, interrupting her fantasy games, and also violating her need for her parents' unconditional love and approval. The very difficult issue, however, is how to judge at the time when 'enough is enough', how to predict the limits of a child's likely progress, particularly given a changing pattern of impairment such as in cerebral palsy.

A second problem of strategy in setting goals may arise from the attempt to use Western standards for the quality of a service: *e.g.* 'a blind child should receive special education in the medium of braille'; 'a child identified as having hearing impairment should see an audiologist within two months'; 'the child's hearing aid should be being worn on each occasion when the child is visited at home'. Such standards are in theory a way of auditing a service because they appear easily measurable. However, they are illusory in any circumstance, let alone in a rural village in a developing country. The audiologist may not conduct rural clinics, and the child may refuse to wear the hearing aid, particularly if s/he has outgrown it and it tends to come loose and whistle, or if the batteries are flat. In any case, these standards are based on the Western requirement for quantitative data, and ignore qualitative aspects of a child's experience; how people in the family and village communicate with the child are more crucial for her/his development.

Standards for services need to reflect how available resources can be used to close the gap between what is provided for a child from a privileged family and what is provided for children of poor families. For example, in both Denmark and India specialist residential blind schools have been closed so as to provide a service to a greater number of children. Staff were retrained in order to provide more intensive short courses to young children, their parents and their teachers, to enable the children to be educated in ordinary schools.

Therefore the service standard suggested in the previous paragraph would have changed to 'all blind children should have basic skills in independent mobility, and in braille reading and numeracy to a level comparable with mainstream first grade children'. This standard could be met for a much larger percentage of blind children in each country than had previously been the case.

The problem with narrow definitions of goals based on methods or standards is that they are 'problem-oriented' rather than 'evolutionary'. In developed countries the emphasis is changing toward family-focused goals for intervention (see Chapter 3). With few professional resources, the appropriate emphasis in developing countries is wider, *i.e.* community-focused, generating strategies for long-lasting attitude change so that children with impairments are enabled to do more and to enjoy a good quality of life through their family members' and neighbours' raised expectations of them, and through their inclusion in and expansion of community activities.

Training of personnel

All the chapters in this book imply changes in the training of rehabilitation professionals intending to work with disabled children in developing countries. There are many instances where project coordinators are appointed because of qualifications gained in a developed country, who are then not well suited to their role because of inappropriate expectations and differences of culture and class from those with whom they work. Where the professional training takes place in a developing country, the content may still be derived from Western models and oriented primarily to alleviating individual impairment, without an understanding of the experience of disabled people and the politics of disablement in developing countries. There are frequently also considerable difficulties in ensuring that students have periods of supervised practice in rural settings. Traditional training models emphasize compartmentalization of professional skills, so that health and education professionals continue to find great difficulty in talking to each other, a continuing problem in developed countries.

So what can be done? First, there is a need to 'demystify' professional skills and to find ways of sharing these with volunteers, community workers and other non-specialists (see Chapters 5 and 9). Professionals have an important role in intervention programmes but often as the trainers, or in the back-up team when technical problems are encountered, rather than as the day-to-day workers. Second, professional training courses should be adapted to enable shared training, to question attitudes about the 'caring professions', to involve parents and disabled people in teaching and curriculum design, and to set professional skills within the relevant context. Third, there is a need to re-examine the core skills being expected of the professionals. Genuine expertise in a speciality is not to be jettisoned; however, any professional in this field would benefit from having skills in counselling, in negotiating, in adult education, and in managing and facilitating change, in order to have a wider and longer-lasting effectiveness. Fourth, the methods of training require scrutiny. The model of learning should reflect the relationship that will need to be developed with disabled children and their families and the community (see also Chapter 9). Teaching through lectures and demonstrations does not ensure understanding; teaching which values the student as a person, and which values their experience (for example through a joint project with a group of disabled people on improving mobility within a school) facilitates flexibility and appropriateness of learning.

Evaluation

There is a paucity of good research concerning disabled children. In some ways we know remarkably little about what approaches to therapy and treatment really 'work'. There are many reasons for this, including the relative rarity and diversity of children's problems, making traditional study designs with large groups of subjects hard to implement. People who have designed an intervention and persuaded a community of its promise can hardly then propose a randomized controlled trial of its efficacy. Deliberate non-treatment would be seen as unethical, and the links among parents would in any case tend to disseminate the ideas which are judged valuable (Robson 1993).

To ask 'What works?' is too restricted a question. A therapy may give some positive results, but is the investment worthwhile for that child at that time? (*e.g.* see Chapter 6). What we need to know is what effect the intervention has on all aspects of the child's life (see Chapter 5). A major limitation of past evaluation studies of intervention with children has been the limited theoretical framework adopted. Frequently aims and measures have focused on short-term child progress in a particular skill, and have ignored significant mediating variables such as the resources of the family or unpredicted outcomes such as raised parental expectations (see Chapters 3 and 8).

The influence of the programme on the wider community is even more difficult to assess. Where resources are few, and little has previously been instituted for children with impairments, parents will usually feel heartened and encouraged by the attention being shown to their child. Community members are often interested in the new developments and are supportive. But how can the quality of community involvement be measured? There are some precedents in studies of community awareness initiatives, noting the removal of barriers to participation of disabled people (McConkey and McCormack 1983). In addition, children's increased activities can be counted: does s/he now go to play outside?; what role is s/he allowed to take in the games?; are games devised by the disabled children being played more frequently?; and so on.

There is a considerable need now for planning of research, to generate and validate appropriate evaluation measures and strategies for disability programmes, in both developing and developed countries. Chapter 4 has presented a structure for the quantitative evaluation of interventions such as a specific treatment or therapy approach. However, the requirements of evaluation cannot be allowed to dominate the responsive development of an appropriate intervention for disabled children. For example, in the case of a community-based rehabilitation (CBR) programme in a particular poor urban community, it will be better to adopt qualitative methods of evaluation (such as a case study approach) than to compromise the richness of the intervention by having to specify narrowly measurable goals. This does not imply sloppiness in evaluation. Concepts such as the reliability and validity of evidence still apply. For example, it will be important in ensuring the reliability of information gathering to consider the gender/class/age of the interviewers. Parents' or disabled children's responses to questions (such as 'What aspect of the programme has been of most help to you?') are likely to differ markedly depending on whether or not the interviewer has an impairment. It will also be necessary to demonstrate the steps taken to overcome social conformity in interviewees' answers in order to establish the validity of information obtained about a programme. It may be suggested that external assessors are less biased and will bring objectivity to the evaluation of a programme; however, they may also bring their own prejudices, and lack the subtlety to judge the quality of the intervention process.

The issues in conducting research with disabled children and their families go further even than this. It is essential to ask 'Who benefits from this research?' The agenda for research is set by governments and other funding bodies. They frame questions in terms of 'What will gain us votes?' or 'Will it give value for money?' Researchers tend to be non-disabled, with a scientific or professional training, and they ask questions about proof of the efficacy of particular programmes or treatments for particular conditions or groupings of impairments. They are thus inclined to miss the point about *disability*. If disabled people and their families are involved in planning intervention projects, then those projects are more likely to reflect their priorities, and their support is likely to be sustained (see Chapter 11). Likewise, if disabled people and their families are involved with researchers in defining research questions and appropriate methods of enquiry, then the research has a greater chance of providing some useful answers (Oliver 1992). For example, in Britain the Office of Population Censuses and Surveys undertook a national disability survey on behalf of the government during the 1980s. Obvious policy initiatives which might have arisen from the results of the survey (*e.g.* concerning income support) have not been taken. The framing of the questions reflected the view that 'disabilty' is a problem experienced by an individual, with no acknowledgement of its social construction (Abberley 1992). Sample questions in the survey included:

- Do you have a scar, blemish or deformity which limits your daily activities?
- Have you attended a special school because of a long-term health problem or disability?
- What complaint causes you difficulty in holding, gripping or turning things?

Whereas these questions could have been asked as follows:

- Do other people's reactions to any scar, blemish or deformity you may have, limit your daily activities?
- Have you attended a special school because of your education authority's policy of sending people with your health problem or disability to such places?
- What defects in the design of everyday equipment like jars, bottles and lids causes you difficulty in holding, gripping or turning them?

A survey which included the latter set of questions would have set an agenda for social and structural change which would have made a real difference to the opportunities open to disabled people, and much of which would not have required major funding to implement.

The question of the purposes of research is an important one in other ways. Projects which are written about tend to be those which report success. This is in part a general problem of publishing, where the professional community wants to see, for example, evidence of child progress represented by a statistically significant difference. In the case of CBR projects in developing countries, there is also the natural desire to celebrate success because of the astonishing achievement of creating a worthwhile project in difficult circumstances. However, in order to learn for the future, the description of 'mistakes' is at least as instructive.

Published examples are few. Ismail (1989) and Nabuzoka (1989) describe problems encountered, such as spending insufficient time in discussing the objectives of an intervention project with parents, so that they expected the rehabilitation worker to do all the work with the child; lack of acceptance of project staff recruited from outside the community in which the project was based; and not identifying carefully which member of the extended family would be the most effective person for ensuring the continuation of the programme. A cautionary example from a developed country was reported by Tannock *et al.* (1992). Exponents of an interaction-based approach to intervention with language-delayed children realized that by encouraging parents to respond so consistently to their children, they had inadvertently limited the children's need to communicate more clearly.

A particular problem in developing countries is that evaluation is often used as part of a decision about future funding. Open discussion of problems can only exist in an atmosphere of cooperation, and evaluation must be part of a joint process of setting directions.

Outcome

What do we know about long-term outcome? This is part of the question of 'What works?' but is rarely asked. Yet it is of sometimes overwhelming importance to parents concerned for their child's future. For example, where parents have a choice of schooling, the questions might be: 'How will she cope with mainstream school?'; and 'Will she get more expert teaching and personal support in a special school?' Studies tend to indicate greater benefits for children, including those with severe degrees of impairment, in attending ordinary school (*e.g.* Casey *et al.* 1988, Cole and Meyer 1991). Yet these are relatively short 'longitudinal' studies, for two years or so (see also Chapter 9). Much longer follow-up is required, including monitoring the support initiatives which schools and communities undertake, changes in teachers' methods and attitudes, opportunities on leaving school, and the views of the young people and their families over time. There are no long-term studies of the outcome of CBR programmes for children in terms of social integration and the permanence of positive change of attitudes in the community.

In developing countries, where a new project is started, frequently young children show dramatic progress and both families and project workers develop high expectations. However, rapid progress can rarely be sustained and there is a strong risk of disillusionment when the reality of a teenager's multiple difficulties is faced. Without a fundamental change in attitude toward disabled people, things may actually be worse than if there had never been an intervention project. However, those studies in developed countries which have followed children with impairments over a significant time span tend to report optimistic outcomes. Carr (1988) has kept contact with a group of young English people with Down syndrome from infancy to young adulthood, many of whom have busy lives and who have been described increasingly by their parents as 'getting easier'. Likewise a group of young Canadians with severe visual impairment, who had at some point been referred for child psychiatric help, were found in the main to be well-adjusted adults, with a better outcome than would have been expected of a similar group of sighted young people so referred (Freeman *et al.* 1989). However, all such studies comment on the very limited opportunities available for disabled young people on leaving school, and the fragmentation of services to adults and their families (*e.g.* Thomas *et al.* 1989, Quine and Pahl 1992).

Learning from developing countries

Many of the chapters in this book have demonstrated that there is much that those in developed countries have to learn from experiences and philosophies originating in developing countries. Striking examples include the integrated community approach of ADD–India, and Project PROJIMO in Mexico where disabled people run their own rehabilitation centre (see Chapter 11; for further examples see also Coleridge 1993). This is altogether less possible in developed countries, where the professional culture is strong and boundaries are jealously guarded. However, more professionals are becoming aware of disabled people's thinking and of human rights initiatives, and are reappraising their approach accordingly.

The UN Convention on the Rights of the Child recognizes children's right to protection, provision and participation. Unlike previous declarations, it is legally binding in international law and has been ratified by almost every country; countries report to a UN-appointed committee their progress toward implementation. Children's ability to make a contribution in their community is recognized more in developing countries than in developed ones. Most of their contribution is informal and traditional, for example, looking after young children and playing with them. The Child-to-Child approach (see Chapters 11 and 13), widely used in developing countries, enables children to tackle issues and problems they perceive as important in their community. Suggestions for activities are contained in activity sheets, and those which focus on children with impairments may include simulations (*e.g.* of what it feels like to be laughed at or ignored). This can develop into an active process of shared problem-solving (Fig. 15.1), in collaboration with a teacher, facilitator or community worker, which can open up new opportunities for both able-bodied and disabled children. It should not be forgotten that in many instances disabled children are themselves providers, for example, bringing up brothers and sisters or earning a living for their family (*e.g.* see Chapters 11, 12).

In developing countries, rehabilitation projects have to learn how to do a lot with very few resources (*e.g.* see Chapter 10). This stimulates clear thinking about how to share professional skills with families and other members of the community. In teaching others, professionals refine their grasp of the essential principles and discover that applications are far more appropriate and creative if arrived at through joint discussion.

However, perhaps the greatest stimulus to new thinking in developed countries can come from consideration of the role of 'the community' in initiating and maintaining change and opportunities for disabled children. In many underdeveloped urban and rural districts, it is impossible to ignore the community, as it is in developed countries. At best, projects for and with disabled people are an integral part of the development strategy for

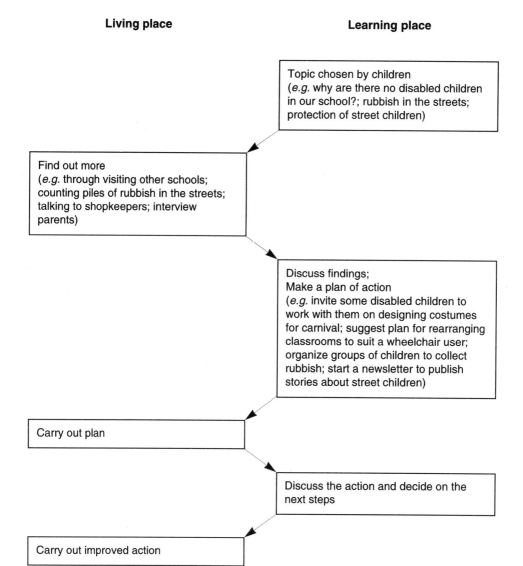

Living place   **Learning place**

Topic chosen by children
(*e.g.* why are there no disabled children
in our school?; rubbish in the streets;
protection of street children)

Find out more
(*e.g.* through visiting other schools;
counting piles of rubbish in the streets;
talking to shopkeepers; interview
parents)

Discuss findings;
Make a plan of action
(*e.g.* invite some disabled children to
work with them on designing costumes
for carnival; suggest plan for rearranging
classrooms to suit a wheelchair user;
organize groups of children to collect
rubbish; start a newsletter to publish
stories about street children)

Carry out plan

Discuss the action and decide on the
next steps

Carry out improved action

Fig. 15.1. The 'Child-to-Child' process.

the whole community, or even the nucleus from which energy is derived to tackle the needs of other groups such as elderly or displaced peoples. Services in developed countries are frequently bogged down in arguments over budgets and responsibilities, and families' wishes for real consultation and for a comprehensive and coordinated approach fall to one side. The chapters in this book should contain more than enough examples to inspire a reappraisal of how better to support disabled children.

REFERENCES

Abberley, P. (1992) 'Counting us out: a discussion of the OPCS disability surveys.' *Disability, Handicap and Society*, **7**, 139–155.

Carr, J. (1988) 'Six weeks to twenty-one years old: a longitudinal study of children with Down's syndrome and their families.' *Journal of Child Psychology and Psychiatry*, **29**, 407–431.

Casey, W., Jones, D., Kugler, B., Watkins, B. (1988) 'Integration of Down's syndrome children in the primary school: a longitudinal study of cognitive development and academic attainments.' *British Journal of Educational Psychology*, **58**, 279–286.

Cole, D.A., Meyer, L.H. (1991) 'Social integration and severe disabilities: a longitudinal analysis of child outcomes.' *Journal of Special Education*, **25**, 340–351.

Coleridge, P. (1993) *Disability, Liberation and Development.* Oxford: Oxfam.

Diamond, S. (1981) 'Growing up with parents of a handicapped child: a handicapped person's perspective.' *In:* Paul, J.L. (Ed.) *Understanding and Working with Parents of Children with Special Needs.* New York: Holt, Rinehart & Winston, pp. 23–50.

Freeman, R.D., Goetz, E., Richards, D.P., Groenveld, M., Blockberger, S., Jan, J.E., Sykanda, A.M. (1989). 'Blind children's early emotional development: do we know enough to help?' *Child: Care, Health and Development*, **15**, 3–28.

Hancock, G. (1989) *Lords of Poverty.* London: Macmillan.

Hanlon, J. (1991) *Mozambique: Who Calls the Shots?* London: James Currey.

Helander, E. (1993) *Prejudice and Dignity: an Introduction to Community-based Rehabilitation.* New York: United Nations Development Project.

Ismail, F.J. (1989) 'Helping pre-school disabled children of low-income urban families to become more independent (Nairobi Family Support Service).' *In:* Serpell, R., Nabuzoka, D., Lesi, F.E.A. (Eds.) *Early Intervention, Developmental Disability and Mental Handicap in Africa.* Lusaka: Psychology Department, University of Zambia, pp. 40–47.

Lynch, E.W., Hanson, M.J. (1992) *Developing Cross-cultural Competence: a Guide for Working with Young Children and Their Families.* Baltimore: Paul Brookes.

McConkey, R., McCormack, B. (1983) *Breaking Barriers: Educating People about Disability.* London: Souvenir Press.

Nabuzoka, D. (1989) 'Individualised programme planning for home-based education of mentally handicapped children in rural areas (CBR pilot projects in Zambia).' *In:* Serpell, R., Nabuzoka, D., Lesi, F.E.A. (Eds.) *Early Intervention, Developmental Disability and Mental Handicap in Africa.* Lusaka: Psychology Department, University of Zambia. pp. 48–58.

Oliver, M. (1992) 'Changing the social relations of research production?' *Disability, Handicap and Society*, **7**, 101–114.

—— (1993) 'Disability and dependency: a creation of industrial societies?' *In:* Swain, J., Finkelstein, V., French, S., Oliver, M. (Eds.) *Disabling Barriers – Enabling Environments.* London: Sage with the Open University, pp. 49–60.

Quine, L., Pahl, J. (1992) 'Growing up with severe learning difficulties: a longitudinal study of young people and their families.' *Journal of Community and Applied Social Psychology*, **2**, 1–16.

Robson, C. (1993) *Real World Research: a Resource for Social Scientists and Practitioner-Researchers.* Oxford: Blackwell.

Ryan, J., Thomas, F. (1980) *The Politics of Mental Handicap.* Harmondsworth, Middlesex: Penguin.

Tannock, R., Girolametto, L., Siegel, L.S. (1992) 'Language intervention with children who have developmental delays: effects of an interactive approach.' *American Journal on Mental Retardation*, **97**, 145–160.

Thomas, A.P., Bax, M.C.O., Smyth, D.P.L. (1989) *The Health and Social Needs of Young Adults with Physical Disabilities. Clinics in Developmental Medicine No. 106.* London: Mac Keith Press.

Werner, D. (1993) *Disabled People in the Struggle for Social Change. Keynote address, Action on Disability and Development, Bangalore, India, April 23, 1993.* Palo Alto, CA: Hesperian Foundation.

229

ACKNOWLEDGEMENTS

We have been supported by many people during the process of editing this book. We would like particularly to thank Merry Cross for her incisive comments on some of the chapters, and Martina Waring for help in chasing elusive references.

INDEX

234

235